Image-Processing Techniques for Tumor Detection

Image-Processing Techniques for Tumor Detection

edited by
Robin N. Strickland
*University of Arizona
Tucson, Arizona*

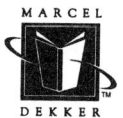

MARCEL DEKKER, INC. NEW YORK · BASEL

ISBN: 0-8247-0637-4

This book is printed on acid-free paper.

Headquarters
Marcel Dekker, Inc.
270 Madison Avenue, New York, NY 10016
tel: 212-696-9000; fax: 212-685-4540

Eastern Hemisphere Distribution
Marcel Dekker AG
Hutgasse 4, Postfach 812, CH-4001 Basel, Switzerland
tel: 41-61-261-8482; fax: 41-61-261-8896

World Wide Web
http://www.dekker.com

The publisher offers discounts on this book when ordered in bulk quantities. For more information, write to Special Sales/Professional Marketing at the headquarters address above.

Copyright © 2002 by Marcel Dekker, Inc. All Rights Reserved.

Neither this book nor any part may be reproduced or transmitted in any form or by any means, electronic or mechanical, including photocopying, microfilming, and recording, or by any information storage and retrieval system, without permission in writing from the publisher.

Current printing (last digit):
10 9 8 7 6 5 4 3 2 1

PRINTED IN THE UNITED STATES OF AMERICA

Preface

The urgent need for computer-assisted detection of tumors and lesions in medical images becomes clear when one considers the state of affairs in X-ray film mammography for breast cancer screening. In the United States it is estimated that there are currently more than 50 million women over the age of 40 at risk of contracting breast cancer. If only one-half of these women are screened by mammographic examination each year—and given that in the United States each breast is viewed from two angles—then the number of X-ray films that must be read by radiologists reaches the staggering total of 100 million per annum. A recent report estimating that somewhere between 10 and 30% of breast lesions are missed during routine screening is therefore not surprising. Motivated by such alarming statistics, researchers are developing computer image processing algorithms for detecting signs of disease. Their goal is to develop screening systems that will provide a second opinion, to prompt the radiologist to take a second look at a suspicious region in the image. Besides mammography, there exists a need for image processing techniques to assist the radiologist in reading chest X-rays, MRI scans, and nuclear medical images. These modalities share the property with mammography that signs of disease are often extremely subtle.

This book is the first ever devoted to the subject of tumor detection using image processing techniques. Many of the chapters discuss image processing algorithms that analyze a specific type of medical image and point to suspected tumors. These are the so-called computer-aided diagnosis (CAD) techniques that act as second-opinion providers. Also represented are image enhancement algorithms that make it more likely that a radiologist will see the tumor. Such algorithms do not perform tumor detection directly, but they certainly can improve detectability.

The book contains 14 chapters arranged into two parts. The first (Chapters 1–5) discusses the background behind diagnostic imaging, image processing methods and their evaluation, and clinical applications. The second part (Chapters 6–14) examines current tumor detection techniques in mammography, chest X-ray, MRI imaging, and nuclear medicine.

This book summarizes the state of the art in image processing methods for detecting tumors in medical images. The intended audience includes electrical engineers, computer scientists, radiologists, and other researchers in the health sciences.

Robin N. Strickland

Contents

Preface   iii

Contributors   vii

1   Tumor Imaging   1
     Harold L. Kundel and Peter B. Dean

2   Evaluating Detection Algorithms   19
     Kevin Woods, Maha Y. Sallam, and Kevin W. Bowyer

3   Clinical Applications: Present and Future   47
     Elizabeth A. Krupinski

4   Statistical Decision Theory and Tumor Detection   71
     Eric Clarkson and Harrison H. Barrett

5   Display, Including Enhancement, of Two-Dimensional Images   101
     Stephen M. Pizer, Bradley M. Hemminger,
     and R. Eugene Johnston

6   Detection of Microcalcifications   131
     Robert M. Nishikawa

7	Evaluation of a Multiscale Enhancement Protocol for Digital Mammography *Ralf Mekle, Andrew F. Laine, and Suzanne J. Smith*	155
8	Detection of Masses in Mammograms *Nico Karssemeijer*	187
9	Region-Based Adaptive Contrast Enhancement *Rangaraj M. Rangayyan, Liang Shen, Yiping Shen, M. Sarah Rose, J. E. Leo Desautels, Heather E. Bryant, Timothy J. Terry, and Natalka Horeczko*	213
10	Computerized Detection of Lung Nodules *Maryellen L. Giger, Samuel G. Armato III, Heber MacMahon, and Kunio Doi*	243
11	Lung: X-ray and CT *Michael F. McNitt-Gray and Matthew S. Brown*	271
12	Optimal Processing of Brain MRI *Hamid Soltanian-Zadeh and Joe P. Windham*	295
13	Brain Tumor Imaging: Fusion of Scintigraphy with Magnetic Resonance and Computed Tomography *Richard J. T. Gorniak, Elissa L. Kramer, and Marilyn E. Noz*	347
14	Image Registration in the Thorax, Abdomen, and Pelvis *Candice L. Aitken, Marilyn E. Noz, and Elissa L. Kramer*	367

Index   407

Contributors

Candice L. Aitken Joint Center for Radiation Therapy, Harvard Medical School, Boston, Massachusetts

Samuel G. Armato III Department of Radiology, The University of Chicago, Chicago, Illnois

Harrison H. Barrett Department of Radiology, University of Arizona, Tucson, Arizona

Kevin W. Bowyer Department of Computer Science and Engineering, University of Notre Dame, Notre Dame, Indiana

Matthew S. Brown Department of Radiology, UCLA School of Medicine, Los Angeles, California

Heather E. Bryant Alberta Program for the Early Detection of Breast Cancer, Calgary, Alberta, Canada

Eric Clarkson Department of Radiology, University of Arizona, Tucson, Arizona

Peter B. Dean Department of Diagnostic Radiology, University of Turku, Turku, Finland

J. E. Leo Desautels Alberta Program for the Early Detection of Breast Cancer, Calgary, Alberta, Canada

Kunio Doi Department of Radiology, The University of Chicago, Chicago, Illnois

Maryellen L. Giger Department of Radiology, The University of Chicago, Chicago, Illnois

Richard J. T. Gorniak Department of Radiology, New York University School of Medicine, New York, New York

Bradley M. Hemminger Department of Radiology, University of North Carolina, Chapel Hill, North Carolina

Natalka Horeczko[†] Alberta Program for the Early Detection of Breast Cancer, Calgary, Alberta, Canada

R. Eugene Johnston Department of Radiology, University of North Carolina, Chapel Hill, North Carolina

Nico Karssemeijer Department of Radiology, University Medical Center Nijmegen, Nijmegen, The Netherlands

Elissa L. Kramer Department of Radiology, New York University School of Medicine, New York, New York

Elizabeth A. Krupinski Department of Radiology, University of Arizona, Tucson, Arizona

Harold L. Kundel Department of Radiology, University of Pennsylvania, Philadelphia, Pennsylvania

Andrew F. Laine Center for Biomedical Engineering, Columbia-Presbyterian Medical Center, New York, New York

S.C. Ben Lo Radiology Department, Georgetown University Medical Center, Washington, D.C.

[†]Deceased.

Contributors

Murray H. Loew   Department of Electrical Engineering and Computer Science Institute for Medical Imaging and Image Analysis, George Washington University, Washington, D.C.

Heber MacMahon   Department of Radiology, The University of Chicago, Chicago, Illnois

Michael F. McNitt-Gray   Department of Radiology, UCLA School of Medicine, Los Angeles, California

Ralf Mekle   Department of Biomedical Engineering, Columbia University, New York, New York

Robert M. Nishikawa   Department of Radiology, The University of Chicago, Chicago, Illinois

Marilyn E. Noz   Department of Radiology, New York University School of Medicine, New York, New York

Stephen M. Pizer   Department of Radiology, University of North Carolina, Chapel Hill, North Carolina

Rangaraj M. Rangayyan   Department of Electrical and Computer Engineering, University of Calgary, Calgary, Alberta, Canada

M. Sarah Rose   Department of Community Health Sciences, University of Calgary, Calgary, Alberta, Canada

Maha Y. Sallam   Intelligent Systems Software, Inc., Clearwater, Florida

Liang Shen   Department of Electrical and Computer Engineering, University of Calgary, Calgary, Alberta, Canada

Yiping Shen   Department of Electrical and Computer Engineering, University of Calgary, Calgary, Alberta, Canada

Suzanne J. Smith   Department of Radiology, Columbia-Presbyterian Medical Center, New York, New York

Hamid Soltanian-Zadeh   Department of Diagnostic Radiology, Henry Ford Health System, Detroit, Michigan; Department of Electric and Computer

Engineering, University of Tehran, Tehran, Iran; and Department of Radiology, Case Western Reserve University, Cleveland, Ohio

Timothy J. Terry Alberta Program for the Early Detection of Breast Cancer, Calgary, Alberta, Canada

Joe P. Windham Department of Diagnostic Radiology, Henry Ford Health System, Detroit, Michigan

Kevin Woods Intelligent Systems Software, Inc., Clearwater, Florida

Image-Processing Techniques for Tumor Detection

1
Tumor Imaging

Harold L. Kundel
University of Pennsylvania, Philadelphia, Pennsylvania

Peter B. Dean
University of Turku, Turku, Finland

I. DEFINITIONS: NEOPLASMS AND TUMORS

The term "tumor," which literally means swelling, can be applied to any pathological process that produces a lump or mass in the body. Tumors are a major manifestation of a vast and varied group of diseases called neoplasms or more commonly cancers. However, many other diseases such as infections can produce tumors, and they are a source of confusion in imaging diagnosis. We will use the term tumor to indicate neoplastic masses.

Neoplasms arise from normal body cells that through a series of transformations lose the capacity to respond to the usual physiological mechanisms that control growth. Uncontrolled growth leads to the formation of a tumor. Slowly growing tumors that lack the capacity to spread to distant sites are called benign, and rapidly growing tumors that can infiltrate surrounding tissues and spread to distant sites (metastasize) are called malignant. Tumors that resemble the parent cell type are classified as well differentiated, whereas tumors that have lost any resemblance to the original cell type are classified as undifferentiated. In general, undifferentiated tumors tend to grow faster than well-differentiated tumors. Tumors growing at a distance from the primary malignant tumor site are called metastases (1). They occur because tumor cells are shed into the surrounding extracellular space and into the blood vessels. The cells in the extracellular space move into the lymphatic system and are trapped in lymph nodes, where they begin to grow, producing lymph node metastases. In a like manner, cells shed into the blood vessels are trapped in other organs, commonly the lungs, liver, brain, lymph nodes, and bone marrow. Diagnostic studies, including surgical biopsies

Table 1 A Typical Assignment of Cancer Stages

Stage	Meaning
0	Atypical cells in a normal anatomical configuration
1	Tumor limited to the local anatomical site
2	Involvement of ipsilateral regional lymph nodes
3	Involvement of contralateral lymph nodes
4	Involvement of a distant site

and images, are used to identify the location and determine the extent of tumors. This information is used to assign a stage to the disease. A general definition of the cancer stages is shown in Table 1. The stage together with an assessment of the degree of differentiation is very important for treatment planning and for determining cancer prognosis.

Every type of cell in the body can be the precursor to a neoplasm, but some types such as those arising from the breast, lung, colon, and prostate are more common. A specific diagnosis is generally made by microscopic examination, which in most cases allows determination of cell type of origin and the degree of malignancy. Neoplasms are generally named after the cell type and tissue from which they originate. The most common ones originate from the epithelial cells and glands that form the inner and outer surface of the body. They are called carcinomas and are given a prefix to indicate the cell type. For example, if the cells tend to form sheets, they are called squamous cell carcinomas from the Latin "squama" meaning scale, and if they form spherical groupings, they are called adenocarcinomas from the Greek "aden" meaning gland. Sarcomas arise from the muscles and connective tissues. Lymphomas arise from the lymphatic tissues, and the enlarged lymph nodes form tumors. Leukemias arise from the blood-forming cells and, in general, do not produce tumors.

II. REASONS FOR IMAGING TUMORS OR POTENTIAL TUMORS

People with tumors or potential tumors are imaged for detection, classification, staging, and comparison. Detection can be subdivided into diagnosis, case finding, and screening, depending on the level of suspicion. People are usually referred for diagnosis because they have signs and symptoms suggestive of cancer. Case finding occurs when a test is performed to find a disease before it becomes clinically evident and, thus, easier to treat and cure. A physician may order or perform a diagnostic test in a person who does not have definite symptoms to be sure that the person is healthy. Case finding should not be confused with population screening, which involves examining a predefined population for one specific disease without performing any other diagnostic examinations. Such a population typically will have a low prevalence of cancer.

Classification ideally consists of making a tissue diagnosis or at least making a determination of whether the tumor is a manifestation of a benign or malignant disease. Benign disease can include both benign tumors and nonneoplastic pathological conditions such as granulomas or hyperplastic cysts. The diagnostician is obligated to classify every suspicious region in an image. If there is uncertainty about the classification, additional diagnostic procedures are done. These generally start with less invasive imaging procedures and proceed to minimally invasive procedures such as endoscopy and arteriography. When minimally invasive procedures are exhausted, needle biopsy or surgical excision can provide a definitive diagnosis. For example, it might not be possible to classify a homogeneous, smoothly marginated mass detected on a mammogram as benign or malignant. Ultrasonographic imaging can then be done to determine whether the mass is a cyst or a solid tumor. If it is a solid tumor, needle biopsy will show that it is benign about 30% of the time (2). Currently, magnetic resonance imaging (MRI) is being studied as a method for improving the classification of breast masses in hopes of decreasing the number of breast biopsies that show benign disease (3). Computer analysis of image features may also play a role in improving disease classification (4).

Staging is performed to determine the extent of the disease, both local and distant. An assessment of local involvement is useful before an excisional surgical procedure to be sure that the entire tumor is included in the resection. Staging is important for the selection of an appropriate treatment regimen and for estimating prognosis. Most statistics about the outcome of cancer treatment are stratified according to the stage of the disease at the start of treatment. Staging usually involves obtaining images or biopsy specimens of regions of the body that are known to have a high probability of harboring metastatic tumor.

Comparison imaging is performed after treatment to determine the effect of treatment and to check for tumor recurrence. The diagnostic problem frequently involves discriminating between changes caused by the treatment and changes caused by recurrent tumor. For example, the radiation therapy of tumors can cause local tissue necrosis that is difficult to distinguish from active tumor (5).

III. DIRECT AND INDIRECT VISUALIZATION OF TUMORS

A tumor can be conceptually modeled as a circumscribed mass of abnormal tissue growing in normal tissue. It has a matrix that can be either textured or homogeneous and a boundary with the normal tissue that can be either fuzzy or distinct. It can be visualized directly if it has either different physical or metabolic properties from the surrounding tissue. When the tumor matrix has the same physical properties as the surrounding tissue, it is said to be "isointense." An isointense tumor is not directly visible, but it may manifest itself indirectly by the alteration of adjacent normal structures such as displaced blood vessels, distorted normal structures, or obstruction of ducts and airways. For example, a lung tumor is suspected when there is persistent collapse (atelectasis) of a lung segment. The tumor may not be visible, but obstruction by a tumor may be the most logical explanation for the segmental lung collapse. Part of the art of radiology consists of recognizing the subtle direct and indirect signs of tumors.

IV. FACTORS THAT INFLUENCE THE APPEARANCE OF TUMORS IN IMAGES

A. Summary

The appearance of a tumor in an image depends on the imaging modality, the image acquisition geometry, the physical parameters of the imaging system, and tumor biology. The imaging modality determines the body property that is mapped into the image. Acquisition geometry determines the spatial relationship of the tumor to surrounding tissues. The physical parameters of the imaging system determine the clarity of details and boundaries, as well as the contrast between the tumor and the surrounding tissue. Tumor biology determines the characteristics of the tumor matrix and the boundary of the tumor with the surrounding normal tissue, as well as the response to physiological probes such as intravascularly administered contrast-enhancing agents and radiopharmaceuticals.

B. Imaging Modality: Anatomical and Functional Imaging

Imaging modalities can be divided into those that show body anatomy and those that show metabolic activity or function. Anatomical imaging modalities such as x-ray imaging, ultrasonography, and MRI apply energy to the body and then map the intensity of the interaction of the energy with the body. For example, x-rays that enter the body can be scattered, absorbed, or directly transmitted. The image shows the distribution of transmitted and scattered x-rays and by inference the distribution of absorbing and scattering material in the body. Ultrasonography sends a beam of sound into the body and records the returning echoes. The echo images show the location of reflecting surfaces in the body. Proton MRI images are more complicated, because they show the distribution of a weighted combination of the density of water protons and two water proton relaxation times called T1 and T2. Varying the weighting factors at the time of image acquisition can produce a great variety of images.

Functional imaging modalities such as radionuclide imaging and magnetic resonance spectroscopy (MRS) show the distribution of metabolic activity in the body. Radionuclide imaging is particularly useful in general tumor imaging for the detection of bone metastases. The mineral content of the bone has to be decreased by 25% to 30% before a change is visible by x-ray imaging. A radionu-

Tumor Imaging

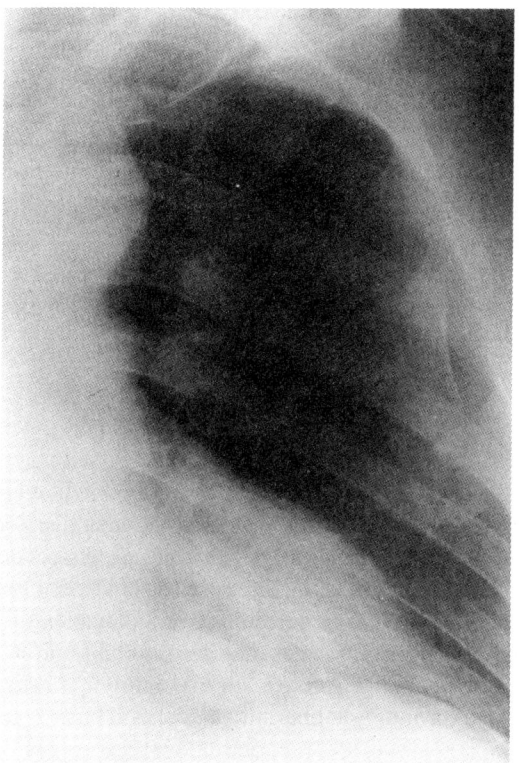

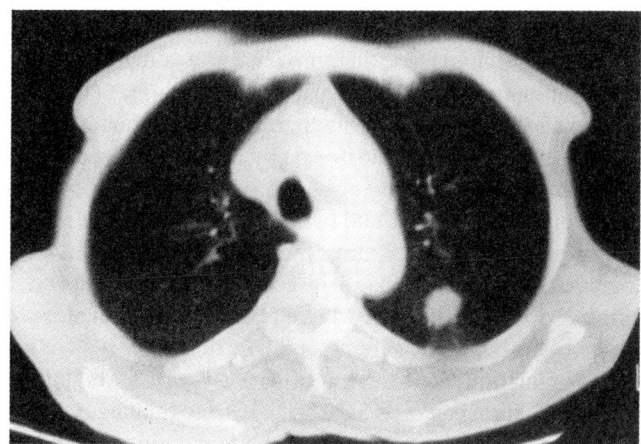

Fig. 1 (A) A planar image of the chest shows a tumor in the left suprahilar region (arrow). The boundaries of the tumor are not well defined, because the shadow of the tumor on the image is a composite of tumor, overlapping pulmonary blood vessels, ribs, and thoracic soft tissues. (B) A cross-section image made through the plane of the tumor. The boundaries of the tumor are now well defined. Notice that it has irregular margins.

clide tracer consisting of a complex of technetium (99^mTc), tin, and a polyphosphate is incorporated into the bone at the metastatic site because of increased metabolic activity associated with bone destruction and attempted repair by the body.

The distinction between anatomical and functional imaging is somewhat artificial, because function can be deduced from sequential images obtained of a moving organ like the heart or by plotting image intensity as a function of time during the passage of a contrast agent through an organ. MRI is being used to study cardiac function (6) and blood flow in breast tumors (7). Doppler ultrasonography is used to image blood flow and experimentally to differentiate tumor blood flow from normal tissue blood flow (8).

C. Image Acquisition Geometry: Planar-Projection vs Cross-Section Imaging

Images can be divided into two major geometric types, planar and cross-section. Planar images are also sometimes called projection images or the words are combined into planar-projection. Most of the x-ray images that are produced in the world are planar images of the chest, axial skeleton, extremities, and breast. Many radionuclide images are also planar. A common metaphor for a planar x-ray image is a shadow of the body cast by a beam of x-rays. It is an unusual shadow, because the body is translucent to x-ray, and the intensity of the emerging beam that produces the shadow depends on x-ray energy, body thickness, and body composition. The final image is a complex sum of the interaction of the x-rays with all of the tissues in the path of the beam. Cross-section imaging was developed to eliminate the ambiguity caused by overlapping structures in planar imaging. Early radiologists developed motion tomography, a technique for visualizing a plane of the body by blurring the planes above and below the plane of interest. This was replaced by x-ray computed tomography (CT) in which a series of thin (typically a few millimeters) planar images (typically 256) made by an x-ray source traveling around the body are used to reconstruct a cross-sectional image of a thin slice of the body. The advantages of CT images relative to planar images are increased image contrast between tissues of differing composition and a relative lack of interference by overlapping shadows. The disadvantages are increased complexity of the examination, increased radiation dose, and increased cost. The advantages of cross-section imaging are illustrated in Figure 1, which shows a planar and a cross-sectional x-ray image of the chest of a person with a tumor in the left lung. The position of the tumor in the chest produces superimposition of pulmonary blood vessels in the planar image. The attenuation of the blood vessels and the tumor combine to produce a composite shadow that has indistinct boundaries in Fig. 1A. The camouflaging effect of the blood vessels is completely overcome in the cross-section image in Fig. 1B.

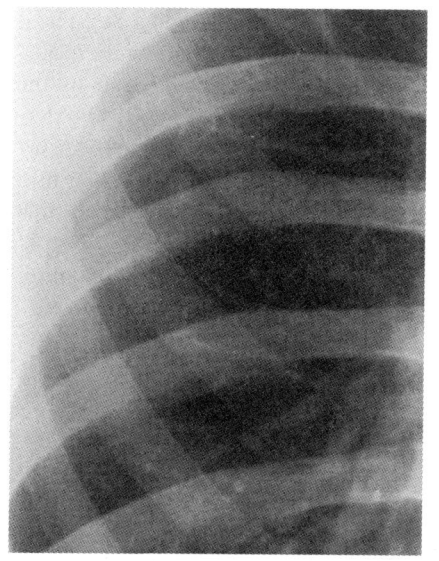 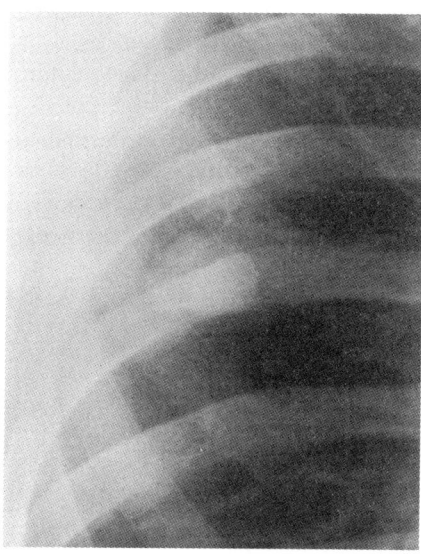

Fig. 2 Effect of tissue anatomy on tumor growth. (A) A 1-cm symmetrical lung nodule. (B) After 2 months, the nodule has enlarged asymmetrically but has not grown across the interlobar fissure.

Despite the advantages of cross-sectional imaging, planar images still predominate in the examination of the chest and breast, because images can be made simply, rapidly, and relatively inexpensively. For example, chest images can be made with a mobile x-ray machine at the bedside of a sick person.

D. Physical Factors

Each imaging modality has fixed and adjustable physical parameters that determine the visibility and sharpness of detail (spatial resolution) and the clarity of boundaries (contrast rendition) (9). Both spatial resolution and contrast rendition are affected by noise. In fact, one of the defining properties of medical images is that they are visibly noisy at normal levels of illumination. The appearance of tumors in images is affected by the adjustable physical parameters of the imaging modality. The most dramatic effects are seen in MRI, in which the image pulse sequence determines the relative weighting of proton density and the T1 and T2 relaxation times. More subtle effects are found in x-ray imaging, in which the peak kilovoltage (kVp) of the x-ray beam affects the tissue contrast. The detection of cancer is improved when planar chest images are obtained at higher kVp (140 vs 75) levels (10). This result is not due to increased contrast of the tumor but to decreased contrast of the surrounding structures such as the ribs that tend to hide tumors (11). The adjustable physical parameters are usually set to achieve some level of image quality specified by a human observer, usually a radiologist. It is altogether possible that parameters that are chosen to meet human specifications may not be optimal for processing the images by computer. Fortunately, the migration to digital imaging, particularly for planar x-ray imaging, makes image data available before they have been processed to meet the requirements of the human observer.

E. Biological Factors

1. Growth Follows the Vascular Supply and Tissue Planes

At first, tumors receive oxygen and nutrients by diffusion from the surrounding extracellular fluid, which is supplied by existing capillaries. As they increase in size, they require an additional blood supply to obtain oxygen and nutrients and, in response to hypoxia, the tumor cells secrete a hormone (tumor angiogenic factor) that stimulates blood vessel growth from surrounding normal tissues (12). The gross morphology of a tumor depends on the rate of growth and the location of available blood vessels in the surrounding normal tissues. Rapidly growing tumors can increase in size faster than blood vessels in the surrounding tissue can proliferate, and cells become hypoxic and then necrotic. Areas of hypoxia and necrosis contribute to variations in the texture of the tumor matrix. The shape of a tumor may also depend on the availability of a blood supply from the normal tissues. Figure 2 is a planar image of a metastatic lung tumor that started as a peripheral nodule and as it grew encountered the pleural fissure between the upper and middle lobe of the lung. The tumor growth stopped at the fissure, creating a flattened profile. More complicated boundary profiles are produced when the tissue planes are more complex or when there is an inflammatory reaction in the surrounding normal tissue.

2. Calcification

Whenever there is tissue injury leading to necrosis, the local physiological conditions favor the deposition of calcium salts. Dystrophic calcification is found commonly in the walls of blood vessels in athersclerosis, in injured heart valves, in necrotic tumors, in healing abscesses, and in granulomas. In the early stages of the development of breast cancers, tiny (10–200 μm) calcifications may form in the tumor. These calcifications typically form within the milk ducts, which are separated from the blood circulation by the basement membrane surrounding the duct. As malignant cells proliferate within the ducts, the ducts enlarge and the central

Tumor Imaging

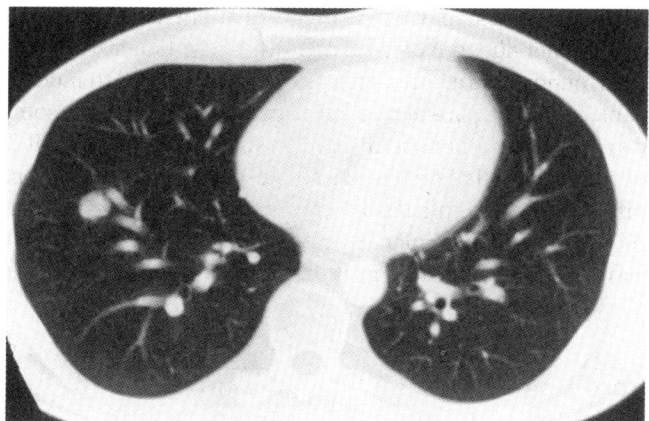

Fig. 3 A CT scan showing a malignant lung tumor. Notice the numerous small circular objects in the lungs. Most of them are cross sections of blood vessels.

core, being the farthest from the blood circulation, begins to undergo necrosis and subsequently calcifies. Microcalcification may be the only sign of malignancy in a mammogram (13) when the noncalcified part of the tumor matrix is isointense to x-rays. Calcification may also be dystrophic in nonmalignant tissue. An important decision made in mammography is the differentiation of malignant from benign calcification (14). As opposed to mammography, calcified lung tumors are usually benign manifestations of healing granulomas caused by tuberculosis or some other infectious disease. Computed tomography can be used to measure the level of calcification and discriminate malignant from benign tumors (15).

3. Secondary Effects: Obstruction and Architectural Distortion

Obstruction of a critical passageway in the body may produce the first symptoms of a tumor and may also provide the only signs of a tumor on an imaging examination. Squamous cell carcinomas of the lung arise from the bronchial endothelium. The growing endobronchial lesions at first partially and then totally obstruct the bronchus in which they are growing. Partial obstruction results in the accumulation of secretions in the lung behind the obstruction. If the secretions become infected, the person develops a pneumonia that may be very resistant to treatment because of the obstruction. Total obstruction results in atelectasis, which consists of a combination of collapse of the airspace and an influx of fluid caused by resorption of the air. In these cases, cross-sectional imaging with CT is generally able to identify the obstructing tumor.

Table 2 Mammographic Features Prompting Biopsy in 300 Successive Nonpalpable Breast Cancers (see Ref. 13)

Mammographic feature	No.	%
Classic signs of malignancy		
Linear/branching calcifications	68	23
Spiculated knobby mass	49	16
Subtotal	117	39
More subtle signs of malignancy		
Other calcifications	57	19
Other masses	69	23
Indirect signs	57	19
Subtotal	183	61
Total	300	100

A tumor that is not growing in the vicinity of a vital passageway may also distort the surrounding tissues, and the distortion may be the only visible sign of a tumor on the imaging examination. Table 2, taken from a report of the mammographic features of 300 consecutive nonpalpable breast cancers, indicates that 19% of the cancers were biopsied because of indirect signs (13). These signs included architectural distortion (9%), a developing density uncharacteristic of a mass (6%), asymmetry (3%), and a single dilated duct (1%).

4. Visualizing Tumors by Means of Contrast-Enhancing Agents

Many diagnostic cross-sectional images are made using intravenous contrast agents to improve the visualization of tumors. The iodinated contrast agents that are used in x-ray imaging and the gadolinium chelates that are used in MRI are freely distributed in the extracellular space of the body but do not cross the blood–brain barrier into the extracellular space of the brain. Right after intravenous administration, the contrast agents are concentrated in the blood, and acquisition of the images can be timed to show the vascular phase. Differences between the vascularity of tumors and the surrounding normal tissue will show as differences in contrast. Tumors can be either more or less vascular than the surrounding tissue, producing either hyper-intensity or hypo-intensity in the image. Sometimes they have an avascular center with a surrounding ring of hypervascularity. The contrast agents rapidly diffuse from the vascular compartment into the extracellular space. Many tumors have an extracellular space that is larger than that of the surrounding normal tissues, and as a consequence they have a higher volume distribution and appear hyper-intense in the image. The matrix of many tumors also contains necrotic, avascular areas into which contrast agents diffuse very slowly producing differences in image contrast with time. The permeability of the blood–brain barrier is increased in the vicinity of most brain tumors, and after the administration of a contrast agent, there may be an increased concentration of the contrast agent relative to the surrounding brain.

V. FEATURES OF MALIGNANT TUMORS SEEN ON IMAGES

A. Some Generalization About the Features of Malignancy

In any tissue, the features of malignancy may be shared by benign neoplasms, non-neoplastic diseases such as infections and granulomas, and occasionally by normal tissues. Some of the features of benign and malignant tumors are shown in Table 3. In general, benign tumors have sharp boundaries and a regular shape, frequently spherical or ovoid. Malignant tumors tend to be irregular in shape with indistinct boundaries and frequently show speculation at the borders. Most of these features indicate rapid growth. Generalizing about calcifications poses a considerable problem, especially for breast cancer. Malignant breast tumors can contain both fine and fairly extensive calcifications. The intraductal, branching calcifications are typically malignant, except when they are smooth and dense, when they can be rather unequivocally called benign. On the other side, most (>80%) clustered calcifications on the mammogram are of benign origin. The very fine, powderish calcifications, which are usually composed of psammoma body calcifications sized approximately 10 μm and visible mammographically as a summation when in larger clusters, are caused by benign processes in two of three instances and by malignant processes in one of three instances.

B. Specific Features of Breast Cancer

The breast is composed of glandular, connective, and adipose (fat) tissue in proportions that vary considerably, not only among women, but also in the same

Table 3 Common Features of Benign and Malignant Tumors Seen on Images

Feature	Benign characteristics	Malignant characteristics
Shape	Regular	Irregular, lobulated
Border	Sharp	Fuzzy, spiculated
Matrix		
Calcification	Dense	Fine
Texture	Smooth	Variegated

woman, depending on her age and the phase of her menstrual cycle. Mammography is excellent for differentiating fat from other soft tissues but cannot differentiate between glandular, connective, and malignant tissues if these are not separated by fat. The interspersed fat, which transmits x-rays more readily than the other tissues, reveals the structure of the more "dense" (more radiopaque) tissues. When a breast cancer has broken through the basement membrane of the ducts and begun to form tumors, it takes one of three characteristic appearances. First, it may appear as a round or oval tumor with slightly indistinct borders. Second, it may appear as a spiculated or stellate tumor with a characteristic radiating border pattern caused by a connective tissue reaction. Finally, in the absence of surrounding fat, the tumor may infiltrate surrounding glandular and connective tissue without producing any easily detectable pattern. The size at which a breast cancer can be differentiated from its surroundings on a mammogram depends on the relative proportion of fat. More fat means that the tumor can be detected at a smaller size, with a lower limit on the order of about 3 mm if there is no surrounding connective or glandular tissue. At the other extreme, if there is no surrounding fat, a tumor may grow to the size of several centimeters and still not be easily detectable on the mammogram, but these larger tumors will always produce a hard lump that can be easily detected by palpation. The normal variation in breast tissue structure will make breast cancers easy to detect in some women and difficult to detect in others. A 1.5-cm tumor can be easily detected in a breast composed predominantly of fat, but a 2.1 cm tumor can be detected only with difficulty in a breast containing relatively little fat.

Although fewer than 20% of clustered breast calcifications are caused by breast cancer, there are certain types of calcifications that are typically associated with breast cancer. These tend to have a typical structure and can often be recognized when the cancer is still in its in situ or preinvasive state. These calcifications (see Sec. IV.E.2) have three typical forms, the granular or crushed stone type, the casting or linear, branching type, and the powderish or amorphous type. Although they are caused by preinvasive growth of breast cancer, there may be invasive breast cancer nearby, which can also cause some of the calcifications to disappear. The powderish type of calcifications is less typical of malignancy, because in most cases these will be associated with benign processes. Because there is no apparent difference between powderish calcifications produced by malignant and benign processes, it is necessary to send all such cases to biopsy. Calcifications have received the most attention in the computer analysis of mammograms, but their importance in the control of death from breast cancer is fairly minor. When left to grow, a very small percentage of breast cancers with calcifications can rapidly lead to fatality, whereas most breast cancer calcifications give an advance warning of several years during which breast cancer fatality can be avoided. On the other hand, most fatal cases of breast cancer result from the stellate (spiculated) tumors, which may be far more difficult to detect than the calci-

Tumor Imaging

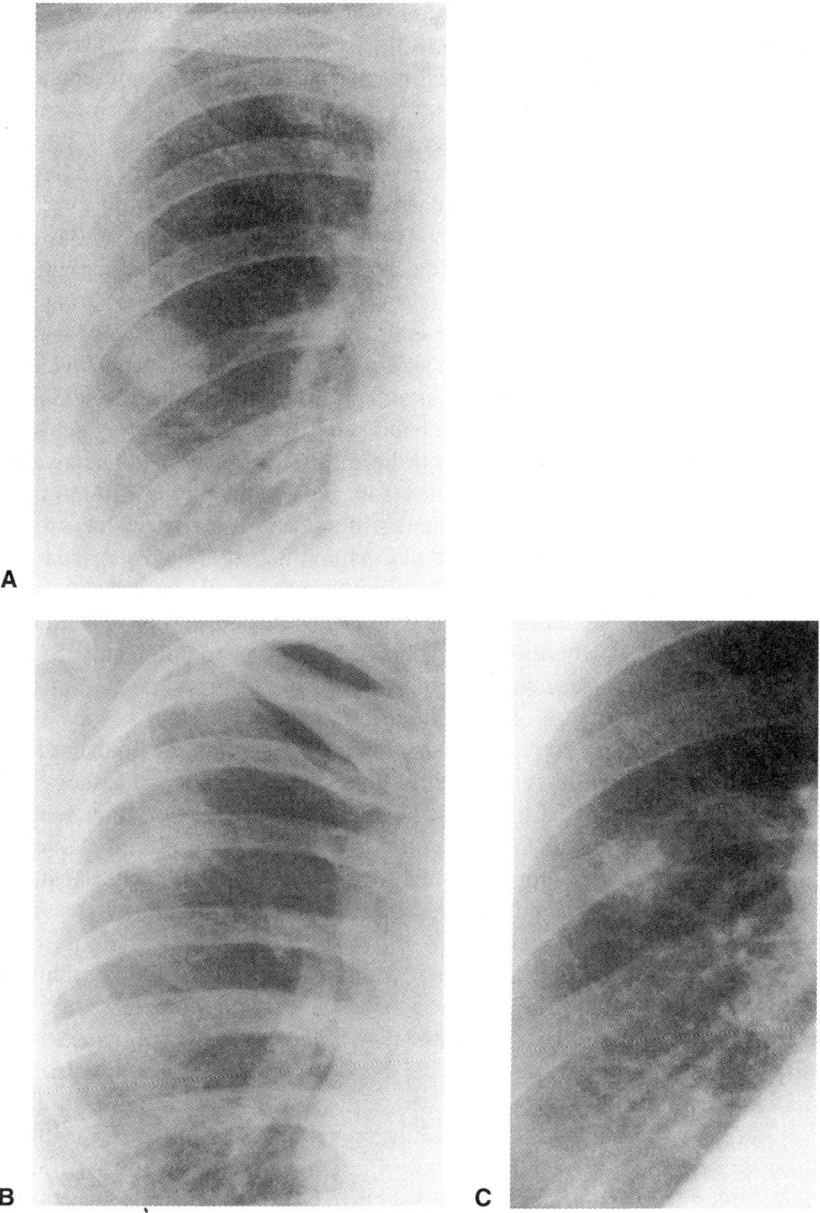

Fig. 4 Three lung masses that are about the same size and located in the midlung. Notice the difference in the distinctness of the tumor boundary with the lung.

fications. It is also easier for radiologists to learn to detect and differentiate breast calcifications than it is for them to learn how to detect small, noncalcified breast cancers.

C. Specific Features of Lung Cancer

Early malignant lung tumors can be found inside the major bronchi (endobronchial lesions) and in the periphery of the lung (nodules). Small endobronchial lesions can be imaged by conventional CT when there is encroachment on the bronchial lumen (16). Virtual bronchoscopy done by reconstructing the bronchial tree from CT scans of the thorax is being explored as a means for identifying early endobronchial lesions (17). Peripheral lung tumors are roughly circular in projection and are generally called nodules. When small and of low contrast, they are very difficult to detect in planar chest images. Nodules less than 1 cm in diameter are rarely detected on planar radiographs, because composite vascular shadows mimic nodules, and radiologists cannot distinguish true nodules from "noise" nodules (18). The situation is improved by cross-section imaging, in which it is possible to detect nodules as small as 3 mm in diameter. Fig. 3 shows a small pulmonary nodule on a CT image. Notice that there are other small circular objects that could be cross-sections of small spherical masses but, in fact, most of them are cross-sections of blood vessels running through the section. Viewing the sections sequentially helps the human observer separate nodules from blood vessels (19).

As a consequence of rapid growth and following the local blood supply, malignant tumors tend to develop irregular shapes, and the boundary with the normal tissue tends to become indistinct as fronds of tumor grow along tissue planes. This produces a boundary that is fuzzy and frequently spiculated. However, the boundary of malignant tumors within the lung can range from sharp to indistinct. Figure 4 shows three rather large malignant lung tumors, an adenocarcinoma and two alveolar cell carcinomas. Notice the character of the boundary, which ranges from very sharp to spiculated and indistinct.

Calcification is one of the features of benign lung tumors. Benign calcification is dense and sometimes irregular (popcorn). Its location in the mass is either central or concentric. Eccentric or stipulated calcification may be associated with malignancy, and frequently it appears as if the tumor has arisen in the neighborhood of a benign lesion and engulfed it.

VI. HUMAN FACTORS THAT INFLUENCE OUR UNDERSTANDING OF THE NATURE OF IMAGE FEATURES

Medical images have three important characteristics: (a) they are transparencies, (b) they are visualized in terms of anatomy and pathology, and (c) the visibility of contrast and detail are limited by noise. Let us briefly consider the implications of each of these for human tumor visualization and image processing. Transparency is a more important property for planar than for cross-section imaging; in fact, it is the reason that cross-section imaging was developed. In planar imaging the superposition of structures located in different planes produces ambiguity in the image. In a chest image two blood vessels in different planes may combine to produce a single nodulelike structure that is mistaken for a tumor. Similarly, as in Fig. 1, a real tumor superimposed on large blood vessels may lose many of its intrinsic features. Most planar image examinations include two views made at approximately right angles, a frontal image (anteroposterior or posteroanterior) and a lateral. Oblique views are sometimes substituted for lateral views as in mammography. The use of two views in a screening study has been controversial, but the incremental increase in tumor detection from the second view has recently been shown to be on the order of 25% to 45% for the detection of tumors smaller than 15 mm with screening mammography (20). There also is a large increase in diagnostic certainty and an associated decrease in false-positive results. Superimposed structures that produce the spurious appearance of a tumor will not be seen on both views. The implication of this for studies of computer-aided diagnosis is that the information supplied by a second planar image should not be neglected.

People with knowledge of anatomy and pathology read images. They describe images using terminology that frequently reflects inferences about anatomy and pathology (21). There are some image-specific terms, but an unambiguous terminology for describing medical images has never been developed. The image is visualized as a surrogate for the patient. A radiologist will report that there is a rib fracture on a chest radiograph. This is a clear statement about the patient but not much of a description of the intrinsic appearance of the image. The radiologist has used the visual clues in the image to build a preferred perception that best fits his or her understanding of the patient. The preferred perception is not necessarily a literal rendition of the image. For example, the clarity of organ boundaries is limited by the noise that is visible in most medical images. Incomplete boundaries may be completed perceptually, because knowledge of anatomy and pathology indicates that they must be there. So when the radiologist describes features in an image, the computer scientist must decide if the features represent the preferred perception (image plus knowledge) or the literal perception (image only). The radiologist may not be able to distinguish one from the other (22).

VII. SCREENING FOR BREAST AND LUNG CANCER

At present, planar x-ray imaging (mammography) is used for screening women older than 40 for breast cancer. Screening for lung cancer using planar imaging has not been very widespread, because a few large clinical trials have not shown that screening reduces lung cancer mortality (23). Recently there has been a re-evaluation of the screening studies that used planar imaging (24) and a movement toward using low-dose CT as a screening method, particularly in Japan where lung cancer is becoming a greater public health problem (25). The screening problem is one of achieving a high true-positive fraction without incurring a large number of costly false-positive results. Computer-aided diagnosis is being applied to both mammography (26) and lung CT (27) to improve cancer detection in the screening environment. Detection, although important for evaluating the technology, is not the criteria for determining whether a cancer-screening program is successful. The effectiveness of screening by CT must eventually be measured as a reduction in cancer mortality.

VIII. CONCLUSIONS: SOME LESSONS FOR THE COMPUTER SCIENTIST

Malignant tumors start small and grow. As they get larger, they become more conspicuous and have more opportunity to show their character. They also produce symptoms and bring the person to a physician. We would like to be able to detect the smallest possible symptomatic malignant tumors and, in the context of screening, the smallest possible asymptomatic tumors. It should be clear that many factors influence the appearance of tumors on images, and although there are some common features of malignancies, there is also a great deal of variation that depends on the tissue and the tumor type. Characteristic features are more likely to be found in large tumors. Small tumors may not have many of the features of malignancy and may even manifest themselves only by secondary effects such as architectural distortion. When studying image processing, it is important to include small asymptomatic tumors in the test material.

REFERENCES

1. CJF VanNoorden, L Meade-Tollin, FT Bosman. Metastasis. Am Scientist 86: 130–141, 1998.
2. G Hermann, C Janus, IS Schwartz, B Krivisky, S Bier, JG Rabinowitz. Nonpalpable breast lesions: Accuracy of prebiopsy mammographic diagnosis. Radiology 165: 323–326, 1987.
3. SG Orel, MD Schnall, CM Powell, et al. Staging of suspected breast cancer: effect of MR imaging and MR-guided biopsy. Radiology 196:115–122, 1995.
4. DJ Getty, RM Pickett, CJ D'Orsi, JA Swets. Enhanced interpretation of diagnostic images. Invest Radiol 23:240–252, 1988.
5. YJ Kim, KH Chang, IC Song, et al. Brain abscess and necrotic or cystic brain tumor: Discrimination with signal intensity on diffusion-weighted MR imaging. AJR 171: 1487–1490, 1998.
6. DC Bloomgarden, ZA Fayad, VA Ferrari, B Chin, MG St. John Sutton, L Axel.

Global cardiac function using fast breath-hold MRI: Validation of new acquisition and analysis techniques. Magn Reson Med 37:683–692, 1997.
7. PS Tofts, B Berkowitz, MD Schnall. Quantitative analysis of dynamic Gd-DTPA enhancement in breast tumors using a permeability model. Magn Reson Med 33: 564–568, 1995.
8. AA Alexander, LN Nazarian, DM Capuzzi Jr, NM Rawool, AB Kurtz, MJ Mastrangelo. Color Doppler sonographic detection of tumor flow in superficial melanoma metastases: Histologic correlation. J Ultrasound Med 17:123–126, 1998.
9. ICRU Report 54, Medical imaging—the assessment of image quality. Bethesda, MD: International Commission on Radiological Units and Measurement, 1995.
10. G Revesz, FJ Shea, HL Kundel. The effects of kilovoltage on diagnostic accuracy in chest radiography. Radiology 142:615–618, 1982.
11. HL Kundel. Peripheral vision, structured noise and film reader error. Radiology 114:269–273, 1975.
12. J Folkman. Seminars in Medicine of the Beth Israel Hospital, Boston. Clinical applications of research on angiogenesis. N Engl J Med 333:1757–1763, 1995.
13. EA Sickles. Mammographic features of 300 consecutive nonpalpable breast cancers. AJR 146:661–663, 1986.
14. L Tabár, PB Dean. Teaching Atlas of Mammograpy. 2nd ed. Stuttgart: George Thieme Verlag, 1985.
15. SS Siegelman, EA Zerhouni, FP Leo, NF Khouri, FP Stitik. CT of the solitary pulmonary nodule. AJR 135:1–13, 1980.
16. Y Saida, Y Kujiraoka, E Akaogi, T Ogata, Y Kurosaki, Y Itai. Early squamous cell carcinoma of the lung: CT and pathologic correlation. Radiology 201:61–65, 1996.
17. RM Summers. Image gallery: A tool for rapid endobronchial lesion detection and display using virtual bronchoscopy. J Dig Imag 11:53–55, 1998.
18. HL Kundel. Predictive value and threshold detectability of lung tumors. Radiology 139:25–29, 1981.
19. SE Seltzer, PF Judy, U Feldman, L Scarff, FL Jacobson. Influence of CT image size and format on accuracy of lung nodule detection. Radiology 206:617–622, 1998.
20. RG Blanks, SM Moss, MG Wallis. Use of two view mammography compared with one view in the detection of small invasive cancers: further results from the National Health Service breast screening programme. J Med Screen 4:98–101, 1997.
21. PJ Friedman. Radiologic reporting: The hierarchy of terms. AJR 140:402–403, 1983.
22. HL Kundel. Perception and representation of medical images. In: Lowe ML, ed. Medical Imaging 1993: Image Processing. SPIE, 1898:1–11, 1993.
23. D Eddy. Screening for lung cancer. Ann Intern Med 111:232–237, 1989.
24. GM Strauss, R.E.G, DJ Sugarbaker. Chest x-ray screening improves outcome in lung cancer. Chest 107:270S–279S, 1995.
25. S Sone, S Takashima, F Li, et al. Mass screening for lung cancer with mobile spiral computed tomography scanner. Lancet 351:1242–1245, 1998.
26. RM Nishikawa, ML Giger, K Doi, CJ Vyborny, RA Schmidt. Computer-aided detection of clustered microcalcifications: An improved method for group detected signals. Med Physics 20:1661–1666, 1993.
27. M Kaneko, K Eguchi, H Ohmatsu, et al. Peripheral lung cancer: screening and detection with low-dose spiral CT versus radiography. Radiology 201:798–802, 1996.

2
Evaluating Detection Algorithms

Kevin Woods and Maha Y. Sallam
Intelligent Systems Software, Inc. Clearwater, Florida

Kevin W. Bowyer
University of Notre Dame, Notre Dame, Indiana

I. INTRODUCTION

This chapter deals with evaluation criteria for software designed to detect abnormalities in medical images. When computer algorithms are designed for applications such as this, strict evaluation criteria are crucial for a number of reasons. The most obvious reason is the need to assess expected system performance. This may be required to gain widespread acceptance or to establish the state of the art. In addition, some means of objective and fair comparison are needed to help determine the relative merit of competing algorithms. A rigorous evaluation also facilitates the development of a robust system. By knowing specifically which situations cause an algorithm to fail, we can begin to isolate and address the causes of the failure. This leads to further development in an effort to correct the problem, handle the error, or enable the algorithm to recognize when failure occurs.

Algorithm evaluation can have a different meaning in a clinical setting. Performance requirements in a day-to-day clinical environment may involve additional or different criteria. In many cases, regulatory approval is necessary before software can be cleared for commercial use. For example, the U.S. Federal Food, Drug, and Cosmetics Act and subsequent amendments to the Safe Medical Device Act give the Food and Drug Administration (FDA) authority to ensure safe and effective devices (1). Many applications involving computerized medical image analysis, such as computer-aided diagnosis (CAD), fall into the medical device category. Here, performance analysis of the computer algorithm alone is not sufficient. The evaluation must consider the effects the computer-generated information ultimately has on decisions involving patient care.

A tumor, or neoplasm, is technically defined as a growth of abnormal tissue that is different in structure from the surrounding tissue. We may only be interested in detecting malignant tumors. However, it is not always possible to easily distinguish between benign and malignant tumors without a biopsy or some other diagnostic test that relies on information not found in the image. Therefore, evaluation criteria are application dependent. If tumor pathology can be predicted with a high degree of accuracy from a visual inspection of the image, it may be desirable to define detection as a task of finding only those tumors that are suspicious for malignancy. If an automated system for detecting tumors is used as a secondary image reader, detecting some number of obviously benign abnormalities may be permissible.

A decision made during a detection task falls into one of four possible categories, shown in Fig. 1. An image region can be called cancerous (positive) or normal (negative), and a decision can either be correct (true) or incorrect (false). There are two types of errors that can be made: false-negative and false-positive errors. A false-negative (FN) error implies that a true abnormality was not detected. A false-positive (FP) error occurs when a detection corresponds to a normal region, and thus falsely identifies the region as abnormal. Two types of correct decisions can also be made: true-positive (TP) and true-negative decisions (TN). A detection that corresponds to an actual abnormality is called a true positive. A true-negative decision simply means a normal region was correctly labeled as being normal.

Sensitivity and specificity are measurements related to the false-negative and false-positive error rates, respectively. The sensitivity is the rate at which tumors are detected (1.0-FN error rate), and so it is referred to as the true-positive rate. Specificity is 1.0-FP error rate. The performance of a process that detects tu-

True State / Computer Decision	IS a cancer	IS NOT a cancer
Called a cancer	True Positive	False Positive
Not called a cancer	False Negative	True Negative

Fig. 1 A decision made during a detection task falls into one of four possible categories. The word "positive" or "negative" corresponds to the decision made, whereas the word true or false denotes whether or not the decision was correct.

mors in medical images, be it a computer system, a human, or a combination of the two, can be completely characterized by its sensitivity/specificity tradeoff. For example, suppose a test set contains 200 images, 100 of which contain cancer and 100 of which do not. If a process detects 80 of 100 tumors, there are 20 false-negative errors. The sensitivity is 80% and the false-negative rate is 20%. If the process also generated 10 false-positive detections, the false-positive rate is about 11.1% (10 of the 90 total detections were false positives). The specificity in this example is 88.9%. When an image may contain more than one distinct abnormality, specificity is often expressed in terms of the average number of false-positive detections per image, which in this example is 0.05. Obviously, 100% sensitivity and specificity (or a false-positive rate of zero) represents perfect performance, the ultimate and usually unrealistic objective.

The first part of this chapter is concerned with performance evaluation of computer detection algorithms alone. This generally involves comparing the computer output with some form of ground truth information for a set of test images and generating some meaningful statistics. We begin with a discussion of detection criteria, which involves how computer detections are characterized as either true positive or false positive. In Sec. III, we describe methods for evaluating and comparing algorithms and discuss some relevant issues. Sec. IV covers several aspects of algorithm evaluation in a clinical environment, including FDA requirements, the elements of a good clinical trial, and techniques for isolating certain aspects of performance. In Sec. V, we summarize what we believe to be the essential aspects of a sound evaluation and make some basic recommendations. Finally, in Sec. VI, we use a case study to illustrate many of the concepts and techniques discussed in this chapter.

II. DETECTION CRITERIA

Perhaps the first issue to deal with concerns the characterization of a computer detection as either true positive or false positive. To do this for a given image, the output of the computer algorithm must be compared with the "ground truth" information associated with the image. How the comparison is performed is somewhat dictated by the intended application of the computer algorithm.

A. Ground Truth

The term "ground truth" is derived from remote sensing applications and essentially means measurements made "on the ground" (near-surface measurements) concerning the objects to be analyzed. The term "gold standard" is sometimes used to mean essentially the same thing. Defining ground truth in biological systems is often complicated. Although applications related to remote sensing, for example, allow measurement of actual distances, height, etc., assessment of most disease processes and symptoms are not always defined in absolute terms. This is particularly applicable to medical image interpretation.

For tumor detection in medical images, ground truth typically would refer to the pathology results from biopsy specimens. For simplicity, we assume that there are no errors in the pathology results. In reality, of course, there is some nonzero error rate in every process. The pragmatic version of the assumption is that the pathology error rate is essentially zero compared with the image analysis error rate. In their simplest form pathology results would classify the specimen as benign or malignant. Regions with tissue found to be malignant would be denoted as positive in the ground truth. Note that other positive regions not subjected to biopsy because they were missed or not found suspicious enough may still be present in the images but not labeled as positive. Follow-up of cases over time can help solve this problem and improve the accuracy of ground truth. For example, in the Digital Database for Screening Mammography (DDSM) project (2) a "normal" set of mammogram images is one that has 4-year follow-up as normal. This reduces the chances of the database containing a "normal" study that actually contains a cancer that is too small or too subtle to be readily detected.

Depending on the application, it may be reasonable to use radiologist interpretation as the basis for establishing ground truth. In this case, truth is defined as the assessment given by an expert radiologist, or possibly, a group of expert radiologists. In its simplest form, this assessment will indicate suspicious regions in an image. Anything that would cause a radiologist to request additional workup or biopsy, regardless of the result, should probably be labeled positive in the ground truth.

In most cases the assessment of the radiologist, and hence ground truth labeling, cannot be limited to simple positive or negative decisions. In screening mammography, for example, the BI-RADS (3) standard for describing the image interpretation allows for one of five overall assessments: (a) negative, (b) benign finding, (c) probably benign, (d) suspicious abnormality, or (e) highly suggestive of malignancy. When radiologist assessment is used to measure performance of a computer system, the ground truth representation must take into account all possible assessments in the context of intended system use. Typically, ground truth is determined by combining radiologist assessment, biopsy results, and case follow-up. Biopsy results are used to determine malignancy, whereas radiologist assessment and follow-up are used to identify benign and nonsuspicious cases not recommended for biopsy.

Regardless of the different types of regions identified in a ground truth, it is always possible to consider a subset of regions as positive while treating the rest of the image as normal for the purpose of evaluating a tumor detection system. Consider a computer application that acts as a second reader for breast cancer detection in screening mammography. A typical screening examination in the United States contains four images, two views of each breast. A radiologist has alternatives to biopsy for suspicious-looking regions and may request additional workup. This workup may include spot compression, additional views of the breast, ultrasound imaging, short-term follow-up, or other methods. Even though additional workup may ultimately convince the radiologist that a biopsy is not necessary, or a biopsy result may be benign, the original screening images were either inconclusive or suspicious enough to warrant extra attention. In this situation, it would make little sense to call a computer prompt a false positive if it points to something on which a radiologist would have required additional workup. To emphasize this point, if a CAD second reader were to prompt only image regions on which the radiologist would ask for additional workup, it could be said to have a zero false-positive rate in a certain context.

In general, a ground truth representation for a particular class of images can be developed by determining the following:

1. All possible findings and how radiologists describe their findings. This task is significantly easier for applications that already have an established interpretation standard.
2. The subset of findings that the ground truth must encode. This will be highly dependent on the intended use of the detection system.
3. A method for recording case assessment in electronic format.
4. A ground truth representation capable of capturing all significant findings and indicating the location and extent of each abnormality in an image.

One of the challenging aspects of establishing medical image ground truth is sometimes the lack of clear separation between possible assessments and important exceptions that may not fit into the framework of the ground truth representation. Another difficulty is the potential for different interpretations among different radiologists for the same case. Carefully following interpretation standards may help overcome some of these difficulties, but some borderline cases will still be problematic. Another important issue is the lack of accuracy in marking the true extent of an abnormality. Although a radiologist may easily indicate the location of an abnormality, providing an accurate outline for that abnormality may be more difficult, especially when the outline is not well defined in the image. In addition, estimating the extent of an abnormality is subjective, and any two radiologists would rarely provide identical estimates.

For the purposes of this discussion, the only ground truth information required is that which denotes the image regions that should be detected. How the ground truth is derived is irrelevant. We only need to know that it is the "gold standard" against which an algorithm will be measured. Once ground truth in-

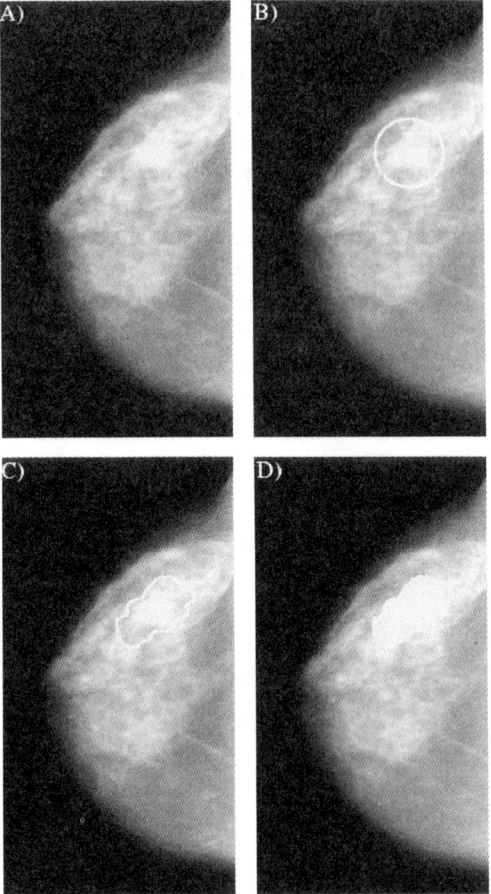

Fig. 2 A mammogram image with a spiculated lesion and three methods for denoting the positive location: (A) the raw image, (B) a circular region defined with a centroid and radius, (C) a region defined with a chain code, and (D) a template image.

formation for a set of test images has been established, characterization of computer detections is quite straightforward. Detections that correspond to positive image regions are true-positive detections. All other detections are false positives. How correspondence is determined is the subject of the next subsection.

Historically, several schemes have been used for ground truth annotation of medical images. Positive image regions are denoted either by some definition of the region boundary or a template image. Some examples are shown in Fig. 2. The

Evaluating Detection Algorithms

MIAS database (4) of mammogram images uses a circle, defined by a center and radius, to denote a positive region. The LLNL/UCSF mammogram database (5) uses template images for ground truth annotation. The DDSM (2) uses a chain code, which permits a more freeform definition of positive regions, and a utility for converting the chain code to a template image.

Depending on the complexity of information given by the ground truth, it is usually possible to convert from a boundary representation to a template image and vice versa. Both methods can encode the same information, but there are advantages to each. Boundary representations require less space to store and can be more flexible than a template image. A boundary representation is easier to use for overlapping abnormalities and abnormal regions that contain different signs of abnormalities (e.g., a tumor with calcifications). On the other hand, from an image-processing point of view, it is generally easier to implement algorithms for comparing computer output to ground truth using template images.

B. Comparing Computer Output to Ground Truth

Specific detection criteria are dictated by the purpose of the intended application. For example, if accurate tumor segmentation is considered important, perhaps for diagnostic reasons or for evaluating intermediate processing results, then some method of measuring segmentation accuracy is useful. However, if the computer system is simply meant to prompt a human user to more closely inspect suspicious image regions (i.e., a second reader system), then some looser evaluation criteria based on tumor localization is more appropriate. Fig. 3 shows some examples of computer detection results overlaid on a positive ground truth region. The perfor-

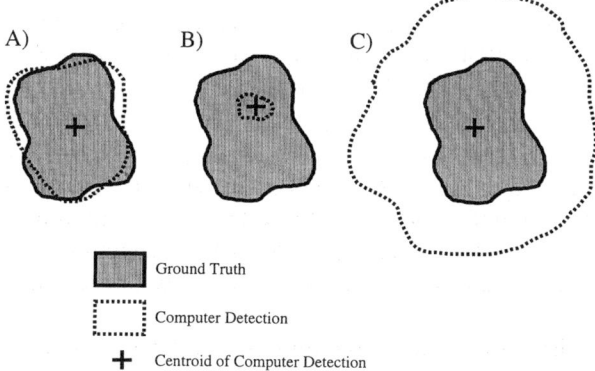

Fig. 3 Comparing computer output with ground truth.

mance of detection algorithms is greatly affected by the detection criteria used to determine the true-positive detection rate (6). Other methods could be used to compare computer output to ground truth, but region overlap and measurements of prompt location are by far the most common.

One method of comparing detection results with the ground truth is to measure the relative amount of a true-positive region that has been detected (or segmented). For example, we could say the computer detection must overlap at least $N\%$ of a ground truth region to be labeled a true positive. One potential problem with this overlap measure is that very large detections, like in Fig. 3C, will be labeled true positives, because 100% of the tumor was detected. This is somewhat misleading, because even though the computer detection is highly sensitive at the pixel level, the specificity is very low. In fact, one could simply generate a single huge detection region for every image. This would guarantee 100% sensitivity and at most one false-positive detection per normal image. Although these numbers sound great, the computer algorithm is useless.

A more accurate detection criteria is one that measures the *mutual* overlap between a computer detection and a positive region. Now, the threshold of $N\%$ mentioned earlier also applies to the relative amount of the computer detection that is overlapped by the ground truth region. So, the detection in Fig. 3C would no longer be a true positive, because the ground truth only overlaps a relatively small percent of the detection. Another way to view this detection criteria is as a measurement of the pixel-level sensitivity and specificity. For example, in Fig. 3B, the pixel-level specificity is 100%, but the pixel-level sensitivity is very low. The main advantage to a mutual overlap detection criteria is that they avoid labeling oversized or undersized detections true positives. One problem is determining how much mutual overlap constitutes a true-positive detection.

For second reader systems that generate prompts, the computer detection can be effectively reduced to a single point. This can be accomplished in any number of ways. For example, the prompt location may be computed as the centroid of the detected region (7), or, if individual pixels have associated probabilities, as the location of maximum likelihood within the detected region (8). Now, all that matters is the location of the prompt. A prompt may be considered a true-positive detection if it lies in or near a positive region, otherwise it is a false positive. The distance between the centroid of a ground truth region and the prompt may also be used. It may be necessary to weight the distance measurement with respect to the size of the ground truth region if tumor size varies greatly. The physical appearance of the prompt, be it an arrow or some other symbol, is probably not critical as long as it is clearly visible. In addition, a single-point prompt is not the only option. Kegelmeyer (9) overlaid the outline of computer-detected regions on the images to prompt radiologists and used an overlap detection criteria to measure sensitivity and specificity.

III. ALGORITHM EVALUATION

Detection algorithms have parameters that can be varied to alter the TP and FP rates. These parameters may correspond to settings for a statistical classifier, threshold values on the algorithm output, or other elements of the detection process. Each set of parameter values may result in a different (TP, FP) pair, called an operating point. In general, as the TP rate of a process increases, so does the FP rate. This is simply because more detections must be generated to increase sensitivity, but some of these extra detections will inevitably be false positives.

In practice, the errors that can be made (false positive and false negative) often have different "costs." For example, it may not be as detrimental to generate a false-positive detection as it is to miss a true abnormality. A false positive may cause a "needless" biopsy, but a false negative allows a cancer to grow. In such cases, "profits" can be maximized by selecting the best available operating point (10). The best parameter settings for an application may well depend on the particular combination of TP and FP rates desired.

Given that detection algorithms can be adjusted to perform at varying levels of sensitivity, it would not seem sufficient to evaluate or compare algorithms on the basis of a single operating point. A couple of well-accepted methods for algorithm evaluation within the context of tumor detection take into account the sensitivity/specificity tradeoff characteristics. Depending on the situation, one or both of these methods may be appropriate.

A. ROC Analysis

Receiver operating characteristic (ROC) analysis is a well-accepted method of evaluation for detection tasks (11,12). An ROC curve is a plot of operating points showing the possible tradeoff between the TP rate vs the FP rate. Two typical ROC curves are shown in Fig. 4. The area under the curve, usually referred to as the A_z index, is an accepted way of evaluating diagnostic performance (11–14). Perfect diagnostic accuracy means a TP rate of 100% (or 1.0) and a FP rate of 0%, and the ROC curve will have an A_z of 1.0. Random guessing would result in an A_z of 0.5.

Analogies for ROC analysis exist in the field of statistics for testing a statistical hypothesis (15). Type I and type II errors correspond to false negatives and false positives, respectively. The probability of committing a type I error, which we are calling the false-negative error rate, is called the level of significance, and is denoted by the Greek letter α. The probability of committing a type II error, which we are calling the false-positive error rate, is denoted by the Greek letter β. The term "power curve" is used instead of ROC curve.

During system development, ROC analysis can be applied to evaluate certain intermediate aspects, or levels, of the computer detection algorithm. For ex-

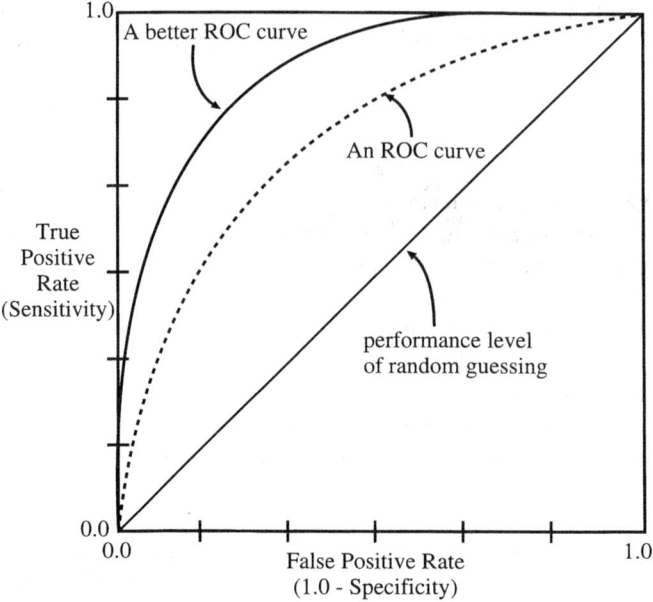

Fig. 4 Two ROC curves and the expected performance from random guessing.

ample, suppose a computer algorithm segments candidate regions from an image, and then each region is classified as normal or abnormal. Segmentation involves pixel-level analysis in which similar neighboring pixels are grouped together into regions. This requires two basic steps: (1) features are computed at each pixel, and (2) a decision is made to either keep or discard a pixel on the basis of the computed features. Segmentation may be as simple as thresholding an image on the basis of intensity, or as complex as sophisticated feature extraction followed by multivariate statistical classification (16). Regardless, the segmentation step can be expressed in terms of a yes/no decision: Is the pixel in question likely to be part of a tumor? Similarly, the region classification task corresponds to a yes/no decision: Is the segmented region likely to be a tumor?

In this example, the performance of the overall system will clearly depend on the sequence of steps used in the pixel-level analysis followed by the region-level classification. Variations of the detection process can be compared to facilitate selection of the optimal components and parameter values. For example, ROC analysis can aid in feature selection by facilitating a comparison of different feature sets extracted at the pixel and region levels. Different classifiers can be compared in the decision-making process of the segmentation and classification steps. An ROC curve can also be useful in selecting parameter values, such as thresholds, by allowing the system developer to visualize the sensitivity/specificity tradeoff associated with different settings.

B. FROC Analysis

It is often not sufficient to simply report the existence of a tumor. Correct localization of the tumor is also required for a true-positive detection. The appropriate method of evaluation in this case is free-response receiver operating characteristic (FROC) analysis (17–20). FROC analysis permits multiple abnormalities per image and requires correct localization of tumors. An FROC curve is a plot of operating points showing the possible tradeoff between the TP rate vs the average number of false positives per image, as shown in Fig. 5.

The ordinate of an FROC plot is the same as for ROC plots, 0% to 100% sensitivity. The abscissa of the FROC plot begins at zero, but the upper limit is open. Realistically, a detection system is not very useful if too many false positives are generated, and for most sufficiently large data sets 100% sensitivity is rarely attainable. For these reasons FROC plots rarely show performance above a few false positives per image. As with ROC curves, the A_z index is useful for evaluating diagnostic performance. The A_z value of an FROC curve, like that of an ROC curve, has a maximum value of 1.0 corresponding to perfect performance. The A_z value is computed by normalizing the area under the FROC curve by the range of the abscissa. For example, the A_z for the FROC curve in Fig. 5 would be computed by dividing the area under the curve by 3.0.

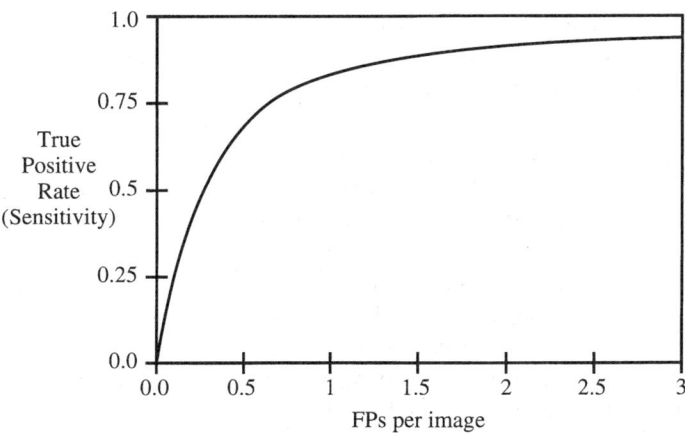

Fig. 5 An FROC curve is a plot of the sensitivity the average number of false positives generated per image.

C. Generating and Comparing ROC and FROC Curves

We should note that ROC and FROC analyses were originally used in psychophysics (21), signal detection (22), and statistical decision making (23). However, the concepts have since been adapted for performance evaluation of computer detection/recognition algorithms. In traditional ROC analysis involving human observer experiments in medical imaging, operating points are generated by requiring the observer to use confidence ratings rather than a strict yes or no answer (12). Typically, the observer would rate a finding on a scale of 1 to 5, or some similar range, where 5 indicates the highest confidence the finding is abnormal, and 1 indicates the lowest confidence (12). The ROC points are generated by considering successively less certain categories of abnormal (i.e., category 5 alone, categories 4 and 5 together, categories 3, 4, and 5 together, etc.) (13).

Generating operating points for computer detection algorithms is usually done by applying a threshold to the algorithm output. This roughly corresponds to the concept of confidence ratings used by human observers. For example, Kegelmeyer (9,24) and Karssemeijer (8) use decision tree classifiers to generate a probability image for each mammogram image. The value at each pixel represents a probability estimate that the pixel is part of an abnormality. The probability image is thresholded at some value, and detections are generated for remaining regions. Numerous operating points are generated by varying the threshold value. In fact, most statistical classifiers produce an output that can be easily thresholded to generate a large number of operating points. Some classifiers may use more complicated methods to generate operating points (25), and detection algorithms involving the combination of multiple classifiers may also require specialized methods (26).

1. Computing A_z Values

The area under an ROC or FROC curve can be computed at least two different ways. One method is to integrate a smoothed curve that has been fitted to the operating points. For ROC curves, the ROCFIT program developed by Metz and colleagues (27) is typically used. For FROC curves, Chakraborty's FROCFIT program seems to be the software of choice (19). These curve-fitting programs assume continuous binormal distributions for ROC and FROC curves. This is why the index A_z is used, because it symbolizes the gaussian underpinnings. This assumption is generally well accepted (11,13,19,20,27).

Because computer algorithms can typically generate an abundance of operating points, a reasonable estimate for the area under ROC and FROC curves can be obtained using the trapezoidal rule. The trapezoidal rule does systematically underestimate areas under the curve. However, if many operating points can be generated, this underestimation becomes negligible. In addition, if competing methods generate a similar number and distribution of operating points, then A_z values for both methods will have approximately the same underestimation, and a comparison will still be valid.

Detection algorithm performance at very low sensitivities or very high FP rates is usually not of practical interest. When large portions of a curve lie outside the range of interest, it may be more useful to analyze only a portion of the ROC or FROC curve (28). An area computed under a portion of a curve needs to be normalized (in the same manner as the FROC measurement) to arrive at an A_z value before applying tests for statistical significance. Consider the FROC curve in Fig. 5, but assume that our application requires the false-positive rate to average less than 1.5 per image *and* the sensitivity must be greater than 75%. This situation is depicted in Fig. 6. First, the area under the curve over the range of interest is estimated (the shaded area in Fig. 6). Next, it is normalized by the maximum possible area over the ranges of interest as in

$$A_z = \frac{A_p}{(TP_2 - TP_1)(FP_2 - FP_1)} \quad (1)$$

where A_p is the area under the curve computed between TP rates TP_1 and TP_2, and FP rates FP_1 and FP_2. In this example, the partial area A_p is normalized by $(1.0 - 0.75)(1.5 - 0) = 0.375$, to get the A_z value.

2. Comparing A_z Values

To compare two A_z values, a critical ratio is computed, and a test for statistical significance is applied. The formula for the test statistic, z, is

$$z = \frac{A_z^1 - A_z^2}{\sqrt{Var(A_z^1 - A_z^2)}} \quad (2)$$

where A_z^1 and A_z^2 are the two estimated A_z values. The variance term in the denominator can be estimated several ways. In the context of comparing computer

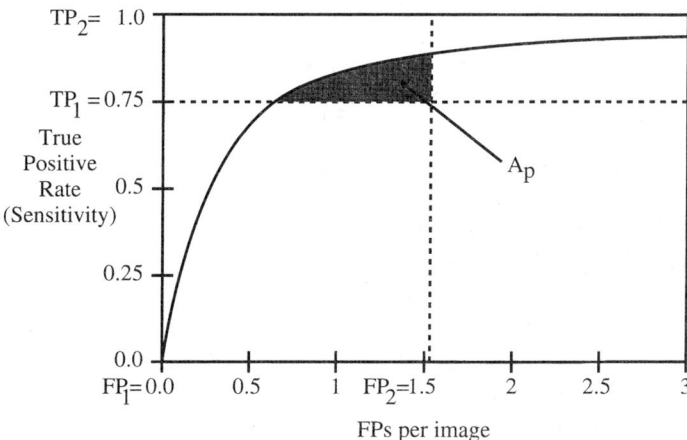

Fig. 6 Computing an A_z value for a portion of an FROC curve.

detection algorithms (or variations of the same algorithm), it is likely that ROC or FROC curves for competing methods will be generated from the same set of test data. Thus, the A_z values will be statistically dependent, and there is a covariance term associated with $Var(A_z^1 - A_z^2)$. Hanley and McNeil (13,14) provide a method for estimating the variance term when ROC curves are derived from the same cases. Alternatively, a jackknife method (29–31) can be used to directly estimate the variance term as:

$$Var(A_z^1 - A_z^2) = \frac{N-1}{N} \sum_{i=1}^{N} [(A_z^1 - A_z^2) - (A_z^{1i} - A_z^{2i})] \qquad (3)$$

where A_z^{1i} and A_z^{2i} represent the A_z values of the two methods obtained by analyzing all images except the ith image, and N represents the total number of images.

A two-tailed test for statistical significance is appropriate, where the null hypothesis is that the two observed A_z values are the same. The alternate hypothesis is that the two A_z values are different. A critical range of $z > 1.96$ or $z < -1.96$ (a level of significance $\alpha = 0.05$) indicates that the null hypothesis can be rejected, and there is sufficient evidence to support the alternate hypothesis.

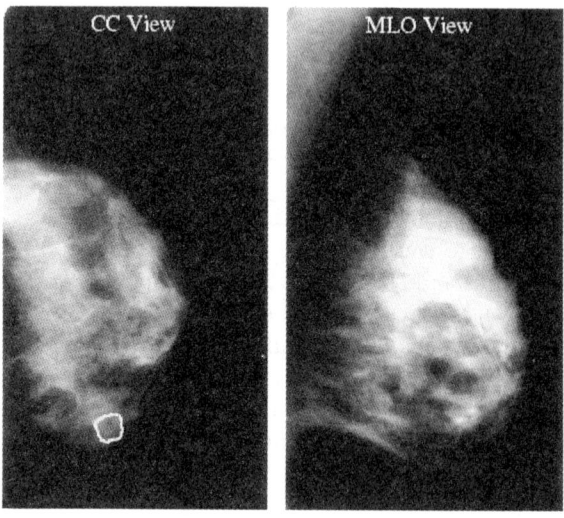

Fig. 7 Case B_3033 from volume cancer_01 of the Digital Database for Screening Mammography (2). In two mammogram views of the same breast, an irregular mass with ill-defined margins is visible in the craniocaudal view but not in the mediolateral oblique view.

D. Levels of Evaluation

Earlier, we discussed the usefulness of pixel-level and region-level evaluation during algorithm development. For overall system evaluation, "image-level" results are typically reported in ROC or FROC form. Some screening or diagnostic applications may include multiple images of the same object. For example, a typical mammogram screening in the United States contains two views of each breast: a craniocaudal view and a mediolateral oblique view. Sometimes a tumor may be detected in one view, but not in the other, as in Fig. 7. The results of the detection algorithm in this situation are perfectly acceptable, because the tumor was indeed detected. Thus, "case-level" performance evaluation may be a reasonable, or even preferred, alternative. Kegelmeyer et al. report the case level sensitivity and specificity of an algorithm for detection of spiculated lesions (9). An FROC curve may be used to plot case-level results. Here, the sensitivity refers to the detection rate of each tumor that is present in the study. If a tumor is visible in multiple images, it need only be detected in one view for a successful case-level result.

IV. CLINICAL EVALUATION

Retrospective testing on previously diagnosed cases is only the first step in testing and refining tumor detection methods for clinical use. To ensure that a system is safe and effective, it must be tested in the operating environment for which it was designed. The intended use of a detection system must be defined before determining appropriate clinical trial design.

The most ambitious use of CAD is as a fully automated system capable of determining the existence of an abnormality on its own. In this scenario, the system is expected to have at least the same performance as an expert in terms of both specificity and sensitivity. Another potential application is to use a system as a prescreener that can reliably eliminate clearly normal cases from further review by a human. In this case, the system should be highly sensitive and should be able to identify a substantial number of normal cases with a high degree of confidence. Given the current state of the art in medical image analysis, perhaps the most realistic current use of a tumor detection system is as an aid to radiologists. This detection system can act as a second reader such that radiologist's performance with the help of the system is better than unassisted performance (9,32–36). A second reader system must have high sensitivity but may not need to be as specific as a prescreening or stand-alone system.

Clinical testing is not only concerned with the effectiveness of a detection system but also with the safety of using that system. Medical image interpretation is a diagnostic tool that results in consequences for patient care. The result of this interpretation may send a patient to biopsy, which is an invasive procedure with lasting implications. In addition to the inevitable trauma and cost, a biopsy that results in a benign finding can, for example, cause problems in reading future diagnostic images of the affected area (37).

Prospective clinical testing is usually complicated because of the large number of variables involved in any trial (38). Careful design is required to achieve meaningful results. Clearly defining the objectives of each experiment is the first step toward a successful design. Interestingly, designing clinical testing protocols for measuring effectiveness and safety of the more sophisticated fully automated system or prescreener may be easier than designing protocols for measuring the effect of using a detection system in conjunction with a radiologist. The main reason for this is the complexity introduced by the interaction between the detection system and the radiologist.

It is often helpful to break down the main objective of a study into several smaller objectives. Designing a single large study with complex interactions between variables and parameters makes it difficult to draw any conclusions based on final results. It is easier to to come up with more conclusive results from smaller experiments. In showing the safety of a tumor detection system, it may be easier to design a protocol aimed at answering the simple question: Does the biopsy rate of a particular radiologist increase by using the system compared with his or her prior biopsy rate? In the context of showing effectiveness, a reasonable question may concern the ability of the tumor detection system to detect tumors missed by radiologists. One way to show this is to apply the tumor detection system to cases with previous images that were originally found to be normal, but for which an abnormality was found on a subsequent examination. If the tumor detection system is able to identify regions in the previous images that correspond to where the tumor was eventually found, then clearly the system has the ability to detect abnormalities missed by a radiologist.

The application and the intended use of the system will play major roles in determining the appropriate design of a clinical study. Also, understanding the current workflow of clinical practice for a particular application is important for a successful design. Once the main objectives have been defined, several smaller studies can be designed to provide evidence that support or refute the basic assumptions. Each smaller study design can go through the following process:

1. Define a central simple question that, when answered, will offer evidence of safety or effectiveness.
2. Design a focused experiment aimed at answering that central question while taking into account the current practice in the clinical environment.
3. Carry out the experiment and collect needed data.
4. Analyze the data to determine whether it supports a positive or negative response to the central question.

V. RECOMMENDATIONS

In addition to using the evaluation criteria and statistical methods for algorithm evaluation presented here, we shall end this chapter with some recommendations for sound research.

A. Train/Test Protocol

One very important aspect of developing a system for tumor detection is the training and testing protocol used for algorithm development and evaluation. In most medical image analysis applications, the availability of high-quality, reliably ground-truthed data is scarce. Among the reasons for this are (a) the time required of a domain expert to provide ground truth information is quite expensive and perhaps difficult to reserve, (b) converting ground truth from what is provided by the domain expert to a suitable computer-usable format is tedious and labor intensive, (c) expensive digitization equipment may be required, and (d) medical institutions are reluctant to provide data that might reveal patient identity, constituting an invasion of privacy. Given a limited set of data that must be used for both algorithm development (e.g., training machine learning algorithms) and evaluation using efficient train/test protocol is very important. It is also important to keep in mind that training data should never be used as test data in any one experiment. Therefore, the best approach is probably some form of cross-validation training and testing.

For cross-validation, the data set is divided into N separate subsets. One subset is held out, and the algorithm is trained using the remaining $N - 1$ subsets and tested on the held-out subset. Next, a different subset is held out, and the train/test cycle is repeated. This process continues until each subset has been used as the test set. Unbiased test results can now be reported on all the data, and, more importantly, training data have never been used to test in any one experiment. The value of N can range from 2 to $M - 1$, where M is the total number of cases available. The case where $N = M - 1$ is called leave-one-out or "round-robin" testing, and in general this process is called N-fold cross-validation. It may be important to consider what the "one" is that is left out. In mammography, it would appropriately be one study consisting of four images.

B. Data Selection and Detection Criteria

One aspect of algorithm evaluation concerns the selection of test data. Performance figures given in the "research" stage are typically much better than in application. Evidence of this has been shown by the University of Chicago's work on mammogram image analysis (39). This is due in part to inadequate or small data sets at the research stage, inconsistent evaluation criteria, and optimistic train/test formulations. To whatever extent possible, the test data should be typical of what could be expected in a real-world environment. This applies with respect to the subtlety of the tumors, variability of image quality, and overall appearance of the images. For example, mammogram images exhibit a wide variety of breast tissue densities and textures. As one would expect, less-dense and less-textured breast images are generally easier to read for humans and computers. So, it is important to include the more difficult cases in a test set, as well as the easier ones (40).

With the abundance of results reported in scientific journals and conference proceedings, it is usually impossible to determine the relative merit of multiple algorithms designed for the same task, because each has been tested on a different set of data. Ideally, researchers should share data to facilitate comparisons among competing algorithms. Because many times privacy constraints prohibit such data sharing, whenever possible test results should be reported for publicly available image databases (2,4,5,41). In fact, identical sets of test images should be used for an unbiased, direct comparison of competing algorithms (41).

Because performance varies greatly depending on how computer detections are scored (6), identical detection criteria should be used when comparing algorithms. Therefore, researchers should specify the parameters of their published work well enough for it to be repeated.

C. Simulated Data

In general, performance evaluation based on simulated data is not acceptable (unless you want to detect simulated abnormalities!). Simulated data can be used effectively as developmental tools. For example, in some problem domains real data are not overly abundant. Chan et al. (42) superimpose simulated microcalcifications onto normal mammograms to optimize the image-processing and signal-extraction parameters used in their detection algorithm. FROC analysis is used to evaluate and compare different combinations of parameters. Once the parameters have been set using the simulated data set, the algorithm is evaluated on real mammogram data. If real data are used for extensive parameter optimization, that same data should not be used for a final evaluation, because this constitutes testing on the training data. Thus, they were able tweak their algorithm without biasing the results.

Another good example of simulated data as a developmental tool is to verify that particular software modules are functioning properly. Karssemeijer (8) uses a schematic model of a spiculated lesion embedded in gaussian noise at various signal–noise ratios (SNR) to verify that feature extraction code behaves as expected on an ideal example of the type of abnormality his algorithm is attempting to detect.

Evaluating Detection Algorithms

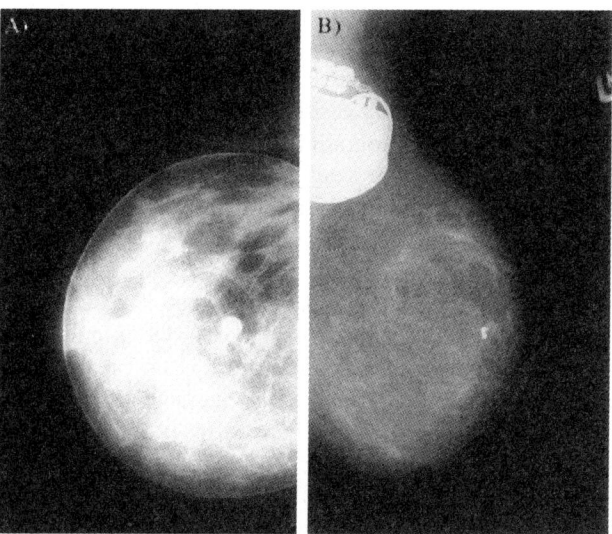

Fig. 8 Examples of atypical mammogram images. (A) Breast implants may be present as in image aorcc of the LLNL/UCSF digital mammogram library (5). (B) A pacemaker is visible in the left MLO view of case B_3084 from volume cancer_01 of the Digital Database for Screening Mammography (2).

D. Failure/Special Case Handling

No algorithm is unbreakable. However, it may be of interest to detect and handle special known circumstances. Problems with image acquisition, such as scanner-induced artifacts or film-feed errors, may cause unexpected results (43). When humans are involved in the process, there is the potential for other problems such as misplaced identification labels, grease pencil markings, scratch and dust artifacts, or films could be fed into a digitizer in different orientations. Inevitably, unusual-looking images will be encountered. Fig. 8 shows some atypical mammogram images that, although rare, do occur in a clinical environment. Handling special circumstances and graceful degradation are important to maintain physician confidence as new applications involving automated tumor detection begin to make their way into everyday practice.

VI. A CASE STUDY

To illustrate some of the concepts and techniques discussed in this chapter, we will step through an example of algorithm development in which some of the evaluation techniques and recommendations were used to guide the process. The algorithm is designed to detect clustered microcalcifications in digital mammogram images. The basic approach is to segment high-contrast candidate regions, extract a set of measurements from the candidates, classify candidates as either "normal" or "calcification," and finally group individual calcifications into clusters.

We have two separate sets of mammogram images for algorithm development and evaluation. One set of the data is used only for algorithm development. In the next two subsections, we will use this training set to select parameters and algorithm components, perform feature selection, and train a classifier. There are no restrictions on how these data are used in the training phase. The second data set is used only for performance evaluation and will not be used in any way until then. This strict separation of training and test data is critical for unbiased results. For both data sets, we have ground truth for all of the clusters and many of the individual calcifications in the form of template images.

A. Algorithm Component Selection

The first algorithm module is meant to segment candidate regions. For this purpose, a filter designed for small, round, bright spots is used. The filter response is a measure of contrast, and true calcifications should give a high response. The filter is convolved with an image, and a threshold is applied to the filtered image to create a binary template. Although this sounds quite straightforward, there are many variations to the basic process, some more subtle than others. For example, there are preprocessing steps meant to segment the breast tissue from the film background and handle image noise. There is the design of the "spot detection" filter and selection of an appropriate threshold parameter.

First, we need to establish the goal of the segmentation module and the detection criteria that will be used to compare the binary template to the ground truth. The purpose of the segmentation module is really to reduce the amount of image data that will be passed on to the more computationally expensive feature extraction module. So, we want to extract as many calcifications as possible (i.e., a high TP rate) while at the same time limiting the number of normal regions that are segmented (i.e., a low average number of FPs per image). Because we are attempting to locate multiple targets in each image, FROC analysis is the appropriate evaluation technique. From previous experience, we know that the segmentation module should have a sensitivity of around 90%. For this reason the FROC curves are evaluated for sensitivities ranging from 85% to 90%, and for FP rates from 0 to 1000 FPs per image.

Accurate segmentation is not crucial at this point, because in our algorithm, the feature extraction module refines the segmentation results. This being the case, the binary regions in the segmentation template are reduced to single-pixel locations by selecting the pixel within each connected region with the highest response to the contrast filter. The single-pixel locations are compared with the ground truth. A pixel location that lies within the boundary of a labeled calcification is considered a true positive, and anything else is a false positive. Because it is practically impossible to provide ground truth for every individual calcification, the FP rate is computed from the segmentation results of normal images only. This avoids counting a segmented region that corresponds to an unlabeled calcification as a false positive.

Now that performance goals and detection criteria have been set, different configurations of the segmentation module can be easily evaluated. Fig. 9 shows FROC curves and A_z values for two variations of the segmentation module using all the training images. The only difference between methods A and B is a preprocessing step for estimating the image noise level. All other parts of the algorithm are identical. So, this experiment clearly isolates the effect of two variations of a preprocessing step and justifies the selection of method B.

The FROC analysis also permits us to specify the operating sensitivity of the segmentation module by means of selection of an appropriate threshold for the filtered image. Because we would like approximately 90% sensitivity, we simply need to select the threshold that generated the operating point closest to this desired performance. From Fig. 9 we see that an average of 350 candidates per image will survive the segmentation process at a sensitivity of 90%. A typical 18-cm by 24-cm mammogram film digitized at a spatial resolution of 50 μm per pixel produces a digital image with more than 17 million pixels. So, this first part of the

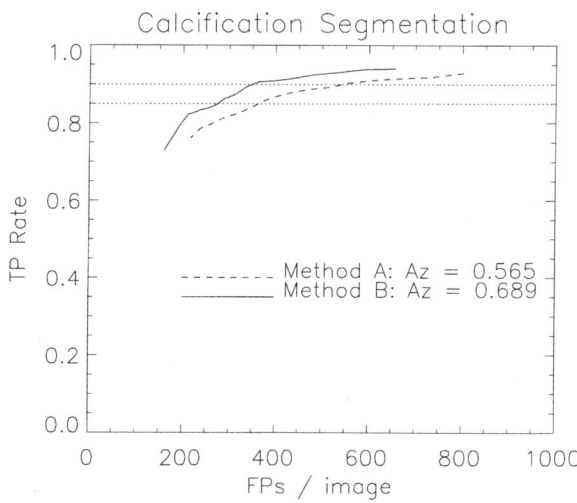

Fig. 9 FROC curves for two variations of a segmentation algorithm. The A_z values are computed over the TP range (85%, 90%), and the FP range (0,1000) FPs per image. This analysis justifies the selection of method B.

detection algorithm reduces the amount of image data from 17 million pixels to about 350 while retaining 90% of calcifications.

B. Feature Selection and Classification

Once the segmentation module has been optimized, we turn our attention to the feature extraction and classification modules. Because localization has already been performed, we are left with a yes/no question: Is the candidate a calcification or not? The performance goal is to retain as many true calcifications as possible (high TP rate) while eliminating as many noncalcifications as possible (low FP rate). This is a typical two-class pattern recognition problem, and the use of ROC analysis techniques is appropriate for evaluation.

The feature extraction routines compute a set of measurements, or features, in the neighborhood of each candidate. On the basis of the set of features, a statistical classifier assigns each candidate a value that indicates the probability that it is a calcification. The operating points for a ROC curve are generated by applying a threshold to the probability associated with each candidate.

This evaluation process requires training data for the classifier and validation data with which to generate ROC curves. We simply divided the training set into two halves with approximately the same numbers of normal and abnormal images. Now, different feature sets, classifiers, and parameter settings can be easily evaluated by generating and comparing ROC curves. Properly conducted experiments can isolate the effect of different variations of the feature extraction and classification process.

Fig. 10 shows ROC curves and A_z values for three different feature sets. The only difference across each experiment is the features extracted for each candidate. All other parts of the process, including classifier training, parameter settings, and validation data, are identical. Feature Set A was the original attempt to distinguish calcifications from normal tissue. We noticed that a good number of false positives were fine linear strips of connective tissue and calcified arteries. Feature Set B is the same as Set A plus an extra feature designed to respond to linear structures. Feature Set C is the same as Set B plus another feature designed to respond to calcified arteries. There is a significant jump in performance going from Feature Set A to Set B. Clearly, the linear structure feature was a worthwhile addition. The calcified artery feature led to a small performance gain, but because it is not computationally expensive, we opted to include it in the final algorithm.

C. Performance Evaluation

Once the algorithm has been sufficiently tweaked on the basis of the training set data, we are ready for performance evaluation. The detection algorithm is applied to the test images using a leave-one-case-out train/test protocol. That is, a single

Evaluating Detection Algorithms

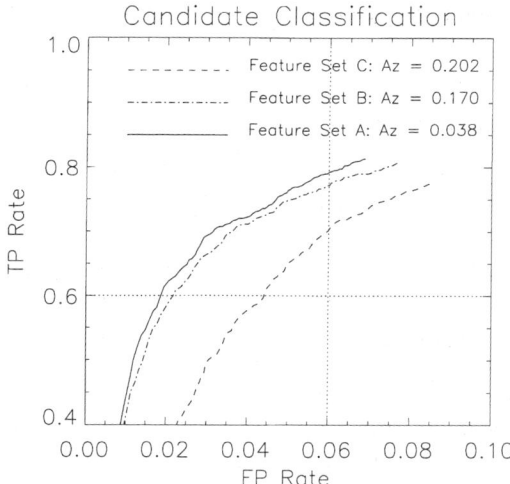

Fig. 10 ROC curves for three different feature sets for microcalcification classification. The A_z values are computed over the TP range (60%,100%), and the FP range (0%,6%).

case is pulled from the test set, the algorithm training is performed with the remaining cases, and test results are generated for the single test case. The process is repeated with each case used as the single test case, and the results are compiled together.

The images are preprocessed and passed through the segmentation, feature extraction, and classification stages. After classification, images are postprocessed by grouping all calcification objects into clusters. A cluster is defined as three or more calcifications within 1 cm^2. The intended use of this detection algorithm is for a CAD second reader system. Therefore, cluster detections are reduced to single-pixel prompt locations computed as the centroid of the individual calcifications within each cluster. If a prompt falls within 1 cm of a true cluster, it is considered a true positive, otherwise it is a false positive.

Performance can be measured at the image or case level using FROC analysis. Each individual operating point in the FROC curves are generated by applying a threshold to the probability associated with each calcification and then running the postprocessing clustering routine. Fig. 11 compares the FROC curves at the case level and image level for the set of test images. As the detection algorithm is further refined, new FROC curves can be compared with those shown in Fig. 11 to determine whether any tangible improvements have been made.

Some changes to the detection algorithm may give better intermediate results but not make a difference in the final evaluation. For example, an improved segmentation step may significantly reduce the number of false-positive objects

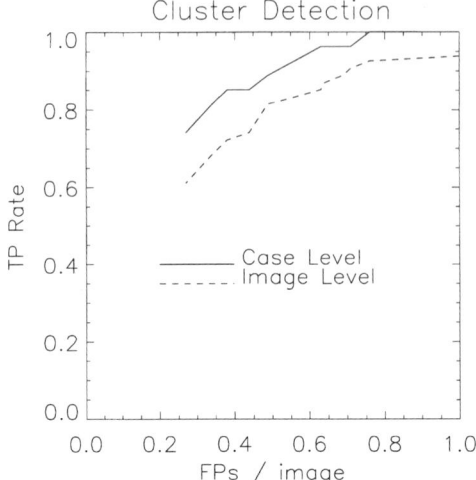

Fig. 11 FROC curves for clustered microcalcification detection at the image and case level.

that reach the classification step. However, most of those extra object removed before classification may have not been classified as calcifications in the previous version of the algorithm. The end results are the same for both versions of the algorithm. The evaluation still provides useful information, because one may now select whichever version of the algorithm is conceptually more appealing or computationally less expensive.

ACKNOWLEDGMENTS

This work has been partially supported by U.S. Army Medical Research and Materiel Command grants DAMD17-94-J-4015 and DAMD17-94-J4328, Sun Microsystems Academic Equipment Grant EDUD-US-950408, and the NASA Florida Space Grant Consortium grant NGT-40015.

REFERENCES

1. "http://www.fda.gov."
2. KW Bowyer, D Kopans, WP Kegelmeyer, Jr, R Moore, M Sallam, K Chang, K Woods. The digital database for screening mammography. Proceedings of the 3rd International Workshop on Digital Mammography. Chicago: Elsevier Science, 1996, pp 431–434.

3. American College of Radiology. Breast Imaging Reporting and Data System (BI-RADS), May 1993.
4. J Suckling, J Parker, DR Dance, S Astley, I Hutt, CRM Boggis, I Ricketts, E Stamatakis, N Cerneaz, SL Kok, P Taylor, D Betal, J Savage. The mammographic image analysis society digital mammogram database. Proceedings of the 2nd International Workshop on Digital Mammography. York, England: Elsevier Science, 1994, pp 375–378.
5. LN Mascio, SD Frankel, JM Hernandez, CM Logan. Building the LLNL/UCSF digital mammogram library with image groundtruth. Proceedings of the 3rd International Workshop on Digital Mammography. Chicago: Elsevier Science, 1996, pp 427–430.
6. LM Yarusso, RM Nishikawa, K Doi. Comparison of objective methods of scoring computer-detected microcalcification clusters in mammograms. Radiol Soc North Am 205(P):217, 1997.
7. KS Woods, CC Doss, KW Bowyer, JL Solka, CE Priebe, WP Kegelmeyer, Jr. Comparative evaluation of pattern recognition techniques for detection of microcalcifications in mammography. Int J Pattern Recognition Artif Intell 7:1417–1436, 1993.
8. N Karssemeijer, GM te Brake. Detection of stellate distortions in mammograms. IEEE Trans Med Imaging 15:611–619, 1996.
9. W Kegelmeyer, J Pruneda, P Bourland, A Hillis, M Riggs, M Nipper. Computer-aided mammographic screening for spiculated lesions. Radiology 191:331–337, 1994.
10. RM Haralick, LG Shapiro. Computer and Robot Vision. Vol. 1. Addison-Wesley, 1992.
11. JA Swets. ROC analysis applied to the evaluation of medical imaging techniques. Invest Radiol 14:109–121, 1979.
12. CE Metz. ROC methodology in radiologic imaging. Invest Radiol 21:720–733, 1986.
13. JA Hanley, BJ McNeil. The meaning and use of the area under a receiver operating characteristic (ROC) curve. Radiology 143:29–36, 1982.
14. JA Hanley, BJ McNeil. A method of comparing the areas under receiver operating characteristic curves derived from the same cases. Radiology 148:839–843, 1983.
15. RE Walpole, RH Myers. Probability and Statistics for Engineers and Scientists. 3rd ed. New York: Macmillan, 1985.
16. K Woods, K Bowyer. A general view of detection algorithms. Proceedings of the 3rd International Workshop on Digital Mammography. Chicago: Elsevier Science, 1996, pp 385–390.
17. JP Egan, GZ Greenberg, AI Schulman. Operating characteristics, signal detectability, and the method of free response. J Acoust Soc Am 33:993–1007, 1961.
18. PC Bunch, JF Hamilton, GK Sanderson, AH Simmons. A free-response approach to the measurement and characterization of radiographic-oberserver performance. J Appl Photogr Eng 4:166–171, 1978.
19. DP Chakraborty. Maximum lilelihood analysis of free-response receiver operating characteristic (froc) data. Med Physics 16:561–568, 1989.
20. DP Chakraborty. Free-response methodology: alternate analysis and a new observer-performance experiment. Radiology 174:873–881, 1990.
21. WP Tanner, Jr., JA Swets. A decision-making theory of visual detection. Psychol Rev 61:401–409, 1954.

22. WW Peterson, TG Birdsall, WC Fox. The theory of signal detectability. IRE Trans PGIT-4:171–212, 1954.
23. A Wald. Statistical Decision Functions. New York: John Wiley & Sons, Inc., 1950.
24. WP Kegelmeyer, Jr., MC Allmen. Dense feature maps for detection of calcifications. In: Digital Mammography: Proceedings of the 2nd International Workshop on Digital Mammography. Vol. 1069 of International Congress Series. York, England: Elsevier Science, 1994, pp 3–12.
25. K Woods, KW Bowyer. Generating ROC curves for artificial neural networks. IEEE Trans Med Imaging 16:329–337, 1997.
26. K Woods, WP Kegelmeyer Jr., KW Bowyer. Combination of multiple classifiers using local accuracy estimates. IEEE Trans Pattern Analysis Machine Intell 19:405–410, 1997.
27. CE Metz. Some practical issues of experimental design and data analysis in radiological ROC studies. Invest Radiol 24:234–245, 1989.
28. DK McClish. Analyzing a portion of the ROC curve. Medical Decision Making 9:190–195, 1989.
29. BJ McNeil, JA Hanley. Statistical approaches to analysis of receiver operating characteristic ROC curves. Medical Decision Making 14:137–150, 1984.
30. DD Dorfman, KS Berbaum, CE Metz. Receiver operating characteristic rating analysis: generalization to the population of readers and patients with the jackknife method. Invest Radiol 27:723–731, 1992.
31. FF Yin, ML Giger, CJ Vyborny, K Doi, RA Schmidt. Comparison of bilateral subtraction and single image processing techniques in the computerized detection of mammographic masses. Invest Radiol 28:473–481, 1993.
32. HP Chan, K Doi, CJ Vyborny. Improvement in radiologists' detection of clustered microcalcifications on mammograms: The potential of computer-aided diagnosis. Invest Radiol 25:1102–1110, 1990.
33. S Astley, I Hutt, S Adamson, P Miller, P Rose, C Boggis, CJ Taylor, T Valentine, J Davies, J Armstrong. Automation in mammography: Computer vision and human perception. Proceedings of the SPIE/IS&T Symposium on Electronic Imaging Science and Technology. vol. 1905. San Jose, CA, Jan 31–Feb 4 1993 pp 716–730.
34. RA Schmidt, RM Nishikawa, K Schreibman, ML Giger, K Doi, J Papaioannou, P Lu, J Stucka, G Birkhahn. Computer detection of lesions missed by mammograhy. In: Digital Mammography: Proceedings of the 2nd International Workshop on Digital Mammography. vol. 1069 of International Congress Series. York, England: Elsevier Science, 1994, pp 289–294.
35. IW Hutt, SM Astley, CRM Boggis. Prompting as an aid to diagnosis in mammography. In: Digital Mammography: Proceedings of the 2nd International Workshop on Digital Mammography. Vol. 1069 of International Congress Series. New York, England: Elsevier Science, 1994, pp 389–398.
36. CJ Vyborny. Can computers help radiologists read mammograms. Radiology 191: 315–317, 1994.
37. KG Marshall. Prevention. how much harm? how much benefit? 3. physical, psychological and social harm. CMAJ 155:169–176, 1996.
38. E Arnold. Clinical Biostatistics: An Introduction to Evidence-Based Medicine. New York: Halsted Press, John Wiley & Sons, Inc., 1995.

39. RM Nishikawa, ML Giger, CE Comstock, J Papaioannou, AM Urbas, K Doi. Performance of a prototype clinical mammography workstation for computer-aided diagnosis (CAD). Radiol Soc North Am 205(P):217, 1997.
40. RM Nishikawa, ML Giger, K Doi, CE Metz, F Yin, CJ Vyborny, RA Schmidt. Effect of case selection on the performance of computer-aided detection schemes. Med Physics, 21:265–269, 1994.
41. RM Nishikawa, RE Johnston, DE Wolverton, RA Schmidt, ED Pisano, BM Hemminger, J Moody. A common database of mammograms for research in digital mammography. In: Proceedings of the 3rd International Workshop on Digital Mammography. New York: Elsevier Science, 1996, pp 435–438.
42. HP Chan, K Doi, CJ Vyborny, KL Lam, RA Schmidt. Computer-aided detection of microcalcifications in mammograms, methodology and preliminary clinical study: Invest Radiol 23:664–671, 1988.
43. MY Sallam, KW Bowyer, K Woods, DB Kopans, RH Moore, WP Kegelmeyer, Jr. The Digital Database for Screening Mammography: lessons learned. Radiol Soc North Am, 205(P):216, 1997.

3
Clinical Applications
Present and Future

Elizabeth A. Krupinski
University of Arizona, Tucson, Arizona

I. INTRODUCTION

One of the main advantages of acquiring radiologic images digitally and displaying them on cathode ray tube (CRT) monitors is that image-processing tools and computer-aided detection (CAD) schemes can be readily implemented. Thus, there has been a proliferation of image processing (1–2) and CAD (3–5) tools developed in the past 20 years. With the advent of digital acquisition technologies in chest imaging (i.e., computed radiography [CR]) and the recent progress in digital mammography, clinical implementation of CAD seems even more probable than in the past. Image-processing tools are often used regularly in certain clinical situations now (e.g., in computed tomography [CT], magnetic resonance imaging [MRI], and ultrasonography [US], where images are digitally acquired and are often displayed on and diagnosed from a CRT monitor), but for the most part CAD tools are used only in experimental situations. Part of the problem with implementing CAD and image-processing tools in the clinical environment is that only a few, limited studies have been conducted to demonstrate reliably their usefulness in improving observer performance. For the most part, results from the use of CAD and image processing in the clinical environment have been equivocal (6–10). Sometimes CAD or image processing aids performance, sometimes it has little or no effect, and sometimes it actually hurts overall performance. Before getting into the specific applications of CAD and the clinical implementation of CAD, a brief explanation of why and how CAD might be useful to the radiologist is in order.

II. PROMPTING/CUEING TO IMPROVE PERFORMANCE

Radiologic images are generally quite complex, especially chest radiographs and mammograms. The detection and recognition of lesions in these images can be difficult because (a) x-ray images are two-dimensional representations in which three-dimensional solid structures are made transparent, requiring an understanding of projective geometry to determine the true depth and location of imaged structures; and (b) lesions, especially nodules or masses, are typically embedded in a background of anatomical noise. The difficulty of the task of finding a lesion in a radiographic image is especially evident when one considers general screening in the clinical setting. If the radiologist has no clinical history and is looking for any possible abnormality, then the entire image must be searched, or read, to make a complete and accurate diagnosis. Even when clinical information is available, the radiologist must read the entire image carefully for the possible presence of other abnormalities in the image.

For general screening studies, error rates (misses) have been estimated to range from 15% to 30% with 2% to 15% false-positive rates (11–16). Many of these missed lesions are, in retrospect, visible on the radiograph and thus are one of the major causes for malpractice suits in radiology (17–21). Malpractice is not the only issue, because missed lesions can result in delayed treatment and possibly increase the severity of the patient's illness. These are just a few of the many reasons why ways have been investigated (including CAD) to aid the human observer in detecting and classifying (i.e., either as a particular type of lesion or as benign vs malignant) lesions in radiographic images.

There have been a number of ways that have been tried over the years to improve observer detection performance. Computer-aided detection is one of the more recent ways tried and differs from past attempts in that a computer is used to analyze the radiographic image and provide detection and/or classification information to the radiologist to incorporate into the final diagnostic decision. The advantage of using computers is that they are objective. An algorithm(s) is developed that uses the same basic criteria for every case it analyzes, and detection results are consistent as long as the algorithm or its thresholds are not changed. Other attempts to improve performance rely more heavily on the human observer. The human observer, however, is much more subjective and variable than the computer. Depending on any number of factors (even time of day!), radiologists will change their decision criteria and the way they search images (22), which can contribute to errors being made.

In general, investigators have found that cueing radiologists to direct their attention to and search a particular area of an image does improve performance. Computer-aided detection does essentially the same thing, but a computer generates the cue and tells the radiologist where to look. The most common type of cueing that has been investigated uses a cue that radiologists generally have available when reading images—the patient's clinical history (e.g., slipped on ice, sore knee) or referral request (e.g., rule out pneumonia). The results of investigations into the effect of history information have, however, been equivocal. Some studies have reported an increase (23–26) in the true-positive rate (e.g., for complex abnormalities other than nodules), but sometimes this gain has been offset by an accompanying increase in the false-positive rate. On the other hand, some studies that have given the radiologist a complete physical description or history of the target abnormality have found that overall performance does not improve (27–29). General consensus does seem to support the belief that clinical history does improve detection performance for many abnormalities.

Kundel et al. have used the radiologists' own eye-position data to cue them to possible lesion locations. A series of experiments demonstrated, by recording the eye position of radiologists as they searched chest images for nodules, that gaze duration is a good predictor of missed nodules (30). Radiologists tended to spend more time fixating nodule locations, even if they did not report detecting a lesion, than they did fixating image locations without nodules. Similar results have also been found with bone and mammography images (31–34). A convenient method for displaying distributions of gaze durations associated with different diagnostic decisions is survival analysis. Fig. 1 shows typical gaze duration distributions associated with true-positive (TP), false-positive (FP), false-negative (FN), and true-negative (TN) decisions for radiologists searching chest images for pulmonary nodules. Fig. 2 shows the same type of distributions for search in mammograms. The characteristic distributions for diagnostic decisions in the two search tasks are quite similar. Note that true-positive and false-positive decisions

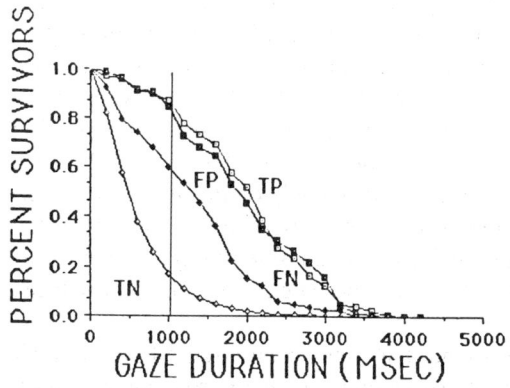

Fig. 1 Distributions of gaze durations (as derived from survival analysis) associated with true-positive (TP), false-positive (FP), false-negative (FN), and true-negative (TN) decisions. The data are from six radiologists searching chest images for pulmonary nodules.

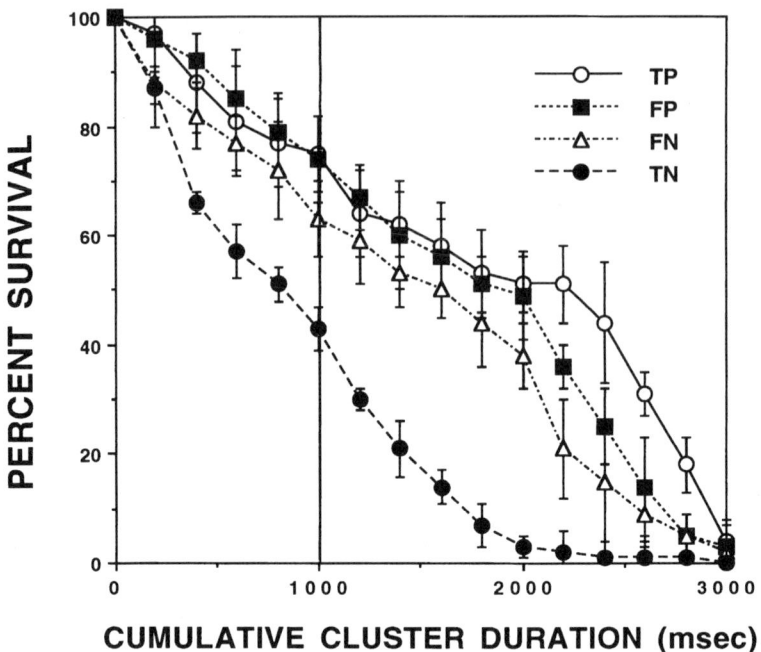

Fig. 2 Distributions of gaze durations (as derived from survival analysis) associated with true-positive (TP), false-positive (FP), false-negative (FN), and true-negative (TN) decisions. The data are from six radiologists searching mammograms for masses and/or microcalcification clusters.

are associated with longer dwell times than true negatives. False-negative decisions fall somewhere in between positive decisions and true-negative decisions, suggesting that the unreported lesion locations are being visually processed to a greater extent (although they are not recognized as lesions) than truly negative areas.

On the basis of the observation that missed nodules receive prolonged dwell, Kundel et al. designed an experiment that fed back areas of prolonged dwell (by circling) to the radiologist for reconsideration (35). A dwell time of 1000 msec (see the vertical line at 1000 msec in Figs. 1 and 2) was chosen as the feedback threshold. Using this threshold, 38% of missed nodules were fed back for reconsideration. Fig. 3 shows an example of a chest image with a single missed nodule circled for feedback. Typically about five image areas were fed back per image. Perceptually based feedback resulted in a 16% increase in performance compared with a control condition in which radiologists looked at the image for a second time but without feedback. The number of true positives increased, and the number of false positives decreased compared with a control second look at the image without feedback.

A series of follow-up experiments (36,37) demonstrated that the feedback circle served to increase the frequency with which the radiologist fixates directly on the nodule and decreases the spread of fixations in the region of interest. Both of these factors would suggest an increased probability that the lesion would be detected and recognized. By progressively decreasing the amount of image area available for viewing outside of the feedback circle (see Figs. 4–6), it was further demonstrated that the circle cue essentially had the effect of focusing attention to such an extent that information outside the circle was essentially blocked off so the observer could concentrate completely within the circle. Performance with the feedback circle present on the chest was essentially equivalent to having all of the area outside the circle removed (see Fig. 7). The problem with perceptually based feedback is that the radiologist has to fixate missed nodules for enough time to pass the feedback threshold. If the radiologist fails to fixate the nodule during the initial search, it will not be fed back for reconsideration. Also, if the radiologist fails to fixate the lesion altogether, it cannot be fed back for reconsideration.

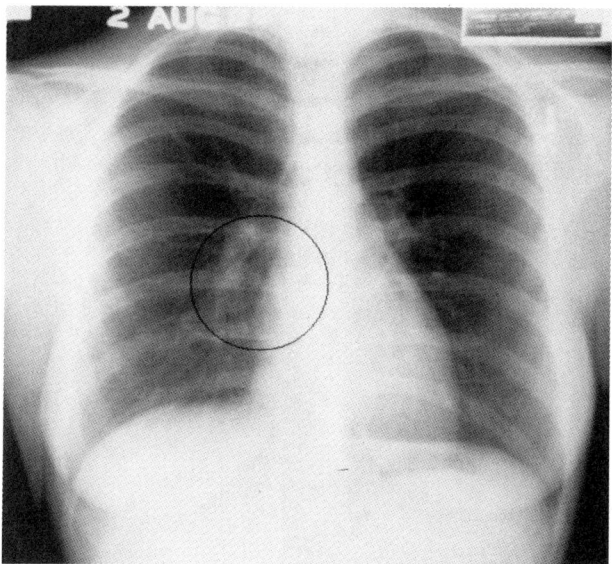

Fig. 3 An example of a feedback circle superimposed over a pulmonary nodule missed during an initial search of the image. Although the nodule was not reported, it was fixated for more than 1000 msec and therefore was fed back for further consideration during a second look at the image.

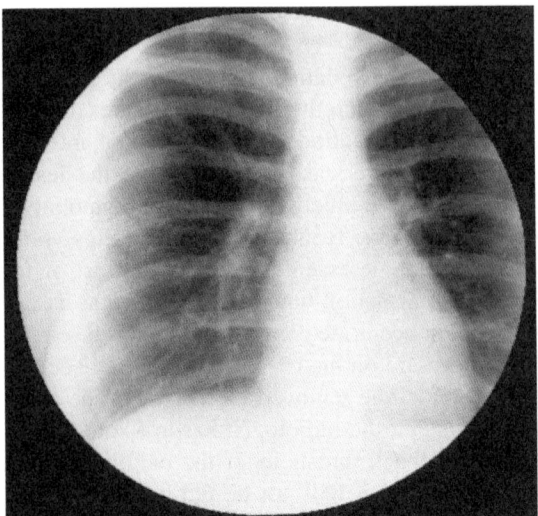

Fig. 4 An example of how image area outside the region of a feedback was reduced to determine the mechanism by which feedback circles improved nodule detection performance. This image has 25% of the image area removed.

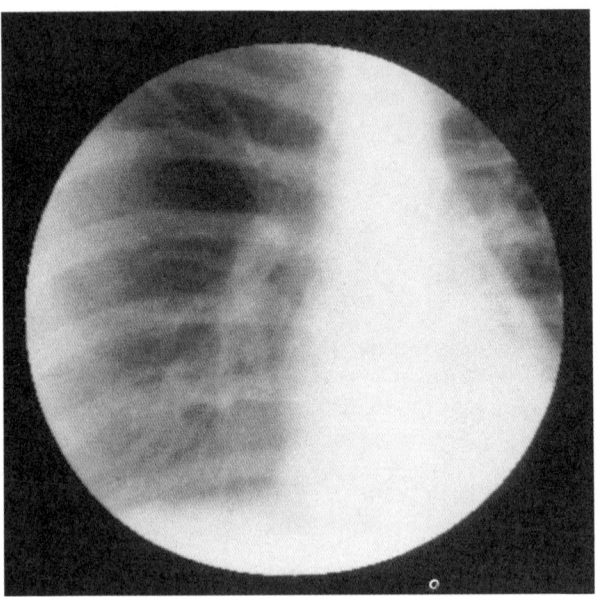

Fig. 5 An example of how image area outside the region of a feedback was reduced to determine the mechanism by which feedback circles improved nodule detection performance. This image has 50% of the image area removed.

Clinical Applications 53

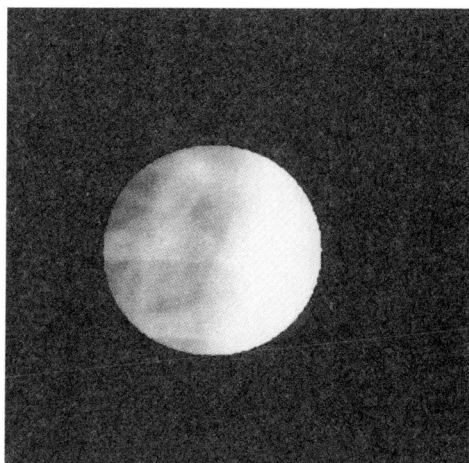

Fig. 6 An example of how image area outside the region of a feedback was reduced to determine the mechanism by which feedback circles improved nodule detection performance. This image has 100% of the image area removed.

There are other ways that have been used to try to improve radiologists' performance. Dual reading has been shown to improve performance (38,39) and is often used clinically, but it is still a rather subjective procedure and requires having two radiologists read the same image. In some clinics, two radiologists are not available for dual readings, and in others dual reading is not a cost-effective procedure. Picture Archiving and Communication Systems (PACS) and teleradiology services are one way to facilitate the use of dual reading and second opinions, but not all hospitals have access to these technologies yet. Computer-aided detection is intended to function in much the same way as a second reader does, but without the cost associated with using a second radiologist.

Checklists have also been used to help radiologists classify lesions (40–42), and in many cases these have been quite useful for correctly classifying lesions as benign vs malignant. The Breast Imaging Reporting And Data System (BIRADS) lexicon was developed by the American College of Radiology as a quality assurance tool to reduce variability in mammographic interpretations and use of terminology. Recent studies (42–44) have demonstrated that the BIRADS lexicon is a useful predictor of malignancy—lesions classified as category 5 have a very high probability of being malignant, and those classified as category 3 have a high probability of being benign on biopsy. The use of checklists such as the BIRADS classification is, however, dependent on the radiologist detecting the lesion in the first place. The usefulness and reliability of

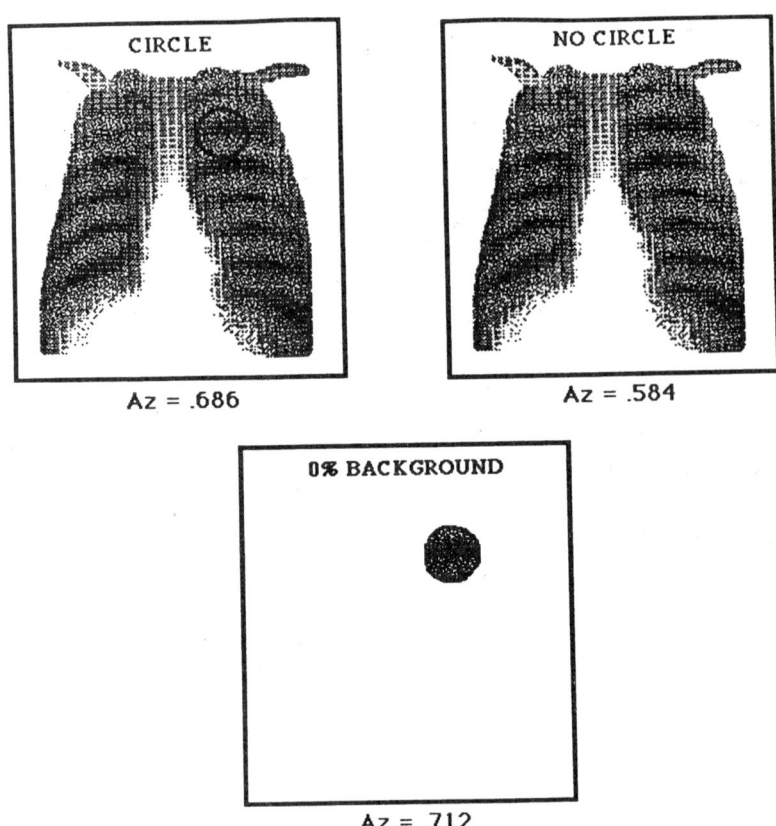

Fig. 7 Examples of conditions in an experiment reducing the amount of background information outside the area of the feedback circle. Performance was measured using receiver operating characteristic Az values.

checklists also depend on the consistency with which they are used by different radiologists and by the same radiologist on different cases. In the case of mammography, even when using the BIRADS system, variation in classification among readers can be quite high, especially for masses (45). The goal of some CAD programs is to detect lesions, then apply checklist-like criteria and assign a probability value as to whether the lesion is benign or malignant. The advantage of CAD over the human observer is again that the computer is objective and will use the image data in a consistent manner using consistent criteria; whereas the human observer can be quite variable from image to image and from one point in time to another.

III. MEDICAL IMAGING AND LESION DETECTION

Much of the work in CAD has been done using mammographic images with microcalcifications and masses as targets of detection (46–50). Most of the early work, and much of the work done now, has focused on detection of microcalcifications and microcalcification clusters. Part of the reason for concentrating on this particular lesion is that microcalcifications are generally fairly high contrast, punctate objects that have very different properties than the surrounding breast tissue. In contrast to microcalcifications, masses tend to be embedded in the surrounding breast tissue and have properties quite similar to the surrounding tissue. Stellate lesions are especially difficult to detect because of their irregular borders and very thin "tendrils" that emanate from the body of the lesion into the surrounding tissue. Currently, detection rates for microcalcifications using CAD tend to be higher than for masses, but there is much work being done to improve detection rates and decrease false-positive rates in both of these area (51,52).

A number of people are also using computer analysis techniques to characterize other potentially useful characteristics of mammograms. For example, there are attempts being made to characterize breast tissue parenchymal patterns using computer algorithms (53,54), because different breast patterns are associated with differing levels of risk for breast cancer developing. Some breast tissue classification systems have been developed for use by radiologists (55), but their use is not universal or standard among those who do use them. Computer-aided detection analysis of parenchymal patterns and detection of subtle lesion patterns within different parenchymal patterns (especially dense breasts) could prove to be quite useful in improving the detection of breast lesions.

The detection of changes in the appearance of the breast, or in the appearance of potential lesions that are being watched mammographically over time for changes in appearance, is also of great interest to mammographers and those developing CAD techniques. The human visual system is very good at detecting change, but subtle differences in size or shape can be difficult to detect, especially because subtle changes require that attention be focused on the locus of change (56). Lapses in attention or distractions, which often occur in reading rooms, can result in subtle lesion changes being missed. A computer does not suffer from lapses in attention or distractions, so changes in lesion shape or size might be more reliably detected using CAD schemes designed for this purpose (57).

In chest radiography, some of the issues for lesion detection and classification are very similar to those in mammography. Radiologists look for changes over time in the appearance of the lungs in some cases, and in other cases they are searching for specific lesions either in the screening situation or in response to a particular patient history or symptoms. As in mammography, however, lesions such as nodules are generally embedded in the complex background of the lungs and are often quite difficult to detect. Other disease patterns such as interstitial lung abnormalities can also be quite difficult to detect and classify. Computer-aided detection has had some success in detecting and characterizing lung lesions and disease entities (58–61), although the success rate is not as high as with microcalcifications in mammograms. One of the major differences between research in CAD for mammography vs chest imaging is that research in chest imaging uses different types (62,63) of images (e.g., digitized film, CR, CT, MRI), whereas CAD for mammography uses almost exclusively mammography images (although there are some exceptions, see Ref. 64, for example).

IV. CRITICAL ISSUES FOR CLINICAL USE OF CAD

Many investigators are working in the area of CAD, using many different approaches to the general problem of detecting and classifying lesions in medical images. A number of chapters in this book deal with some of the successes in the development of CAD systems for mammographic and lung lesions and go into the details of the various procedures implemented. It is safe to say, however, that the clinical success of any CAD system depends on a number of issues in addition to the basic one of how well a particular CAD system detects and/or classifies lesions (i.e., what are the true-positive and false-positive rates). It is obvious that the CAD information provided must be relatively reliable. True-positive rates need to be high and false-positive rates need to be low. Too many false positives per image will result in radiologists not trusting and becoming frustrated with the system. Too few true positives will have the same result. Ideally, one would like the CAD system to confirm what has been detected by the human observer and to point out the very subtle lesions that are missed, without pointing out too many irrelevant locations.

For the most part, CAD systems have been and still are evaluated in terms of what the true-positive and false-positive rates are, independent of if and how a radiologist uses the CAD information in the diagnostic decision process. It is only recently that studies are being conducted that actually include the radiologist in the evaluation process and use CAD as a second reader or prescreening tool during the diagnostic process (65–67). The results of these studies are so far generally positive. In one study (65), when CAD was compared with double reading, there were no statistically significant differences in sensitivity and specificity for CAD-assisted reading compared with the double-reading consensus of two independent radiologists. CAD also seems to be especially useful in helping radiologists classify correctly lesions as benign vs malignant. Chan et al. (67) and Jiang et al. (66) both found that radiologists performed significantly better when CAD information on the probability of malignant vs benign was provided. Radiologists recommended more malignant lesions for biopsy and fewer benign ones when

Clinical Applications 57

CAD was used compared with standard clinical reading without CAD. Methods to enhance digitally displayed mammograms (68,69) also seem to improve (or at least bring to the level of film screen) detection performance compared with digitally displayed but unenhanced images.

It is worth noting, however, that not all studies have found CAD to be helpful in improving performance. Mugglestone et al. (70) compared reading mammograms with and without lesion prompts. Each case had three prompts—one for the true lesion and two false-positive prompts on 87% of the abnormal cases, and three false positives with the lesion unprompted for 13% of the abnormal cases. The normal cases all had three false-positive prompts. It was found that the addition of prompts did not improve significantly the number of lesions detected. There was a slightly lower false-negative rate with prompts, but this was accompanied by an associated rise in the false positives on both normal and abnormal cases. For a secondary analysis, the cases were divided into easy and difficult cases. Prompting did not aid performance in either case, which is unexpected in the difficult cases, because these are the ones one would expect CAD prompting to be most effective in. The authors conclude that overall, prompting has an interfering effect, because it has little influence on the true-positive rate and actually may increase the false-positive rate.

The more general finding, however, that CAD improves performance of radiologists is not surprising. CAD is a form of cueing, and as noted previously, it has been demonstrated that cueing in general, whether it be by perceptual feedback, clinical history, or CAD, does improve performance. There is also extensive evidence in the psychology literature that supports the beneficial effects of cueing on performance (71–73). However, there are a number of issues that need to be looked at for CAD to be a useful and productive tool in the clinical environment.

A. Display

At this time, image display is probably the most critical issue for clinical implementation of CAD. For chest radiography this is not as much a problem as it is for mammography. Many departments use computed radiography to acquire chest images, and although they are generally printed to film, they can be displayed on a CRT monitor directly. The same is true for CT and MRI images of the chest/lungs. There is no need to digitize films (unless traditional screen/film images are acquired), so the CAD algorithms can work directly on the digitally acquired image data. Computer-aided detection information can then be displayed directly on the image when it appears on the CRT monitor. Radiologists can either diagnose the images from the monitor, or they can diagnose the images from film and use the monitor display for viewing the CAD prompts.

In mammography, however, screening images are not acquired or displayed digitally at this time. Stereotactic images are acquired and displayed digitally, but these images are used during biopsies once the lesion has been detected and diagnosed rather than for screening purposes. There is also much excitement surrounding the advances being made in the development of systems for full-field digital acquisition of mammograms (74–76). The problem in this area, however, is that digital image acquisition for mammography is much farther advanced than digital displays for mammography. Conventional screen/film combinations used in mammography have an extremely high spatial resolution: 5% MTF at a frequency of almost 20 lp/mm is typical. If this high limiting spatial resolution had to be reproduced in a digital image for the typical mammography format of 20.3 × 25.4 cm, a digital matrix of 8120 × 10,160 pixels would be required (77)! Some studies (78,79) have suggested that a pixel matrix of at least 2048 × 2560 is the minimum spatial resolution required for digital mammography. This figure is more realizable than the former for direct translation of film to digital resolution, but it is not clear yet whether it is really sufficient. Monitors are currently available with resolutions of 2048 × 2560 and fairly high luminance levels (e.g., 140 ftL), but there have been no formal studies assessing diagnostic performance using digitally acquired mammograms displayed on these high-resolution monitors. Because digital mammograms will likely be acquired at a higher resolution than 2048 × 2560, better monitors than currently available will be needed for display, especially if it is found that radiologists need to see the entire image at once at full resolution (i.e., rather than relying on zoom and pan functions to access the full resolution data for viewing specific regions of interest).

Obviously, CAD for mammography would be most efficiently displayed directly on digitally acquired mammograms displayed on a high-resolution monitor. Currently, this is not possible. Mammograms must be digitized, and then the CAD prompts must be displayed on the lower resolution digitally displayed images. The digitization step itself is a major bottleneck in the process at this time. For each examination, at least four films need to be digitized (right and left breast, craniocaudal and mediolateral views) to be analyzed by the CAD system. Depending on the digitizer, this takes at least 5 minutes, often longer, per case. In a high-volume clinic, it could be very difficult, time-consuming, and impractical to digitize every case and have it examined by CAD for a second opinion. At our institution we have the ImageChecker CAD system from R2 Technology, Inc. (Los Altos, CA), and we are able to process about one-third of the daily case load without interfering significantly with the normal flow of activities and reading schedules.

B. Invalid Cues or False-Positive Rates with CAD

As noted previously, there is quite a bit of evidence both in the psychological and radiological literature that cueing or prompting observers to attend to specific image locations aids detection performance. There are, however, some potential problems with prompting that could influence the effectiveness of CAD prompt-

Clinical Applications 59

ing when used in the clinical environment. Although already mentioned, it is worth mentioning again that radiologists must have confidence in the fact that whatever CAD system they are using, the CAD prompts are for the most part accurate (i.e., have a very high true-positive rate and a relatively low false-positive rate). On the one hand, it is a matter of reliability and the observer's confidence in what they are being shown. On the other hand, there is substantial evidence that cueing accuracy can affect performance. Research in psychology (80–82) has demonstrated quite reliably that valid spatial cues (i.e., those that correctly indicate target locations) provide more benefits in terms of correct identification rates and recognition times than do invalid cues. Invalid cues, which falsely indicate locations that do not contain a target, result in increased response times and increased false-positive reports.

The invalid cue could potentially be a problem, although possibly minor, with CAD. So far no CAD system is 100% perfect (i.e., 100% true positives with 0% false positives). With microcalcifications, the true-positive rates are very high (>90%), but there are still false positives. Much work is being done to reduce the false-positive rates, and much progress is being made. However, it seems unlikely that a 0% false-positive rate with 100% true-positive rate will ever be reached, given the wide variety of features in a mammographic image that resemble microcalcifications or masses. The key is to get the false-positive rates low enough that the radiologist does not get frustrated with an overabundance of false reports and can easily disregard obviously false locations. According to the mammographers at our institution, the microcalcification false-positive rate with the R2 ImageChecker is low enough that they have a very high degree of confidence in this part of the CAD system. They have also noted that for the most part, the false-positive microcalcification prompts are easily disregarded, because they tend to indicate obvious things such as obviously benign macrocalcifications or minor nicks and scratches on the original film image. This observation agrees nicely with studies in the psychology literature on the effects of nontarget similarity and difficulty on target detection (83,84). It is possible that many of these false positives will disappear altogether once digitally acquired mammograms can be displayed directly on CRT monitors!

C. The Influence of CAD on Image Search

The mammographers at our institution also noted another potential problem with CAD, because they have so much confidence in the ability of the CAD system to correctly identify the microcalcification clusters, they tend to find themselves "skimming" the original film mammogram (no CAD information) instead of conducting a thorough microcalcification search. To see if this is really the case, a recent study by Krupinski (85) recorded the eye position of radiologists as they scanned mammograms in a CAD situation. Mammographic cases with masses and/or microcalcification clusters were digitized and analyzed by the ImageChecker CAD system. Half of the readers were experienced mammographers and half were fourth-year residents. Observers were instructed to search the original film images, provide an initial diagnosis, then access and view the CAD information whenever they wanted to and provide a revised diagnosis. Fig. 8 shows

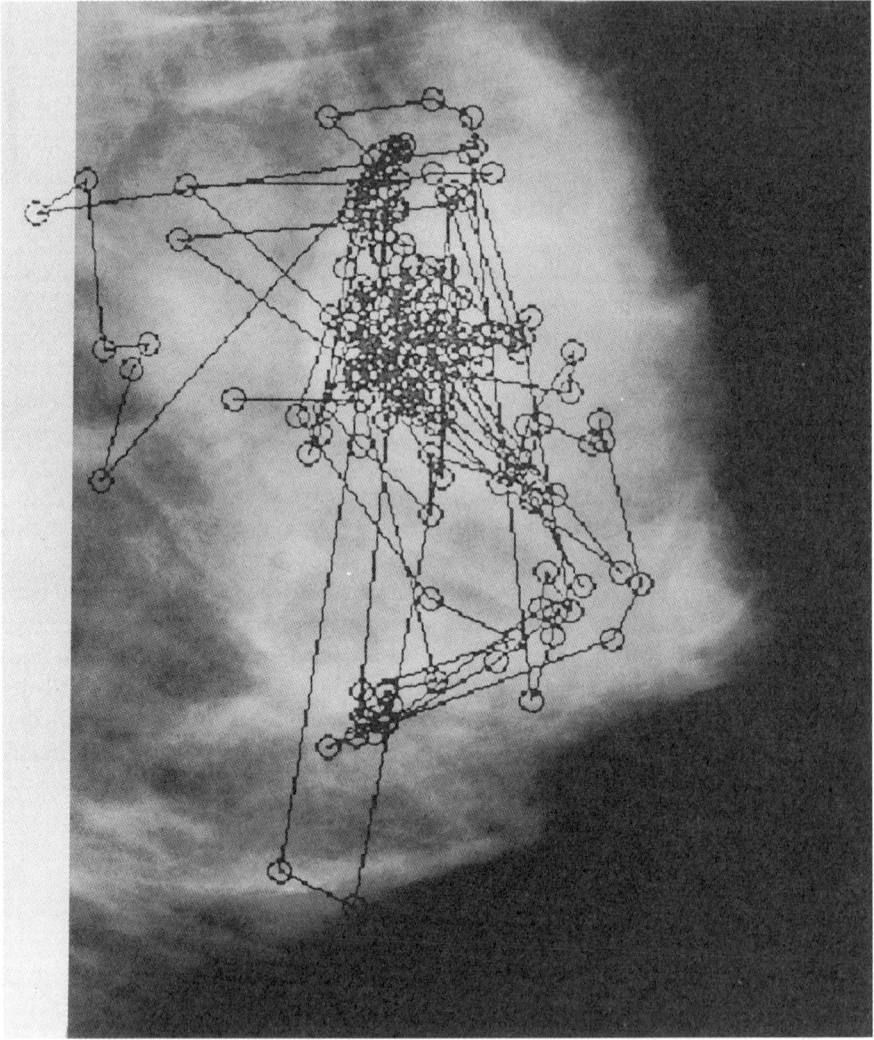

Fig. 8 An example of a mammographer's eye-position pattern during search for masses and/or microcalcifications. Each small circle represent a fixation or location where the eye landed during search.

Clinical Applications

a typical eye-position pattern of an experienced mammographer searching a mammogram for masses and microcalcifications.

On average, the mammographers accessed the CAD images after 104 sec of search, and the residents accessed it after 86 sec of search. The mammographers then spent 49 sec on average searching the CAD and original images, and the residents spent 63 sec. By correlating dwell times with decisions, it was found that the median dwell time for mammographers on false negatives (unreported lesions) before the CAD image was revealed was 1383 msec. The residents had a pre-CAD median false-negative dwell time of only 921 msec. After CAD was revealed and the false-negative locations were prompted, the mammographers had a median dwell on those locations of 524 msec and the residents had a median dwell of 737 msec. For the mammographers 50% of the original false negatives were reported as lesions after CAD, and 33% of the false negatives were reported by the residents. In this study all the false-negative areas were prompted.

True positives had a median dwell of 1743 msec and 1801 msec before CAD for mammographers and residents, respectively. Median dwells on these areas were 187 msec and 329 msec, respectively, for mammographers and residents after CAD was revealed. With respect to false positives, the mammographers had a median dwell of 1681 msec on false positives before CAD and 328 msec after CAD. The residents had a median dwell on false positives of 1829 before CAD and 490 msec after CAD.

These results suggest a number of interesting conclusions and implications for CAD use. The first is that there may be a significant difference in how CAD is used, depending on the experience of the observer. For the most part CAD will probably be more useful for the general radiologist than for the expert mammographer. The results of this study suggest, however, that the radiologists with less mammographic experience seemed to rely more heavily on the CAD information than did the mammographers and that this reliance on CAD affected their visual search behaviors. The residents tended to access the CAD images sooner than the mammographers and spent less time dwelling on false-negative locations before CAD was revealed. After CAD was revealed, the residents' dwells on the false-negative areas were longer than those of the mammographers, but their false-negative to true-positive conversion rate was lower (33% vs 50%) than the mammographers. It would seem that a thorough search of the image before CAD is presented is extremely beneficial with respect to CAD having its desired effect. Perceptually speaking, it seems as if the more a suspicious region is fixated and visually processed before CAD is presented, the easier it is to recognize that suspicious region as actually positive after CAD reinforces the suspicion by prompting it as a lesion.

The finding that lesions detected before CAD is presented receive extended dwell but receive very little dwell once CAD is presented is also interesting. This result confirms the idea that CAD is a good way to confirm the radiologists' suspicion if the level of suspicion was high enough to report the lesion in the initial search before CAD. The very short dwells on these lesions after CAD is presented suggest that the radiologists are basically giving a quick double-checking glance to these already detected areas just to make sure the CAD location and their originally detected location are one in the same. The interesting thing is that the false positives showed this same trend—extended dwell on the suspected location before CAD and relatively short dwell duration after CAD. With the false positives, however, the dwells after CAD were short but slightly longer than for the true positives. With respect to performance, the mammographers changed 50% of their false positives to true negatives after CAD was presented, and the residents changed 25% of their decisions. These results suggest a benefit of CAD that is rarely talked about—the influence of CAD on the radiologists' false positives. Because CAD and the radiologist report the same false-positive areas only about one-third of the time (86), it is not surprising that the radiologists would spend more time looking at an area that they called positive but that the computer did not. This is especially true if the radiologist has faith in CAD's performance and expects it to be right most of the time. By double-checking areas that the radiologist called positive, but CAD did not, the experienced mammographer seems better able to modify the initial incorrect decision than the less-experienced resident. The effect is not complete, however, because even the experienced mammographers changed only 50% of their false-positive reports to true negatives. If general radiologists are found to perform more like residents than expert mammographers, they too may have trouble changing their false-positive calls even if CAD does not confirm their suspicions.

D. Satisfaction of Search (SOS) and CAD

Satisfaction of search (SOS) is a phenomenon first reported by Tuddenham (87) and subsequently studied by others (88–91), in which the radiologist fails to report multiple lesions on a radiograph after one lesion has already been detected. Tuddenham suggested that radiograph interpretation involves a "search for meaning." If a lesion is detected during search, then this "search for meaning" is satisfied, and the radiologist may prematurely halt search and fail to detect further lesions. Hence the term satisfaction of search. Although this phenomenon has not yet been studied specifically with respect to visual search, CAD and detection performance, two studies (70,85) do suggest that SOS might occur with CAD. Mugglestone et al. (70) found that radiologists tended to concentrate mostly on prompted areas of mammograms and to ignore unprompted areas. Unprompted lesions tended to be fixated minimally and were often missed. Krupinski (85) also found this to be true. Before CAD was presented, radiologists had a median true negative dwell time of about 700 msec. After CAD was presented, true negative dwell times fell to about 150 msec, and the number of fixation clusters outside areas indicted by CAD was minimal. Radiologists often went back to check areas that they had called positive that CAD did not, but they did not spend much time on other areas outside the CAD-indicated regions of interest.

The findings from both of these studies suggest that a sort of SOS effect may be occurring with CAD. The presence of the CAD prompts tends to draw the radiologists' attention to the prompted areas and tends to inhibit them from searching unprompted areas. Because CAD does not have a 100% detection rate (neither does the radiologist), there are lesions that will be unprompted by CAD and undetected by radiologists in an initial search of the image. In fact, Krupinski and Nishikawa (86) found that about 5% of microcalcification clusters go undetected by both CAD and radiologists when both search the same mammogram. If there truly is an SOS effect associated with CAD, these unprompted lesions may remain undetected if the radiologists do not conduct a thorough search of the image even after CAD has been presented. Therefore, although having faith in CAD's performance is certainly required if CAD is to be implemented and used in the clinical situation, it should not be blind faith. Radiologists need to recognize that CAD is not a perfect second reader and that they still should give an image a good second search even after CAD has been presented. This is especially true if, as mammographers at our institution noted, it is found that it is all too easy to give an image a cursory initial search then access the CAD information for the prompts. The ImageChecker does have a built-in delay, but that does not ensure that the radiologist will conduct a thorough search of the image while waiting out the delay.

IV. CONCLUSIONS

The potential for CAD is immense. It should prove to be an important aid to the mammographer in the near future. As noted, the main factor inhibiting its wide-scale use in the mammography clinic is that all the mammographic films have to be digitized before CAD systems can analyze them. The CAD results must then be displayed on a CRT monitor rather than the original film image, requiring the radiologist to make comparisons between the two displays. Both of these factors make the use of CAD at this point rather time-consuming, especially the digitization phase. In a large-volume clinic, it will be extremely difficult and time-consuming to process every case for CAD analysis. Even though the detection rates are high and false-positive rates relatively low, especially for microcalcifications, time delays will make the clinical use of CAD less attractive. With the advent of digital mammography and future development of CRT displays that can handle mammographic images, this problem should be solved. CAD will work directly on the digital data and will display the detection prompts directly on the image as it is displayed on a high-resolution monitor. Hopefully, this is a scenario that can be realized within the next 5 to 10 years.

In chest radiography, clinical use of CAD may not be as widespread as in mammography. Lung cancer still has the highest incidence of all cancers, especially in men. However, people are generally not screened as regularly for lung cancer as women are for breast cancer. In addition, chest images are acquired routinely for many other purposes than screening for lung cancer, and chest imaging often represents the highest volume case type in many hospitals. In our hospital, chest imaging accounts for almost 80% of all radiographic images acquired. Thus, it may be impractical to use CAD on every chest image acquired. In combination with a clinical history or presenting symptoms, however, judicious use of CAD for detection of lung nodules might be useful and feasible. The same scenario would hold for use of CAD for detection and classification of interstitial disease or other abnormalities amenable to CAD analysis. Ideally, one might want to see a "package" CAD system developed that operates on many types of lesions much as the ImageChecker does for masses and microcalcifications in mammography. If the detection algorithms could work in parallel with sufficient speed, they could work directly on the digital data from a CR system. If the chest images are then viewed directly on a CRT monitor, the CAD prompts could be accessed quite easily and superimposed over the image. If CR images are still printed to film, one could still view the CAD images on the CRT and refer back to the film image, which is what is currently done with the ImageChecker system in mammography.

Most of the potential problems with using CAD that were noted earlier can be avoided with judicious use of CAD systems. As long as radiologists recognize the limitations of CAD and their own limitations, the use of CAD will serve quite nicely as a reliable second reader. Radiologists need to integrate CAD into their normal reading procedure, without changing their normal search and detection behaviors to any great extent. Careful and thorough search of images and lesions will be necessary no matter how accurate CAD systems get. Computer-aided detection detection rates will eventually be quite high for both microcalcification clusters and masses in mammography and probably for lesions in other types of images as well. Computer-aided detection programs to provide probabilities of benign vs malignant are also getting more reliable and accurate and will be quite useful in many circumstances. However, in the final analysis it is the radiologist who is responsible for collecting, analyzing, and weighing all the available data and coming up with a diagnostic decision and suggesting a course of treatment.

REFERENCES

1. SR Bolle, T Sund, J Stromer. Receiver operating characteristic study of image preprocessing for teleradiology and digital workstations. J Dig Imag 10:152–157, 1997.
2. N Oda, H Nakata, H Watanabe, K Terada. Evaluation of automatic-mode image processing method in chest computed radiography. Acad Radiol 4:558–564, 1997.

3. NF Vittitoe, JA Baker, CE Floyd. Fractal texture analysis in computer-aided diagnosis of solitary pulmonary nodules. Acad Radiol 4:96–101, 1997.
4. CM Kocur, SK Rogers, LR Myers, T Burns. Using neural networks to select wavelet features for breast cancer diagnosis. IEEE Engin Med Biol May/June:95–102, 1996.
5. ML Giger, RM Nishikawa, M Kupinski, U Bick, M Zhang, RA Schmidt, DE Wolverton, CE Comstock, J Papaioannou, SA Collins, AM Urbas, CJ Vyborny, K Doi. Computerized detection of breast lesions in digitized mammograms and results with a clinically-implemented intelligent workstation. In: HU Lemke, MW Vannier, K Inamura, eds. Computer Assisted Radiology and Surgery. New York: Elsevier Science, 1997, pp 325–330.
6. MD Mugglestone, R Lomax, AG Gale, ARM Wilson. The effect of prompting mammographic abnormalities on the human observer. In: K Doi, ML Giger, RM Nishikawa, RA Schmidt, eds. Digital Mammography '96. New York: Elsevier Science, 1996, pp 87–96.
7. EA Krupinski. An eye-movement study on the use of CAD information during mammographic search. Paper presented at the 7th Far West Image Perception Conference, Tucson, AZ, Oct 16–18, 1997.
8. JH Hendriks, R Holland, H Rijken, B Thoosen, J Van Dijck, KF O'shaughnessy. A pilot study on computer aided diagnosis-assisted reading compared to double reading in screening for breast cancer. Radiology 205 (P):216, 1997.
9. Y Jiang, RM Nishikawa, RA Schmidt, CE Metz, K Doi. Improving breast cancer diagnosis with computer-aided diagnosis (CAD): An observer study. Radiology 205 (P):274–275, 1997.
10. EA Krupinski, M Evanoff, T Ovitt, JR Standen, TX Chu, J Johnson. The influence of image processing on chest radiograph interpretation and decision changes. Acad Radiol 5:79–85, 1998.
11. RT Heelan, BJ Flehinger, MR Melamed. Non-small cell cancer: Results of the New York screening program. Radiology 151:289–293, 1984.
12. HL Kundel. Perception errors in chest radiology. Semin Respir Med 10:203–210, 1989.
13. JR Muhm, WE Miller, RS Fontan, DR Sanderson, MA Uhlenhopp. Lung cancer detection during a screening program using four-month chest radiographs. Radiology 148:609–615, 1983.
14. LW Bassett, V Manjikian, RH Gold. Mammography and breast cancer screening. Surg Clin North Am 70:775–800, 1990.
15. LW Bassett, RH Gold. Breast Cancer Detection: Mammography and Other Methods in Breast Imaging. New York: Grune & Stratton, 1987.
16. RE Bird, TW Wallace, BC Yankaskas. Analysis of cancers missed at screening mammography. Radiology 184:613–617, 1992.
17. L Berlin. Malpractice and radiologists. AJR 135:587–591, 1980.
18. L Berlin. Does the "missed" radiographic diagnosis constitute malpractice? Radiology 123:523–527, 1977.
19. AE James. Medical/Legal Issues for Radiologists. Chicago: Precept Press, 1987.
20. KA Kern. Causes of breast cancer malpractice litigation: A 20-year civil court review. Arch Surg 127:542–546, 1992.

21. RL Kravitz, JE Rolph, K McGuigan. Malpractice claims data as a quality improvement tool. I. Epidemiology of error in four specialties. JAMA 266:2087–2092, 1991.
22. AG Gale, D Murray, K Millar, BS Worthington. Circadian variation in radiology. In: AG Gale, F Johnson, eds. Theoretical & Applied Aspects of Eye Movement Research. Amsterdam, The Netherlands: Elsevier Science, 1984, pp 305–312.
23. TW Parker, CA Kelsey, RD Moseley, FA Mettler, JF Garcia, DE Briscoe. Directed vs free search for nodules in chest radiographs. Invest Radiol 2:152–155, 1982.
24. KS Berbaum, EA Franken, KL Anderson, DD Dorfman, WE Erkonen, GP Farrar, JJ Geraghty, TJ Gleason, ME MacNaughton, ME Phillips, DL Renfrew, CW Walker, CG Whitten, DC Young. Influence of clinical history on visual search with single and multiple abnormalities. Invest Radiol 28:191–201, 1993.
25. KS Berbaum, EA Franken, DD Dorfman, T Barloon, SR Ell, CH Lu, W Smith, MM Abu-Yousef. Tentative diagnoses facilitate the detection of diverse lesions in chest radiographs. Invest Radiol 7:532–539, 1986.
26. UO Aideyan, K Berbaum, WL Smith. Influence of prior radiologic information on the interpretation of radiographic examinations. Acad Radiol 2:205–208, 1995.
27. RG Swensson, SJ Hessel, PG Herman. Radiographic interpretation with and without visual search: Visual search aids the recognition of chest pathology. Invest Radiol 17:145–151, 1982.
28. RG Swensson, GH Theodore. Search and nonsearch protocols for radiographic consultation. Radiology 177:851–856, 1990.
29. LA Cooperstein, BC Good, EA Eelkema. The effect of clinical history on chest radiograph interpretations in a PACS environment. Invest Radiol 25:670–674, 1990.
30. HL Kundel, CF Nodine, EA Krupinski. Searching for lung nodules: Visual dwell indicates locations of false-positive and false-negative decisions. Invest Radiol 24:472–478, 1989.
31. CH Hu, HL Kundel, CF Nodine, EA Krupinski, LC Toto. Searching for bone fractures: A comparison with pulmonary nodule search. Acad Radiol 1:25–32, 1994.
32. EA Krupinski, PJ Lund. Differences in time to interpretation for evaluation of bone radiographs with monitor and film viewing. Acad Radiol 4:177–182, 1997.
33. EA Krupinski. Visual scanning patterns of radiologists searching mammograms. Acad Radiol 3:137–144, 1996.
34. CF Nodine, HL Kundel, SC Lauver, LC Toto. The nature of expertise in searching mammograms for breast lesions. SPIE Medical Imaging Proc 2712:89–94, 1996.
35. HL Kundel, CF Nodine, EA Krupinski. Computer-displayed eye position as a visual aid to pulmonary nodule interpretation. Invest Radiol 25:890–896, 1990.
36. EA Krupinski, CF Nodine, HL Kundel. A perceptually based method for enhancing pulmonary nodule recognition. Invest Radiol 28:289–294, 1993.
37. EA Krupinski, CF Nodine, HL Kundel. Perceptual enhancement of tumor targets in chest x-ray images. Perception Psychophysics 53:519–526, 1993.
38. CA Beam, DC Sullivan, PM Layde. Effect of human variability on independent double reading in screening mammography. Acad Radiol 3:891–897, 1996.
39. EL Thurfjell, KA Lernevall, AAS Taube. Benefit of independent double reading in a population-based mammography screening program. Radiology 191:241–244, 1994.
40. DJ Getty, RM Pickett, CJ D'Orsi, JA Swets. Enhanced interpretation of diagnostic images. Invest Radiol 23:240–252, 1988.

Clinical Applications

41. AG Gale, EJ Roebuck, P Riley, BS Worthington. Computer aids to mammographic diagnosis. Br J Radiol 60:887–891, 1987.
42. SG Orel, DC Sullivan, TJ Dambro. BIRADS categorization as a predictor of malignancy. Radiology 205(P):447, 1997.
43. L Liberman, FB Squires, AF Abramson, J Glassman, EA Morris, DD Dershaw. Positive predictive value of BI-RADS final assessment categories. Radiology 205(P): 446, 1997.
44. JY Lo, JA Baker, ED Frederick, PJ Cornguth, CE Floyd. Predicting breast lesion malignancy and invasion using the BI-RADS mammography lexicon. Radiology 205(P):447, 1997.
45. WA Berg, C Campassi, MJ Sexton, P Langenberg, JM Destouet, HR Singh. Analysis of sources of variation in mammographic interpretation. Radiology 205(P):447, 1997.
46. H Yoshida, RM Nishikawa, ML Giger, K Doi. Optimally weighted wavelet packets for detection of clustered microcalcifications in digital mammograms. In: K Doi, ML Giger, RM Nishikawa, RA Schmidt, eds. Digital Mammography '96. New York: Elsevier, 1996, pp 317–322.
47. SS Buchbinder, IS Leichter, P Bamberger, R Lederman, SI Fields, DJ Behar. Analysis of clustered microcalcifications using a single numerical classifier extracted from mammographic digital images. Radiology 205(P):402, 1997.
48. D Meersman, P Scheunders, D Van Dyck. Detection of microcalcifications using neural networks. In: K Doi, ML Giger, RM Nishikawa, RA Schmidt, eds. Digital Mammography '96. New York: Elsevier, 1996, pp 287–290.
49. NA Petrick, H Chan, B Sahiner, MA Helvie, S Sanjay-Gopal, MM Goodsitt. Computer-aided detection of breast masses: Evaluation of a fuzzy morphological classifier. Radiology 205(P):216, 1997.
50. BR Groshong, WP Kegelmeyer. Evaluation of a Hough transform method for circumscribed lesion detection. In: K Doi, ML Giger, RM Nishikawa, RA Schmidt, eds. Digital Mammography '96. New York: Elsevier, 1996, pp 361–366.
51. GM teBrake, N Karssemeijer. Detection of stellate breast abnormalities. In: K Doi, ML Giger, RM Nishikawa, RA Schmidt, eds. Digital Mammography '96. New York: Elsevier, 1996, pp 341–346.
52. RM Nishikawa, ML Giger, CE Comstock, J Papaioannou, AM Urbas, K Doi. Performance of a prototype clinical mammography workstation for computer-aided-diagnosis (CAD). Radiology 205(P):217, 1997.
53. Z Huo, ML Giger, OI Olopade, DE Wolverton, B Weber, W Zhong, PG Tahoces, SI Narvid, T Baker, S Cummings, K Doi. Computer-aided diagnosis: Breast cancer risk assessment from mammographic parenchymal patterns in digitized mammograms. In: K Doi, ML Giger, RM Nishikawa, RA Schmidt, eds. Digital Mammography '96. New York: Elsevier, 1996, pp 191–194.
54. CE Priebe, JL Solka, RA Lorey, GW Rogers, WL Poston, M Kallergi, W Qian, LP Clarke, RA Clark. The application of fractal analysis to mammographic tissue classification. Cancer Lett 77:183–189, 1994.
55. JN Wolfe. Breast patterns as an index of risk for developing breast cancer. Am J Roentgenol 126:1130–1139, 1976.
56. RA Rensink, JK O'Regan, JJ Clark. To see or not to see: The need for attention to perceive changes in scenes. Psychol Sci 8:368–373, 1997.

57. S Sanjay-Gopal, H Chan, B Sahiner, NA Petrick, TE Wilson, MA Helvie. Evaluation of interval change in mammographic features for computerized classification of malignant and benign masses. Radiology 205(P):216, 1997.
58. F Mao, W Qian, LP Clarke. Fractional dimension filtering for multiscale lung nodule detection. Proc SPIE Medical Imaging 3034:449–456, 1997.
59. XW Xu, H MacMahon, ML Giger, K Doi. Adaptive feature analysis of false positives for computerized detection of lung nodules in digital chest images. Proc SPIE Medical Imaging 3034:48–436, 1997.
60. T Ishida, K Ashizawa, S Katsuragawa, H MacMahon, K Doi. Computerized analysis of interstitial lung diseases on chest radiographs based on lung texture, geometric-pattern features and artificial neural networks. Radiology 205(P):395, 1997.
61. S Kido, J Ikezoe, S Tamura, H Nakamura, C Kuroda. A computerized analysis system in chest radiography: evaluation of interstitial lung abnormalities. J Digital Imaging 10:57–64, 1997.
62. B Zhao, AP Reeves, DF Yankelevitz, CI Henschke. Three-dimensional multi-criteria iterative segmentation of helical CT images of pulmonary nodules. Radiology 205(P):168, 1997.
63. S Toshioka, K Kanazawa, N Niki, H Satoh, H Ohmatsu, K Eguchi, N Moriyama. Computer-aided diagnosis system for lung cancer based on helical CT images. Proc SPIE Medical Imaging 3034:975–984, 1997.
64. U Behrens, J Teubner, CJG Evertsz, M Walz, H Jurgens, HO Peitgen. Computer assisted dynamic evaluation of contrast-enhanced breast-MRI. In: HU Lemke, MW Vannier, K Inamura, eds. Computer Assisted Radiology '96. New York: Elsevier, 1996, pp 362–367.
65. JH Hendriks, R Holland, H Rijken, B Thoonsen, J Van Dijck, KF O'shaughnessy. A pilot study on computer aided diagnosis-assisted reading compared to double reading in screening for breast cancer. Radiology 205(P):216, 1997.
66. Y Jiang, RM Nishikawa, RA Schmidt, CE Metz, K Doi. Improving breast cancer diagnosis with computer-aided diagnosis (CAD): An observer study. Radiology 205(P):274, 1997.
67. H Chan, B Sahiner, MA Helvie, CP Paramugul, JS Newman, S Gopal. Effects of computer-aided diagnosis (CAD) on radiologists' classification of malignant and benign masses on mammograms: An ROC study. Radiology 205(P):275, 1997.
68. RN Strickland, LJ Baig, WJ Dallas, EA Krupinski. Wavelet-based image enhancement as an instrument for viewing CAD data. In: K Doi, ML Giger, RM Nishikawa, RA Schmidt, eds. Digital Mammography '96. New York: Elsevier, 1996, pp 441–446.
69. M Kallergi, LP Clarke, W Qian, M Gavrielides, P Venugopal, CG Berman, SD Holman-Ferris, MS Miller, RA Clark. Interpretation of calcifications in screen/film, digitized, and wavelet-enhanced monitor-displayed mammograms: A receiver operating characteristic study. Acad Radiol 3:285–293, 1996.
70. MD Mugglestone, R Lomax, AG Gale, ARM Wilson. The effect of prompting mammographic abnormalities on the human observer. In: K Doi, ML Giger, RM Nishikawa, RA Schmidt, eds. Digital Mammography '96. New York: Elsevier, 1996, pp 87–92.

71. CW Eriksen, JD St. James. Visual attention within and around the field of focal attention: A zoom lens model. Perception Psychophysics 40:225–240, 1986.
72. BJA Krose, B Julesz. The control and speed of shifts of attention. Vision Res 29: 1607–1619, 1989.
73. A Treisman. Verbal cues, language, and meaning in selective attention. Am J Psychol 77:206–219, 1964.
74. JD Cox, SR Sharma, RB Schilling. Advanced digital mammography. In: HU Lemke, MW Vannier, K Inamura, eds. Computer Assisted Radiology and Surgery '97. New York: Elsevier, 1997, pp 11–16.
75. H Liu, LL Fajardo, J McAdoo, G Halama, A Jalink. Development of a detector-scanning, radiation-shielding technique for large field digital mammography: Technical characteristics of the system. Radiology 205(P):302, 1997.
76. MJ Yaffe. Technical aspects of digital mammography. In: K Doi, ML Giger, RM Nishikawa, RA Schmidt, eds. Digital Mammography '96. New York: Elsevier, 1996, pp 33–42.
77. H Roehrig, EA Krupinski, WJ Dallas. Necessary spatial resolution in digital mammography. In: HU Lemke, MW Vannier, K Inamura, eds. Computer Assisted Radiology and Surgery '96. New York: Elsevier, 1996, pp 53–59.
78. HP Chan, CJ Vyborny, H MacMahobn, CE Metz, K Doi, EA Sickles. Digital mammography: ROC studies of the effects of pixel size and unsharp-mask filtering on the detection of subtle microcalcifications. Invest Radiol 22:581–589, 1987.
79. N Karssemeijer, JTM Frieling, JHCL Hendricks. Spatial resolution in digital mammography. Invest Radiol 24:234, 1989.
80. JF Juola, H Koshino, CB Warner. Tradeoffs between attentional effects of spatial cues and abrupt onsets. Perception Psychophysics 57:333–342, 1995.
81. MI Posner. Orienting of attention. Q J Exp Psychol 32:3–25, 1980.
82. J Jonides. Voluntary versus automatic control over the mind's eye's movement. In: JB Long, AD Baddeley, eds. Attention and Performance. Hillsdale, NJ: Erlbaum, 1981, pp 187–203.
83. G Chastain, M Cheal, DR Lyon. Attention and nontarget effects in the location-cuing paradigm. Perception Psychophysics 58:300–309, 1996.
84. R Ward, J Duncan, K Shapiro. Effects of similarity, difficulty, and nontarget presentation on the time course of visual attention. Perception Psychophysics 59:593–600, 1997.
85. EA Krupinski. An eye-movement study on the use of CAD information during mammographic search. Paper presented at the 7th Far West Image Perception Conference, Tucson, AZ Oct 16–18, 1997.
86. EA Krupinski, RM Nishikawa. Comparison of eye position versus computer identified microcalcification clusters on mammograms. Med Phys 24:17–23, 1997.
87. WJ Tuddenham. Visual search, image organization and reader error in roentgen diagnosis: Studies of the psychophysiology of roentgen image perception. Radiology 78:694–704, 1962.
88. KS Berbaum, EA Franken, DD Dorfman, SA Rooholamini, MH Kathol, TJ Barloon, FM Behlke, Y Sato, CH Lu, GY El-Khoury, FW Flickenger, WJ Montgomery. Satisfaction of search in diagnostic radiology. Invest Radiol 25:133–140, 1990.

89. KS Berbaum, EA Franken, DD Dorfman, EM Miller, EA Krupinski, K Kreinbring, RT Caldwell, CH Lu. Cause of satisfaction of search effects in contrast studies of the abdomen. Acad Radiol 3:815–826, 1996.
90. S Samuel, HL Kundel, CF Nodine, LC Toto. Mechanism of satisfaction of search: Eye position recordings in the reading of chest radiographs. Radiology 194:895–902, 1995.
91. KS Berbaum, EA Franken, DD Dorfman, EM Miller, RT Caldwell, DM Kuehn, ML Berbaum. Role of faulty search in the satisfaction of search effect in chest radiography. Acad Radiol 5:9–19, 1998.

4
Statistical Decision Theory and Tumor Detection

Eric Clarkson and Harrison H. Barrett
University of Arizona, Tucson, Arizona

I. INTRODUCTION

Statistical decision theory is the branch of mathematics and statistics that deals with the task of choosing among competing hypotheses based on a finite amount of data that contain some randomly varying components. In medical imaging the problem of tumor detection is an example of this kind of task. The data in this case are the output of a digital imaging device, either the raw data or the image that results from a reconstruction algorithm. The competing hypotheses are that the tumor is absent or the tumor is present in the patient. The randomness in the data has three sources, noise from the imaging system itself, anatomical and other variations in the patient population, and random variations in tumor characteristics.

The imaging-system noise, or measurement noise, is due to the random nature of the physical processes that produce the data. This means that even if we created many images by using the same system on one patient, there would be random variations in the data sets that we collect. The sources of this type of noise are often well known. From this knowledge, the statistics of the measurement noise can be modeled by familiar probability distributions, such as the Poisson or gaussian distributions.

The anatomical or background noise is mainly due to random variations in the normal anatomical structure from one patient to the next. The statistics of large-scale variations, such as organ shapes and skeletal structure, are difficult to model mathematically (1,2). The statistics of small-scale variations, such as the texture of a particular tissue type, is often modeled by correlated gaussian distributions (3–6). There are also texture synthesis algorithms that can produce ensembles of simulated backgrounds for Monte Carlo studies of the effects of small-scale structural variations (7).

Random variations in some tumor characteristics, such as size and location, are easily modeled with known probability distributions. For example, the location of a tumor may be uniformly distributed within a certain specified region of the anatomy. Variations in other tumor characteristics, such as shape and texture, are more difficult to model analytically, and Monte Carlo calculations with simulated ensembles may be necessary to account for them.

For the purposes of this chapter an observer is a human or a computer algorithm that uses the noisy output data from an imaging system that views a patient and decides whether a tumor is present in that patient. The observer is not allowed to equivocate, and there can be no random element in the decision process. The latter condition implies that, given a data set that is identical to a previous one, the observer will make the same decision the second time around. To some extent human observers violate this last condition. This is often accounted for by assuming that there is an internal noise component to the human decision-making process. We will not deal with this complication here.

Given an imaging system, patient ensemble, tumor parameters, and an observer, we would like to calculate the performance of the observer in the tumor detection task. To do this we must first define a figure of merit, a function that assigns a number to each observer for the given task, that corresponds to detection performance. Then we can devise ways to compute this number to some degree of approximation for the given observer. We will consider some of the commonly used figures of merit from statistical decision theory and discuss their applicability to various tumor-detection tasks.

II. DATA AND OBSERVERS

The output of a digital imaging system is always a finite list of numbers. This is true even when we consider the output to be a reconstructed image derived from the raw data. For example, a gray-level image is a list of numbers, one for each pixel, that determine the gray levels. It is convenient to think of these numbers as the components of a data vector **g**. We will assume that **g** has M components and write

$$\mathbf{g} = \begin{bmatrix} g_1 \\ g_2 \\ \vdots \\ g_M \end{bmatrix}$$

Of course, a radiologist would not have much use for this vector, preferring an image instead.

Statistical Decision Theory

In signal detection theory we are often concerned with mathematical manipulations of the data that lead to a decision on the presence or absence of a signal. A tumor produces a signal in the data, some change in the components of the data vector relative to the data components we would expect from a tumor-free patient, and we want to distinguish this change from the variations in the data vector caused by noise.

Along with the signal and the data we need an observer. The observer could be a radiologist looking at an image, but in this chapter we will concentrate on mathematical observers. A mathematical observer, which is usually a computer program, uses the data vector to compute a single number and decides whether the tumor is present or absent on the basis of whether that number exceeds a threshold. This number is often called the observer's test statistic, and it may be an extremely complicated function of the data. The two mathematical observers we will discuss the most are the ideal observer and the Hotelling observer.

The ideal observer has full knowledge of the statistics of the data under both tumor-present and tumor-absent hypotheses. The test statistic that the ideal observer uses is called the likelihood ratio and is simply the ratio of the probability density functions under the tumor-present and tumor-absent hypotheses evaluated at the given data vector. By many commonly used measures of observer performance in the tumor detection task, some of which will be discussed later, the performance of the ideal observer is the best possible. A drawback of the ideal observer is that it is often very difficult to compute the likelihood ratio.

If we restrict ourselves to linear observers, those whose test statistic is a linear function of the data, then a commonly used figure of merit for the performance of the observer is the signal-to-noise ratio (SNR) of the test statistic, which will be defined later. The linear observer that maximizes the SNR is called the Hotelling observer (8). Similarly, the test statistic for this observer is often called the Hotelling test statistic. It is considerably easier to compute this test statistic than the likelihood ratio. A drawback of the Hotelling observer is that, for non-gaussian statistics, the SNR may not be an accurate reflection of the performance of the observer in the actual signal detection task.

The reason we are interested in these two observers is that their performance on the tumor detection task is a measure of how useful the imaging system itself is for this task. For example, if the ideal observer for a given imaging system and tumor detection task performs very badly, then all other observers, including a radiologist looking at a reconstructed image, will also have poor performance on this particular task. The ideal observer for a given imaging system and tumor detection task sets an upper bound on the performance of any observer using that system for that task. Thus, the ideal observer performance can be used to optimize system parameters for a particular task or set of tasks. On the other hand, the performance of a Hotelling observer with certain detection tasks is often a good predictor of human performance at those tasks. In addition, because the Hotelling test statistic is also usually easier to compute and analyze than the likelihood ratio, it may be used for system optimization when the ideal observer performance is too difficult to compute. Of course, in both cases we must specify exactly how the performance of an observer is being measured for these statements to be meaningful. In the next few sections we will introduce ideal observers, Hotelling observers, and some measures of observer performance.

III. IDEAL OBSERVERS

In this section we will introduce the bayesian risk and show how it leads to the ideal observer. Reality is represented by one of two hypotheses H_0 and H_1. Under H_0 the tumor is absent, whereas under H_1 the tumor is present. The observer is trying to determine which hypothesis is correct, given one data vector from the imaging system. This observer must choose one of two decisions, D_0 or D_1. With D_0 the observer is declaring that the tumor is absent, whereas with D_1 that it is present. As noted earlier, we assume that the observer will make the same decision if presented with the same data vector at a later time.

A. Minimizing the Bayesian Risk

Of course, the observer's decision may be correct or incorrect. This implies the existence of certain conditional probabilities for the various combinations of hypothesis and decision. The probability that the observer decides that the tumor is present when it is actually present will be denoted by $\Pr(D_1 \mid H_1)$ and is called the true-positive fraction (*TPF*). The false-positive fraction (*FPF*) is the probability that the observer declares the tumor present when it is actually absent, $\Pr(D_1 \mid H_0)$. The probability of deciding the tumor is absent when it is actually present is $\Pr(D_0 \mid H_1)$, the false-negative fraction (*FNF*). Finally, the true-negative fraction (*TNF*) is the probability of declaring the tumor to be absent when it is actually absent, $\Pr(D_0 \mid H_0)$. These numbers are determined by the imaging system, detection task, and the observer, and they always satisfy the constraints

$$\Pr(D_1 \mid H_1) + \Pr(D_0 \mid H_1) = 1$$
$$\Pr(D_1 \mid H_0) + \Pr(D_0 \mid H_0) = 1$$

These equations follow from the fact that the observer cannot equivocate.

The two other relevant probabilities are $\Pr(H_0)$, the probability that the tumor is actually absent, and $\Pr(H_1) = 1 - \Pr(H_0)$, the probability that it is present. These prior probabilities reflect the prevalence of the type of tumor that we are trying to detect in the patient population that we are studying.

Statistical Decision Theory

For each combination of decision and hypothesis there is an associated cost. For example, the cost of a false-positive outcome is c_{10}. The three other costs, c_{11}, c_{01}, and c_{00}, are defined similarly and are thought of as elements of a cost matrix C:

$$C = \begin{bmatrix} c_{00} & c_{01} \\ c_{10} & c_{11} \end{bmatrix}$$

Generally we would expect c_{10} and c_{01} to be high, because they are the costs for incorrect decisions, whereas c_{11} and c_{00} would be low, or even negative, being the costs for correct decisions. We will assume that $c_{10} > c_{00}$ and $c_{01} > c_{11}$. The Bayes risk is the average cost and is given by

$$R = c_{11} \Pr(D_1 \mid H_1) \Pr(H_1) + c_{01} \Pr(D_0 \mid H_1) \Pr(H_1)$$
$$+ c_{10} \Pr(D_1 \mid H_0) \Pr(H_0) + c_{00} \Pr(D_0 \mid H_0) \Pr(H_0)$$

Note that in this expression each cost value is multiplied by the probability that that cost will be incurred. The cost matrix is usually difficult to determine in practice. Fortunately, for our purposes, the exact values of the entries of this matrix are not needed.

Using the constraints on the conditional probabilities noted earlier, we may write the Bayes risk in the form

$$R = c_{01} \Pr(H_1) + c_{00} \Pr(H_0)$$
$$+ (c_{10} - c_{00}) \Pr(D_1 \mid H_0) \Pr(H_0) - (c_{01} - c_{11}) \Pr(D_1 \mid H_1) \Pr(H_1)$$

Now consider an observer for the tumor-detection task and let Γ be the region in data space that consists of all possible data vectors. This region may be separated into two disjoint regions Γ_0 and Γ_1. The region Γ_0 consists of all data vectors that lead the observer to declare D_0, tumor absent, whereas Γ_1 is all data vectors that lead to D_1, tumor present. Associated with the hypotheses, H_0 and H_1 are probability density functions for the data $pr(\mathbf{g} \mid H_0)$ and $pr(\mathbf{g} \mid H_1)$, respectively. Then $\Pr(D_1 \mid H_0)$ is the integral of $pr(\mathbf{g} \mid H_0)$ over the region Γ_1, whereas $\Pr(D_1 \mid H_1)$ is the integral of $pr(\mathbf{g} \mid H_1)$ over Γ_1. In terms of these density functions, the Bayes cost may therefore be written as

$$C = c_{01} \Pr(H_1) + c_{00} \Pr(H_0)$$
$$+ \int_{\Gamma_1} [(c_{10} - c_{00}) \Pr(H_0) pr(\mathbf{g} \mid H_0) - (c_{01} - c_{11}) \Pr(H_1) pr(\mathbf{g} \mid H_1)] d\mathbf{g}$$

In this last expression, the observer controls Γ_1 only. Everything else on the right side of this equation is independent of the observer. The observer that minimizes the Bayes risk is the one that chooses Γ_1 to be exactly that region of Γ

where the integrand is negative. This observer declares the tumor to be present (D_1) if

$$\frac{pr(\mathbf{g}\,|\,H_1)}{pr(\mathbf{g}\,|\,H_0)} > \frac{(c_{10} - c_{00})\Pr(H_0)}{(c_{01} - c_{11})\Pr(H_1)}$$

and declares the tumor absent (D_0) if

$$\frac{pr(\mathbf{g}\,|\,H_1)}{pr(\mathbf{g}\,|\,H_0)} \leq \frac{(c_{10} - c_{00})\Pr(H_0)}{(c_{01} - c_{11})\Pr(H_1)}$$

The test statistic on the left in these inequalities is the likelihood ratio, and is denoted by $\Lambda(\mathbf{g})$. The decisions of the observer using this ratio may be summarized as

$$\Lambda(\mathbf{g}) \underset{D_1}{\overset{D_0}{\lessgtr}} \Lambda_0$$

where Λ_0 is a threshold that depends on the cost matrix and the prior probabilities. The likelihood ratio itself is independent of these details, which is fortunate, because they are often unknown.

B. Minimum Error Detector

The total probability of error for a given observer and tumor detection task is given by

$$P_e = \Pr(D_0\,|\,H_1)\Pr(H_1) + \Pr(D_1\,|\,H_0)\Pr(H_0)$$

This is the Bayes risk if the cost matrix is

$$\mathbf{C} = \begin{bmatrix} 0 & 1 \\ 1 & 0 \end{bmatrix}$$

Therefore, the observer that minimizes the total probability of error is the ideal observer with the decision threshold given by the ratio of prior probabilities:

$$\Lambda_0 = \frac{\Pr(H_0)}{\Pr(H_1)}$$

If we use the equations

$$pr(\mathbf{g}\,|\,H_1)\Pr(H_1) = \Pr(H_1\,|\,\mathbf{g})pr(\mathbf{g})$$
$$pr(\mathbf{g}\,|\,H_0)\Pr(H_0) = \Pr(H_0\,|\,\mathbf{g})pr(\mathbf{g})$$

this can be reformulated in terms of posterior probabilities as follows. Declare the tumor present if the probability that the tumor is present, given the data, is greater than the corresponding probability that the tumor is absent: $\Pr(H_1\,|\,\mathbf{g}) > \Pr(H_0\,|\,\mathbf{g})$.

If the reverse is true, $\Pr(H_1 \mid \mathbf{g}) \le \Pr(H_0 \mid \mathbf{g})$, then declare the tumor to be absent.

C. Maximum Likelihood Detector

If we have no knowledge of the prior probabilities on the hypotheses, then we may as well assume that $\Pr(H_0) = \Pr(H_1) = \frac{1}{2}$. This gives the decision threshold $\Lambda_0 = 1$. The decision process for this observer may be rephrased in terms of likelihood functions. The observer declares the tumor present if the likelihood of the data given that the tumor is present is greater than the corresponding likelihood given that the tumor is absent: $pr(\mathbf{g} \mid H_1) > pr(\mathbf{g} \mid H_0)$. If the reverse is true, $pr(\mathbf{g} \mid H_1) \le pr(\mathbf{g} \mid H_0)$, then this observer declares the tumor to be absent. In other words, pick the hypothesis that gives the maximum likelihood for the given data vector.

D. Ideal Observers

Each of the three observers we have just discussed computes the likelihood ratio and declares the tumor present if $\Lambda(\mathbf{g}) > \Lambda_0$, and the tumor absent if $\Lambda(\mathbf{g}) \le \Lambda_0$, for some threshold Λ_0. Any observer that follows this or an equivalent procedure is called an ideal observer. For example, it is often more convenient to calculate the log of the likelihood ratio, $\lambda(\mathbf{g}) = \log \Lambda(\mathbf{g})$, and compare the result to the threshold $\lambda_0 = \log \Lambda_0$. An observer who does this is an ideal observer. If $L(r)$ is any monotonically increasing function of the non-negative real variable r, then the observer who computes $\tilde{\lambda}(\mathbf{g}) = L(\Lambda(\mathbf{g}))$ and compares the result to the threshold $\tilde{\lambda}_0 = L(\Lambda_0)$ is also an ideal observer.

We have seen that minimizing the Bayes risk, minimizing the total probability of error, or maximizing the likelihood of the data all lead to the same decision statistic, the likelihood ratio. Either the Bayes risk or the probability of error could be used as a measure of ideal-observer performance, and therefore as a measure of the performance of the imaging system for the given tumor detection task. One drawback to this approach, however, is that the cost matrix and prevalence are often unknown. Later we will see that there is an alternative measure of observer performance that is also maximized by ideal observers and that only depends on the statistical properties of the imaging system data.

IV. HOTELLING OBSERVERS

A linear observer computes a test statistic that is linear in the data:

$$\tau(\mathbf{g}) = \mathbf{w}^T \mathbf{g} = \sum_{m=1}^{M} w_m g_m$$

where $\mathbf{w}^T$ indicates the transpose of the vector $\mathbf{w}$. This vector is often called the template for the given linear observer. We will see examples later where the ideal observer is linear, but in general the ideal observer will perform nonlinear operations on the data vector to arrive at a decision.

At this point we introduce the following notation for expectation values of an arbitrary function of the data $\omega(\mathbf{g})$ under the two hypotheses:

$$\langle \omega \rangle_0 = \langle \omega(\mathbf{g}) \rangle_0 = \int_\Gamma \omega(\mathbf{g}) pr(\mathbf{g} | H_0) d\mathbf{g}$$

$$\langle \omega \rangle_1 = \langle \omega(\mathbf{g}) \rangle_1 = \int_\Gamma \omega(\mathbf{g}) pr(\mathbf{g} | H_1) d\mathbf{g}$$

The variances of $\omega(\mathbf{g})$ under each hypothesis are defined in the usual way by

$$var_0(\omega) = \langle (\omega - \langle \omega \rangle_0)^2 \rangle_0$$
$$var_1(\omega) = \langle (\omega - \langle \omega \rangle_1)^2 \rangle_1$$

Using this notation, the SNR of the linear observer is given by

$$SNR_\tau^2 = \frac{[\langle \tau \rangle_1 - \langle \tau \rangle_0]^2}{\frac{1}{2} var_1(\tau) + \frac{1}{2} var_0(\tau)}$$

In fact, this expression applies even when $\tau(\mathbf{g})$ is not a linear function of the data. The numerator is a measure of the change in the observer's test statistic when a tumor is present, whereas the denominator is a measure of the strength of the noise in the test statistic.

For a linear observer we may compute the SNR explicitly. The components of a signal vector $\mathbf{s}$ in the data can be defined as the difference of means

$$s_m = \langle g_m \rangle_1 - \langle g_m \rangle_0$$

The signal vector is a measure of the change in the data when a tumor is present. We may also define the elements of the average covariance matrix $\mathbf{K}$ for the data by means of the equation

$$K_{mn} = \tfrac{1}{2} \langle (g_m - \langle g_m \rangle_0)(g_n - \langle g_n \rangle_0) \rangle_0 + \tfrac{1}{2} \langle (g_m - \langle g_m \rangle_1)(g_n - \langle g_n \rangle_1) \rangle_1$$

The average covariance is a measure of the strength of the noise in the data and the correlations between the different data components. In terms of these quantities, the SNR for the linear observer using the template $\mathbf{w}$ is given by

$$SNR_\tau^2 = \frac{(\mathbf{w}^T \mathbf{s})^2}{\mathbf{w}^T \mathbf{K} \mathbf{w}}$$

Statistical Decision Theory

The Hotelling observer is the linear observer that maximizes this SNR. This observer uses the Hotelling template $\mathbf{w}_H$ to compute the test statistic

$$\tau_H(\mathbf{g}) = \mathbf{w}_H^T \mathbf{g} = (\mathbf{K}^{-1}\mathbf{s})^T \mathbf{g} = (\mathbf{K}^{-1/2}\mathbf{s})^T (\mathbf{K}^{-1/2}\mathbf{g})$$

and then compares the result to a threshold. The Hotelling observer therefore needs to know only the first- and second-order statistics of the data under each hypothesis, as opposed to the ideal observer, who must know the complete probability densities. The operation of multiplying a vector by $\mathbf{K}^{-1/2}$ is called prewhitening, and the Hotelling observer is said to be using a prewhitened matched filter on the data.

The SNR for the Hotelling observer is called the Hotelling trace and is given by (8–10)

$$\text{SNR}_H^2 = \mathbf{s}^T \mathbf{K}^{-1} \mathbf{s} = (\mathbf{K}^{-1/2}\mathbf{s})^T (\mathbf{K}^{-1/2}\mathbf{s})$$

Therefore, the Hotelling trace is the square magnitude of the prewhitened signal in the data. This quantity could also be used as a measure of the performance of the imaging system on the given detection task. It is usually easier to compute than other measures of performance, and, in certain circumstances, it correlates well with human observer performance (5,11–14). It has the drawback that, when the statistics of the data are not gaussian, it may not correlate well with the ideal performance of the system when it is used to detect tumors.

V. OBSERVER PERFORMANCE

Let us return to the case of an arbitrary observer, one who is not necessarily an ideal observer or a linear observer. The region Γ_1 in the data region Γ that corresponds to decision D_1 for this observer can always be described as the set of data vectors $\mathbf{g}$ that satisfy $\tau(\mathbf{g}) > \tau_0$ for some test statistic $\tau(\mathbf{g})$ and threshold τ_0. There are, in fact, many functions that fulfill this requirement. To find the function $\tau(\mathbf{g})$ that a particular observer is using, we can vary the threshold τ_0 and keep track of the how the region Γ_1 depends on this variable. If we determine Γ_1 for all values of τ_0, then $\tau(\mathbf{g})$ is determined up to a monotonic transformation. This is the best we can do because, if $L(r)$ is a monotonic function as earlier, then an observer who uses $L(\tau(\mathbf{g}))$ with the threshold $L(\tau_0)$ makes the same decisions as the one using $\tau(\mathbf{g})$ and τ_0.

Suppose, then, that a given observer is using the test statistic $\tau(\mathbf{g})$ to make decisions about the presence or absence of tumors. Because $\mathbf{g}$ is a random vector under each hypothesis, we may regard τ as a random variable under each hypothesis. The probability density for τ under the tumor absent hypothesis is a function $pr(\tau \mid H_0)$, whereas under the tumor present hypothesis, it is a different function

$pr(\tau \mid H_1)$. The conditional probabilities that appear in the Bayes risk depend on the threshold τ_0 and are given by

$$TPF(\tau_0) = \Pr(D_1 \mid H_1) = \int_{\tau_0}^{\infty} pr(\tau \mid H_1) d\tau$$

$$FPF(\tau_0) = \Pr(D_1 \mid H_0) = \int_{\tau_0}^{\infty} pr(\tau \mid H_0) d\tau$$

$$FNF(\tau_0) = \Pr(D_0 \mid H_1) = \int_{-\infty}^{\tau_0} pr(\tau \mid H_1) d\tau$$

$$TNF(\tau_0) = \Pr(D_0 \mid H_0) = \int_{-\infty}^{\tau_0} pr(\tau \mid H_0) d\tau$$

Because, as already noted, these quantities always satisfy the constraints $TPF + FNF = 1$ and $TNF + FPF = 1$, only two of them need to be determined, say TPF and FPF, to find values for all four. In the literature TPF is also called the sensitivity or the probability of detection, TNF the specificity, and FPF the false-alarm rate. One of these numbers, or some combination of them, could be used as a figure of merit for the observer, but they all depend on the threshold τ_0, which is often somewhat arbitrary. This dependence can be removed by averaging over the threshold.

A. The ROC Curve and the Area Under the Curve

A figure of merit that is often used and does not suffer from dependence on the threshold is the area under the receiver operating characteristic (ROC) curve (15–22). This scalar is usually called the AUC. The ROC curve is generated by varying the threshold and plotting the points $(FPF(\tau_0), TPF(\tau_0))$. This curve therefore gives us the probability of detection of the tumor for each value of the false-alarm rate. Because $TNF = 1 - FPF$, the ROC curve may also be regarded as a plot of sensitivity versus specificity as the threshold is changed. The ROC curve starts at the point $(1, 1)$ for small values of τ_0 and moves toward $(0, 0)$ as τ_0 is increased. If the observer's decisions are no better than those made by flipping a coin, then the corresponding ROC curve will move along the diagonal of the unit square that has these two points at its corners, and the AUC will be $\frac{1}{2}$. It is desirable for the ROC curve to stay near the top of this square until it approaches the point $(0, 1)$ and then drop down to the origin. This corresponds to a TPF near 1 for almost all FPF, and an AUC near 1.

Statistical Decision Theory

The AUC for the observer using the test statistic $\tau(\mathbf{g})$ is given by

$$AUC_\tau = -\int_{-\infty}^{\infty} TPF(\tau) \frac{d}{d\tau}[FPF(\tau)]d\tau$$

This AUC may also be calculated from the probability density functions for τ under the two hypotheses via the double integral

$$AUC_\tau = \int_{-\infty}^{\infty} \int_{\tau}^{\infty} pr(\tau | H_0) pr(\tau' | H_1) d\tau' \, d\tau$$

From this expression it can be shown that, if another observer uses $\tilde{\tau}(\mathbf{g}) = L(\tau(\mathbf{g}))$, and $L(r)$ is a monotonically increasing function, then $AUC_\tau = AUC_{\tilde{\tau}}$. Therefore, equivalent observers give the same value for the AUC.

We define the characteristic functions of τ under each hypothesis as

$$\Psi_0(\xi) = \langle \exp(-2\pi i \xi \tau) \rangle_0$$
$$\Psi_1(\xi) = \langle \exp(-2\pi i \xi \tau) \rangle_1$$

It is often easier to work with these functions when calculating the AUC. With $\mathcal{P}$ used to indicate the Cauchy principal value of the integral, the relevant formula is (23)

$$AUC_\tau = \frac{1}{2} + \frac{1}{2\pi i} \mathcal{P} \int_{-\infty}^{\infty} \psi_1(\xi) \psi_2^*(\xi) \frac{d\xi}{\xi}$$

The AUC of an observer can also be estimated by simulating a two-alternative forced-choice (2AFC) experiment. An observer performing a 2AFC study is presented with a sequence of pairs of data sets, one from the tumor-present population and one from the tumor-absent population and must choose, for each pair, which data set corresponds to the tumor-present patient. To do this for a mathematical observer, pairs of sample data vectors are drawn randomly from the tumor-absent and tumor-present populations. The test statistic is computed for each data vector in the pair, and the tumor is declared to be present in the sample that gives the largest value for the test statistic. If we use a large number of sample pairs, then the fraction of decisions that are correctly made by the observer is a good estimate of the AUC for that observer on the given task. Thus, the AUC is directly related to a real-world measure of detection performance.

B. Ideal Observer AUC

We now specialize to the ideal observer and see how these formulas for the AUC can be simplified for this case. These simplifications all follow from the fact that, with $\Lambda(\mathbf{g})$ equal to the likelihood ratio, $pr(\Lambda | H_1) = \Lambda pr(\Lambda | H_0)$. Green and Swets call this the Gertrude Stein law, because it tells us that the likelihood ratio of the likelihood ratio is the likelihood ratio (24,25). Therefore, if the probability density for Λ under one hypothesis is known, it is also known for the other hypothesis. As a result of this relation, we can show that AUC_Λ may be computed from the false alarm rate by means of (26)

$$AUC_\Lambda = 1 - \frac{1}{2}\int_0^\infty [FPF(\Lambda)]^2 d\Lambda$$

It must be emphasized that Λ in this formula must be the likelihood ratio for it to be true. Of course, any other ideal observer will have the same value for the AUC.

Some other useful expressions may be derived by defining the moment generating functions

$$M_0(\beta) = \langle \exp(\beta\lambda)\rangle_0 = \langle \Lambda^\beta \rangle_0$$
$$M_1(\beta) = \langle \exp(\beta\lambda)\rangle_1 = \langle \Lambda^\beta \rangle_1$$

From the Gertrude Stein Law it follows that $M_1(\beta) = M_0(\beta + 1)$, so we need to compute only one of these functions. In terms of $M_0(\beta)$, the AUC for an ideal observer is

$$AUC_\Lambda = \frac{1}{2} + \frac{1}{2\pi i} \mathcal{P} \int_{-\infty}^\infty M_0(i\alpha) M_0(1 - i\alpha) \frac{d\alpha}{\alpha}$$

By moving the contour of integration, this can also be written as (23)

$$AUC_\Lambda = 1 - \frac{1}{2\pi}\int_0^\infty \left|M_0\left(\frac{1}{2} + i\alpha\right)\right|^2 \frac{d\alpha}{\alpha^2 + \frac{1}{4}}$$

This form is often convenient, because there is no Cauchy principal value involved, and the integrand is nonnegative. The integral, after dividing by 2π, represents how far AUC_Λ deviates from its maximum possible value of 1.

From the Gertrude Stein law and the fact that the expectation of 1 is always 1, it follows that $M_0(0) = M_1(-1) = 1$ and $M_0(1) = M_1(0) = 1$. These equations imply the existence of a function $G(\beta)$ that satisfies

$$M_0(\beta) = \exp\left[\beta(\beta - 1)G\left(\beta - \frac{1}{2}\right)\right]$$
$$M_1(\beta) = \exp\left[\beta(\beta + 1)G\left(\beta + \frac{1}{2}\right)\right]$$

We will call $G(\beta)$ the likelihood generating function (23). If we know this function, then the statistics of the likelihood ratio under the two hypotheses are completely determined. In particular, the ideal-observer AUC may be written as

$$AUC_\Lambda = 1 - \frac{1}{2\pi}\int_0^\infty \exp\left[-2\left(\alpha^2 + \frac{1}{4}\right)\text{Re}\, G(i\alpha)\right] \frac{d\alpha}{\alpha^2 + \frac{1}{4}}$$

Statistical Decision Theory

This shows us that the behavior of the likelihood generating function on the imaginary axis determines the AUC for an ideal observer.

C. Signal/Noise Ratios

The AUC of an observer is often converted to a SNR, which can vary from 0 to ∞, with larger values corresponding to better tumor-detection performance. For an ideal observer we have

$$SNR_{AUC} = 2\,\text{erf}^{-1}(2AUC_\Lambda - 1)$$

The symbol erf^{-1} in this expression stands for the inverse error function. The reason for calling this number a SNR will become clear later.

Another SNR in common use is derived from the mean and variance of the log-likelihood under each hypothesis by means of:

$$SNR_\lambda^2 = \frac{[\langle\lambda\rangle_1 - \langle\lambda\rangle_0]^2}{\frac{1}{2}var_0(\lambda) + \frac{1}{2}var_1(\lambda)}$$

It might be thought that SNR_Λ would be just as reasonable a choice as SNR_λ for a figure of merit, but in fact SNR_Λ has some peculiar properties that make it unsuitable for this purpose. For example, in many cases, including some discussed later, SNR_Λ will increase to some maximum value and then decrease as the contrast between the tumor and background is increased (26). A reasonable measure of detection performance would increase monotonically as a function of contrast. Just like AUC_Λ, SNR_λ can be computed if either $M_0(\beta)$ or the likelihood generating function is known. All that is needed are the following formulas for moments of λ under the two hypotheses:

$$\langle\lambda^k\rangle_0 = \left[\frac{d^k}{d\beta^k} M_0(\beta)\right]_{\beta=0}$$

$$\langle\lambda^k\rangle_1 = \left[\frac{d^k}{d\beta^k} M_0(\beta)\right]_{\beta=1}$$

A third SNR is derived from the value of the likelihood generating function at the origin (23):

$$SNR_{G(0)} = \sqrt{2G(0)} = \sqrt{-8 \log M_0(\tfrac{1}{2})}$$

In terms of the probability densities for Λ under the two hypotheses, $G(0)$ is given by

$$G(0) = -4 \log \int_{-\infty}^{\infty} \sqrt{pr(\Lambda \mid H_0)pr(\Lambda \mid H_1)}\, d\Lambda$$

This integral can be used to show that $G(0)$ is always a positive quantity. Just like the AUC, $G(0)$ is invariant under a monotonic transformation: if Λ is replaced throughout this integral by $\tilde{\lambda} = L(\Lambda)$ as earlier, then the value of the integral is unchanged. We can also compute $G(0)$ directly from the original probability densities for the data by using

$$G(0) = -4 \log \int_\Gamma \sqrt{pr(\mathbf{g} | H_0) pr(\mathbf{g} | H_1)} \, d\mathbf{g}$$

This integral is invariant under invertible transformations of the data. In other words, if the data are processed in a reversible way, then the value of $G(0)$ will not change. This is also true of AUC_Λ.

By definition AUC_Λ can be retrieved from SNR_{AUC} by using

$$AUC_\Lambda = \tfrac{1}{2} + \tfrac{1}{2} \operatorname{erf}(SNR_{AUC})$$

An often used, and sometimes good, approximation for AUC_Λ is

$$AUC_\Lambda \approx \tfrac{1}{2} + \tfrac{1}{2} \operatorname{erf}(SNR_\lambda)$$

This approximation is exact, when λ is normally distributed under both hypotheses. If λ is approximately normal, then we would expect this approximation to give a good estimate for AUC_Λ. We have found that

$$AUC_\Lambda \approx \tfrac{1}{2} + \tfrac{1}{2} \operatorname{erf}(SNR_{G(0)})$$

is also a good approximation in all of the examples examined so far. This approximation is derived by replacing $G(i\alpha)$ with $G(0)$ in the last integral expression given earlier for AUC_Λ. It is also exact when λ is normally distributed. We have found, in some examples where the exact value of AUC_Λ can be computed, that the $SNR_{G(0)}$ approximation is usually better than the SNR_λ approximation, and it is also easier to compute when $M_0(\beta)$ is known (26).

As a figure of merit for the performance of an imaging system in tumor detection tasks, AUC_Λ has several advantages. It does not depend on the cost matrix, prevalence, or threshold, only on the statistics of the data coming out of the system as it views the tumor-absent and tumor-present patient ensembles. It does not depend on the particular reconstruction being used to generate images, because the ideal observer uses the raw data. Finally, AUC_Λ gives an upper bound for the percentage of correct decisions for any observer on a 2AFC test with the given patient ensembles. For these reasons we would like to be able to compute AUC_Λ for realistic imaging systems, tasks, and noise models. As we will see later, this can be difficult, but even computations in simplified cases can be revealing about the strategies used by ideal observers and their performance on tumor detection tasks.

VI. SKE/BKE

SKE/BKE stands for signal known exactly/background known exactly. This type of task is the easiest to analyze and therefore the least realistic. However, as we will see, the ideal observers that arise from such tasks use techniques for tumor detection that are common in the literature. As we proceed to more realistic tasks, we will see that this is not specific to the SKE/BKE paradigm.

A. Example 1: Normal Noise with the Signal in the Mean

In this example the probability density when the tumor is absent is given by

$$pr(\mathbf{g} \mid H_0) = [(2\pi)^M \det(\mathbf{K})]^{-1/2} \exp[-\tfrac{1}{2}(\mathbf{g} - \mathbf{b})^T \mathbf{K}^{-1}(\mathbf{g} - \mathbf{b})]$$

The mean of $\mathbf{g}$ is the fixed background data vector $\mathbf{b}$, and $\mathbf{K}$ is the covariance matrix for the noise. The effect of the tumor on the data is to shift the background vector from $\mathbf{b}$ to $\mathbf{b} + \mathbf{s}$. This means that the probability density when the tumor is present is given by

$$pr(\mathbf{g} \mid H_1) = pr(\mathbf{g} - \mathbf{s} \mid H_0)$$

An ideal observer computes the log-likelihood,

$$\lambda(\mathbf{g}) = \mathbf{s}^T \mathbf{K}^{-1} \mathbf{g} + \tfrac{1}{2} \mathbf{b}^T \mathbf{K}^{-1} \mathbf{b} - \tfrac{1}{2}(\mathbf{b} + \mathbf{s})^T \mathbf{K}^{-1}(\mathbf{b} + \mathbf{s})$$

and compares this number with a threshold λ_0. If we remove the terms from $\lambda(\mathbf{g})$ that do not depend on $\mathbf{g}$, we get an equivalent observer who computes

$$\tilde{\lambda}(\mathbf{g}) = \mathbf{s}^T \mathbf{K}^{-1} \mathbf{g}$$

and compares this to a threshold $\tilde{\lambda}_0$. We can recognize this last expression as the prewhitened matched filter, which implies that the ideal observer is identical to the Hotelling observer in this example.

The moment generating function under the tumor-absent hypothesis is given by

$$M_0(\beta) = \exp[\tfrac{1}{2} \beta(\beta - 1) \mathbf{s}^T \mathbf{K}^{-1} \mathbf{s}]$$

From this expression, we see that $G(\beta) = \tfrac{1}{2} \mathbf{s}^T \mathbf{K}^{-1} \mathbf{s}$, a constant. We then have immediately the $G(0)$ SNR:

$$SNR_{G(0)} = (\mathbf{s}^T \mathbf{K}^{-1} \mathbf{s})^{1/2}$$

which is also the Hotelling trace. For this example we have exact agreement between the various SNRs:

$$SNR_{AUC} = SNR_{G(0)} = SNR_\lambda$$

If the covariance is diagonal, then an ideal observer computes a weighted inner product of the data with the signal:

$$\tilde{\lambda}(\mathbf{g}) = \sum_{m=1}^{M} \frac{g_m s_m}{\sigma_m^2}$$

The weights σ_m^2 are the variances in each data channel. This could be called a weighted matched filter. If the weights all equal σ^2, then an ideal observer uses the simple matched filter:

$$\tilde{\lambda}(\mathbf{g}) = \left(\frac{1}{\sigma^2}\right) \sum_{m=1}^{M} g_m s_m$$

In each case the filter is optimal, as measured by the AUC, for the SKE/BKE task and the normal noise model with the given covariance. We cannot expect such filters to be optimal in other circumstances.

B. Example 2: Independent Exponential Noise with Signal in the Mean

Exponential noise is related to speckle noise in ultrasonographic imaging (27–30). If the data are distributed as independent exponential random variables and the signal changes the mean of each data component, then the relevant probability distributions are given by

$$pr(\mathbf{g} \mid H_0) = \prod_{m=1}^{M} \frac{1}{b_m} \exp\left(-\frac{g_m}{b_m}\right)$$

$$pr(\mathbf{g} \mid H_1) = \prod_{m=1}^{M} \frac{1}{b_m + s_m} \exp\left(-\frac{g_m}{b_m + s_m}\right)$$

A more realistic model of speckle noise would include correlations between the data components, but that is beyond the scope of this work. In this and the following examples, we will assume that the components of the signal $\mathbf{s}$ are all positive. If some component of $\mathbf{s}$ vanished, then the corresponding component of the data vector $\mathbf{g}$ would not contribute to the likelihood ratio in any of these examples and thus would not affect the figures of merit that we are considering. Negative components of $\mathbf{s}$ could be accommodated with a little more notation.

Statistical Decision Theory

The log-likelihood observer for this task computes the quantity

$$\lambda(\mathbf{g}) = \sum_{m=1}^{M} \frac{s_m g_m}{b_m(b_m + s_m)} + \sum_{m=1}^{M} \log\left(\frac{b_m}{b_m + s_m}\right)$$

Removing the data-independent terms gives an ideal observer who computes

$$\tilde{\lambda}(\mathbf{g}) = \sum_{m=1}^{M} g_m \left[\frac{s_m}{b_m(b_m + s_m)}\right]$$

This observer uses a weighted matched filter similar to the case of normal noise with a diagonal covariance matrix, except that the weights in the denominators in this expression depend on the signal. The variance of g_m is $\sigma_{0m}^2 = b_m^2$ under H_0 and $\sigma_{1m}^2 = (b_m + s_m)^2$ under H_1. The weights are $b_m(b_m + s_m) = \sqrt{\sigma_{0m}^2 \sigma_{1m}^2}$ (i.e., the geometric averages of the variances under the two hypotheses for each data component). Note that the Hotelling observer in this example would use the arithmetic averages of the variances for the weights. Therefore, the ideal observer and Hotelling observer are not identical, even though both are linear observers. This shows that the Hotelling observer does not, in general, maximize the AUC among the class of linear observers.

All of the SNRs for this example are most easily expressed in terms of the inverse contrast ratios $\rho_m = b_m/s_m$. The moment generating function under the tumor absent hypothesis is given by

$$M_0(\beta) = \prod_{m=1}^{M} \frac{(1 + \rho_m)^{1-\beta} \rho_m^\beta}{1 + \rho_m - \beta}$$

From this expression, or by direct calculation of the relevant expectations, we can find SNR_λ:

$$SNR_\lambda = \sqrt{2} \; \sum_{m=1}^{M} \left(\frac{1}{\rho_m} - \frac{1}{1 + \rho_m}\right)$$

From this equation it follows that $SNR_\lambda \leq \sqrt{2M}$ always. This saturation effect is somewhat counter intuitive, because we expect the detectability to increase without bound as the contrast increases (i.e., as $\rho_m \to 0$ for all m).

From the moment generating function evaluated at $\beta = 1/2$ we find that

$$G(0) = 2 \sum_{m=1}^{M} \log\left[\frac{(1 + 2\rho_m)^2}{4\rho_m(1 + \rho_m)}\right]$$

This expression shows that $SNR_{G(0)}$ increases without bound as the contrast increases. The moment generating function also leads to an exact expression for the ideal observer AUC. If we define two functions of the inverse contrasts by

$$A_1(\rho) = \prod_{m=1}^{M} \rho_m(1 + \rho_m)$$

and

$$A_2(\rho) = \sum_{n=0}^{M} \left[(1 + 2\rho_n) \prod_{\substack{m=1 \\ m \neq n}}^{M} (1 + \rho_m + \rho_n)(\rho_m - \rho_n) \right]^{-1}$$

then the ideal observer AUC is given by (26)

$$AUC_\Lambda = 1 - \frac{1}{2} A_1(\rho) A_2(\rho)$$

We can use this equation to show that SNR_{AUC} also increases without bound as the contrast increases. Therefore, we would expect $SNR_{G(0)}$ to more accurately approximate SNR_{AUC} than SNR_λ does, at least for high contrasts.

In the case in which all of the contrasts are the same, $\rho_1 = \ldots = \rho_m = \rho$, we can show that this expectation is fulfilled. An alternative derivation leads to an exact expression for the ideal-observer is AUC in this case that is given by (26)

$$AUC_\Lambda = \left(\frac{1 + \rho}{1 + 2\rho} \right)^M \sum_{k=0}^{M-1} \frac{(M + k - 1)!}{k!(M - 1)!} \left(\frac{\rho}{1 + 2\rho} \right)^k$$

In Fig. 1 this expression is compared with the approximations derived from SNR_λ and $G(0)$ for $M = 3$. Note that the $G(0)$ approximation is very good throughout the range of contrasts, whereas the SNR_λ approximation fails as the contrast increases. For a fixed contrast, the agreement between the exact AUC_Λ and both approximations improves as M is increased, as we would expect from the central limit theorem. However, for a given M the SNR_λ approximation will always fail for large enough contrasts. Of course, we are usually interested in the performance of a system in low-contrast situations, so this kind of defect in the SNR_λ approximation may not be a drawback in practice. It does, however, make us somewhat suspicious of the SNR_λ approximation for non-gaussian noise models.

C. Example 3: Poisson Noise with the Signal in the Mean

In SPECT imaging, among others, a major source of noise arises from the fact that the detectors count photons (31). The Poisson noise model is almost always valid in this situation. When the signal affects the mean, the Poisson model gives us the

Statistical Decision Theory

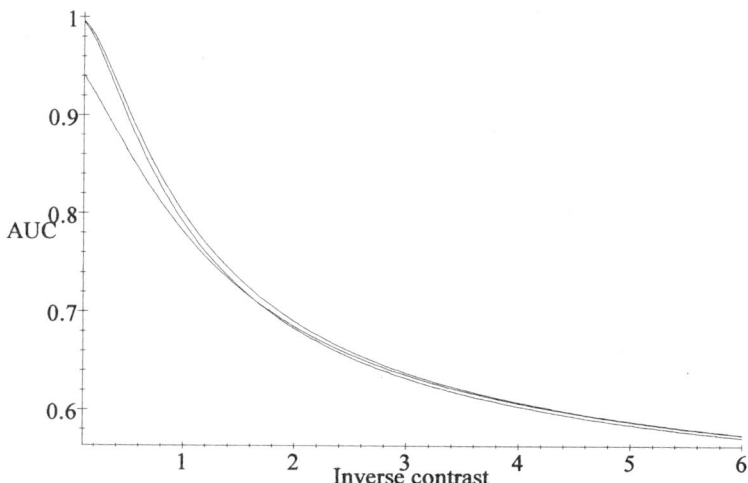

Fig. 1 Exact AUC_Λ, and the SNR_λ and $SNR_{G(0)}$ approximations, for independent exponential noise with three detectors. On the left side of the graph, the exact curve is below the $SNR_{G(0)}$ curve and above the SNR_λ curve. The exact and SNR_λ curves cross as we move to the right. The inverse contrast ratio is background/signal.

probability distributions

$$\Pr(\mathbf{g} \mid H_0) = \prod_{m=1}^{M} \frac{\exp[g_m \log(b_m) - b_m]}{g_m!}$$

$$\Pr(\mathbf{g} \mid H_1) = \prod_{m=1}^{M} \frac{\exp[g_m \log(b_m + s_m) - b_m - s_m]}{g_m!}$$

under the two hypotheses. Note that **g** is a discrete random variable, because it represents the number of photons counted.

The log-likelihood in this example is given by

$$\lambda(\mathbf{g}) = \sum_{m=1}^{M} g_m \log\left(\frac{b_m + s_m}{b_m}\right) - \sum_{m=1}^{M} s_m$$

Removing data independent terms gives an ideal observer who calculates the quantity

$$\tilde{\lambda}(\mathbf{g}) = \sum_{m=1}^{M} g_m \log\left(\frac{b_m + s_m}{b_m}\right) = \sum_{m=1}^{M} g_m \phi_m$$

Again, we find that the ideal observer uses a weighted matched filter. In this case, we have $\sigma_{0m}^2 = b_m$ and $\sigma_{1m}^2 = b_m + s_m$, and the weights are $\left[2 \log\left(\frac{\sigma_{1m}}{\sigma_{0m}}\right)\right]^{-1}$. As in the previous example, the ideal observer here is linear, but it is not identical to the Hotelling observer.

As usual, we can compute all of the SNRs from the moment generating function $M_0(\beta)$, which in this case is given by

$$M_0(\beta) = \exp\left(-\beta \sum_{m=1}^{M} s_m\right) \exp\left[\sum_{m=1}^{M} b_m \exp(\beta \phi_m) - b_m\right]$$

The value of $G(0)$ can be computed from this expression as

$$G(0) = 4 \sum_{m=1}^{M} \left[\frac{1}{2}(2b_m + s_m) - \sum_{m=1}^{M} \sqrt{b_m(b_m + s_m)}\right]$$

The quantity in square brackets is the arithmetic average of b_m and $b_m + s_m$ minus the geometric average of the same two numbers. The SNR of the log-likelihood is given by

$$SNR_\lambda = \sqrt{2} \frac{\sum_{m=1}^{M} s_m \phi_m}{\sqrt{\sum_{m=1}^{M} (2b_m + s_m)\phi_m^2}}$$

Both of these figures of merit are unbounded as the signal strength increases.

The exact value for the AUC of the ideal observer can be computed for this example, but the resulting expression is rather complicated. To compare the approximations to this AUC to exact values, we will consider the special case where $b_1 = \ldots = b_m = b$ and $s_1 = \ldots = s_m = s$. The ideal-observer AUC is then given by (26)

$$AUC_\Lambda = 1 - \exp[-M(2b + s)]\left[\sum_{k=0}^{\infty} \sum_{l=0}^{k-1} \frac{M^{k+1} b^k (b+s)^l}{k!l!} + \frac{1}{2} \sum_{k=0}^{\infty} \frac{M^k b^k (b+s)^k}{k!k!}\right]$$

In Fig. 2 this expression is plotted as a function of Ms for $Mb = 0.1$, along with the approximate expressions derived from SNR_λ and $G(0)$. In this figure, we can see that each approximation is better than the other in some range of contrasts. For significantly larger values of Mb, the total mean background count, the three curves are indistinguishable.

D. Example 4: Independent laplacian Noise with the Signal in the Mean

If a medical image is passed through a high-pass filter, the resulting image often has a histogram that can be well approximated by the laplacian distribution (32,33). If the signal passes through the filter and changes the mean of the result-

Statistical Decision Theory

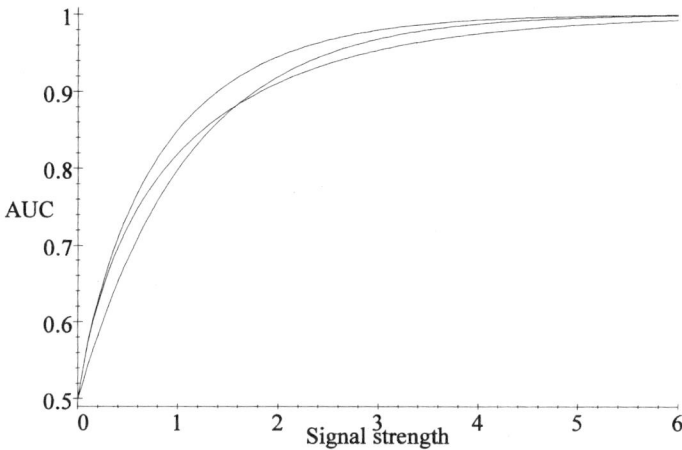

Fig. 2 Exact AUC_Λ, and the SNR_λ and $SNR_{G(0)}$ approximations, for Poisson noise with total mean background level of 0.1 photons. On the left side of the graph, the exact curve is below the SNR_λ curve, which is in turn below the $SNR_{G(0)}$ curve. The exact and SNR_λ curves cross as we move to the right. Signal amplitude is measured in mean number of photons.

ing gray level histogram, then the probability densities under the two hypotheses are given by

$$pr(\mathbf{g}|H_1) = \prod_{m=1}^{M} \frac{1}{2c_m} \exp\left[-\frac{1}{c_m}|g_m - b_m|\right]$$

$$pr(\mathbf{g}|H_2) = \prod_{m=1}^{M} \frac{1}{2c_m} \exp\left[-\frac{1}{c_m}|g_m - b_m - s_m|\right]$$

We are again assuming the statistical independence of the pixel values, which is unlikely to be true in real images. The numbers c_m are related to the variance at each pixel.

The log-likelihood for this task is

$$\lambda(\mathbf{g}) = \sum_{m=1}^{M} \frac{1}{c_m}[\,|g_m - b_m| - |g_m - b_m - s_m|\,]$$

By removing data independent terms we get an ideal observer who computes.

$$\tilde{\lambda}(\mathbf{g}) = \sum_{m=1}^{M} \frac{2}{c_m}[\min\{g_m, b_m + s_m\} - \min\{g_m, b_m\}]$$

In analogy with the morphological correlation, to be discussed later, this test statistic might be called a morphological matched filter. In fact, the quantity $\tilde{\lambda}(\mathbf{g})$ may be computed by means of a thresholding operation. Define a modified data vector $\tilde{\mathbf{g}}$ by applying thresholds above and below:

$$\tilde{g}_m = \begin{cases} b_m & \text{if } g_m \leq b_m \\ g_m & \text{if } b_m \leq g_m \leq b_m + s_m \\ b_m + s_m & \text{if } b_m + s_m \leq g_m \end{cases}$$

Then this ideal observer computes

$$\tilde{\lambda}(\mathbf{g}) = \sum_{m=1}^{M} \frac{2}{c_m} [\tilde{g}_m - b_m]$$

$$= \lambda'(\mathbf{g}) - \sum_{m=1}^{M} \frac{2b_m}{c_m}$$

The observer who uses $\lambda'(\mathbf{g})$ for a test statistic is also ideal. This test statistic is linear in the modified data vector $\tilde{\mathbf{g}}$, although the thresholding operations that lead to $\tilde{\mathbf{g}}$ are nonlinear. Thresholding is a common operation in morphological filtering, but it arises here from the ideal observer for this particular noise model.

The performance of this ideal observer is most easily expressed in terms of the contrast parameters $\theta_m = s_m/c_m$. The moment generating function is given by

$$M_0(\beta) = \prod_{m=1}^{M} \frac{1}{2} \left[1 - \frac{1}{2\beta - 1} + \exp[(2\beta - 1)\theta_m]\left(\frac{2\beta}{2\beta - 1}\right) \right] \exp[-\beta\theta_m]$$

From this expression we have immediately:

$$G(0) = 4 \sum_{m=1}^{M} \left[\frac{1}{2} \theta_m - \log\left(1 + \frac{1}{2} \theta_m\right) \right]$$

Finding the SNR of the log-likelihood is a more tedious computation, but the end result is

$$SNR_\lambda = \frac{2 \sum_{m=1}^{M} [\theta_m - 1 + \exp(-\theta_m)]}{\sqrt{\sum_{m=1}^{M} [3 - 2\exp(-\theta_m) - 4\theta_m \exp(-\theta_m) - \exp(-2\theta_m)]}}$$

Statistical Decision Theory

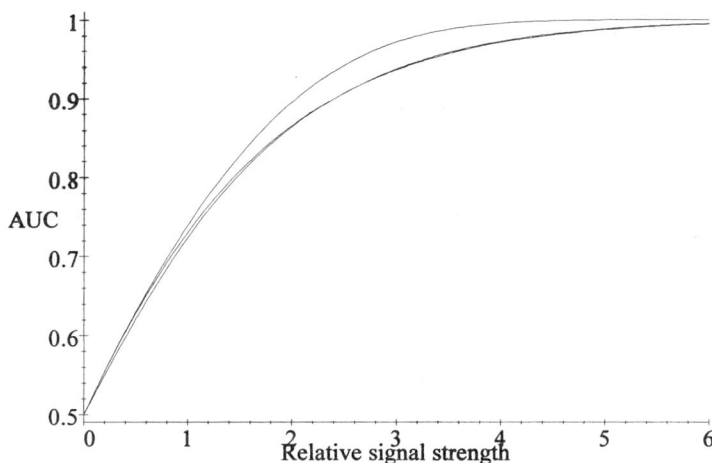

Fig. 3 Exact AUC_Λ and the SNR_λ and $SNR_{G(0)}$ approximations for independent Laplacian noise with one detector. On the left side of the graph the exact curve is below the $SNR_{G(0)}$ curve, which is in turn below the SNR_λ curve. The exact and $SNR_{G(0)}$ curves cross as we move to the right.

The exact AUC for the ideal observer can be reduced to the integral [26]

$$AUC_\Lambda = 1 - \frac{1}{2\pi}\left(\frac{1}{2}\right)^{2M} \exp\left(-\sum_{m=1}^{M} \theta_m\right)\left[\int_0^\infty \left(\frac{1}{\alpha}\right)^{2M} \prod_{m=1}^{M} \right.$$
$$\left. \times [\sin(\alpha\theta_m) + 2\alpha \cos(\alpha\theta_m)]^2 \frac{d\alpha}{\alpha^2 + \frac{1}{4}}\right]$$

which could be evaluated numerically for given parameter values. At this time an exact value for this integral is not known in general. For the $M = 1$ case (one detector) we find that, with $\theta = \theta_1$,

$$AUC_\Lambda = 1 - \frac{1}{2}\exp(-\theta)\left(1 + \frac{\theta}{2}\right)$$

In Fig. 3, this expression is compared with the approximations derived from the $M = 1$ versions of SNR_λ and $G(0)$. The approximation from $G(0)$ is better, especially in the midrange values of the contrast.

VII. SKE

In most cases in medical imaging the background data vector is not known exactly because of anatomical variations in the population. To proceed in this situation we need a probability density function $pr_b(\mathbf{b})$ on the background data vectors that arise from the individuals in the population under study. In the case in which a known signal shifts the background data vector from $\mathbf{b}$ to $\mathbf{b} + \mathbf{s}$, the probability functions for the data under the tumor-absent and tumor-present hypotheses are given by

$$pr(\mathbf{g} \mid H_0) = \int pr_n(\mathbf{g} \mid \mathbf{b}) pr_b(\mathbf{b}) d\mathbf{b}$$

$$pr(\mathbf{g} \mid H_1) = \int pr_n(\mathbf{g} \mid \mathbf{b} + \mathbf{s}) pr_b(\mathbf{b}) d\mathbf{b} = \int pr_n(\mathbf{g} \mid \mathbf{b}) pr_b(\mathbf{b} - \mathbf{s}) d\mathbf{b}$$

The conditional probability density $pr_n(\mathbf{g} \mid \mathbf{b})$ in this expression arises from the random variations in the data caused by measurement noise in the imaging system. An ideal observer looking for this signal computes the likelihood ratio $\Lambda(\mathbf{g})$, or some equivalent statistic, and compares the result with a threshold.

A. Example 5: Normal Noise and Normal Background Variation

Suppose that, for a fixed background, the data vector $\mathbf{g}$ is normally distributed about a mean $\mathbf{b}$ with covariance $\mathbf{K}_n$. Assume also that the background data vectors are themselves normally distributed with mean $\overline{\mathbf{b}}$ and covariance $\mathbf{K}_b$. Then, under the tumor-absent hypothesis, $\mathbf{g}$ is normally distributed with mean $\overline{\mathbf{b}}$ and covariance $\mathbf{K} = \mathbf{K}_n + \mathbf{K}_b$. Under the tumor-present hypothesis, the data covariance is the same and the mean is $\overline{\mathbf{b}} + \mathbf{s}$. This case therefore reduces to Example 1, and the ideal observer uses a prewhitened matched filter. In simulation studies, $\mathbf{K}_n$ is often a diagonal matrix that is known from theoretical considerations, whereas $\mathbf{K}_b$ can be estimated from the collection of noise-free sample data sets.

B. Linear Observers

If either the noise or the background variation are not normal, then the performance of the ideal observer by any of the figures of merit discussed earlier becomes difficult to compute. In fact, simply computing the log-likelihood for a particular data vector can be a difficult task, because computing both $pr(\mathbf{g} \mid H_1)$ and $pr(\mathbf{g} \mid H_2)$ involves approximating a large dimensional integral. For this reason we are often forced to fall back to linear observers to get figures of merit that can be computed in a reasonable amount of time. Assume, as in the preceding, that the linear observer uses the test statistic $\tau(\mathbf{g}) = \mathbf{w}^T \mathbf{g}$ for some template vector $\mathbf{w}$.

Statistical Decision Theory

To find useful expressions for the AUC of a linear observer, we introduce the characteristic functions for the data under each hypothesis

$$\Psi_1(\xi) = \langle \exp(-2\pi i \xi^T \mathbf{g}) \rangle_1$$
$$\Psi_2(\xi) = \langle \exp(-2\pi i \xi^T \mathbf{g}) \rangle_2$$

The AUC of the linear observer can now be computed by means of an integral along the line through the origin in ξ-space that is parallel to the template $\mathbf{w}$: (23)

$$AUC_\tau = \frac{1}{2} + \frac{1}{2\pi i} \mathcal{P} \int_{-\infty}^{\infty} \Psi_1(\mathbf{w}\xi) \Psi_2^*(\mathbf{w}\xi) \frac{d\xi}{\xi}$$

If the conditional probability density for the data given the background satisfies $pr_n(\mathbf{g} | \mathbf{b}) = pr_n(\mathbf{g} - \mathbf{b})$ for some noise probability density $pr_n(\mathbf{n})$, then the AUC for the linear observer reduces to

$$AUC_\tau = \frac{1}{2} + \frac{1}{2\pi i} \mathcal{P} \int_{-\infty}^{\infty} |\Psi_n(\mathbf{w}\xi)|^2 |\Psi_b(\mathbf{w}\xi)|^2 \exp(2\pi i \mathbf{w}^T \mathbf{s} \xi) \frac{d\xi}{\xi}$$

Even this expression is difficult to evaluate analytically, except in the normal-normal case discussed already. Because both of these integrals are one-dimensional, numerical evaluation of them for a given template would not be difficult. When $\mathbf{w}^T \mathbf{s} = 0$, the integrand is an odd function, because the square magnitude of a characteristic function is always and even function. This implies that the integral vanishes and therefore $AUC_\tau = 0.5$, which we expect because the observer in this situation would not see the signal. On the other hand, if $\mathbf{w}^T \mathbf{s} \neq 0$, then the component of the template $\mathbf{w}$ that is orthogonal to the signal $\mathbf{s}$ can have an effect on AUC_τ by means of the noise and background characteristic functions. Once again, this shows that setting the template equal to the signal, a common practice, is not likely to be optimal.

C. Hotelling Observer

If the data vector $\mathbf{g}$ has a large number of components, which it does in medical imaging, then the central limit theorem may imply that the random variable τ is normally distributed. If this is a valid inference, then AUC_τ can be approximated by computing the SNR of τ and using the error function relation noted earlier. The optimal linear observer in this approximation would use the template $\mathbf{w}$ that maximizes the SNR of τ. This is, of course, the Hotelling observer. In the absence of a practical way to compute the AUC of the ideal observer, the resulting Hotelling trace can be used as a figure of merit for an imaging system used in this task.

VIII. BKE

It may be the case that the background is known exactly, from a previous image for example, but the signal is not. Tumors can grow and change shape, for example, or we may know the tumor size and shape but not know its location or orientation. If we use the vector θ to represent the unknown parameters of the tumor, then the data probability densities under the two hypotheses are

$$pr(\mathbf{g}\,|\,H_1) = pr_n(\mathbf{g}\,|\,\mathbf{b})$$

$$pr(\mathbf{g}\,|\,H_2) = \int pr_n(\mathbf{g}\,|\,\mathbf{b} + \mathbf{s}(\theta))pr_\theta(\theta)d\theta$$

We are again assuming that the signal changes the background from $\mathbf{b}$ to $\mathbf{b} + \mathbf{s}(\theta)$. In the second of these equations, $pr_\theta(\theta)$ is some prior probability on the unknown parameters of the tumor. We assume that this prior has been chosen on the basis of some knowledge (or lack of knowledge) of the type of tumor we are interested in.

The likelihood ratio in this situation may be expressed as a weighted integral of simple likelihood ratios that are parametrized by θ (34):

$$\Lambda(\mathbf{g}) = \int \Lambda_b(\mathbf{g}\,|\,\theta)pr_\theta(\theta)d\theta$$

The weighting function is just the prior probability density on θ, and the simple likelihood ratios are given by

$$\Lambda_b(\mathbf{g}\,|\,\theta) = \frac{pr_n(\mathbf{g}\,|\,\mathbf{b} + \mathbf{s}(\theta))}{pr_n(\mathbf{g}\,|\,\mathbf{b})}$$

If there are a small number of unknown parameters, then evaluating this integral may be quite feasible. We will consider some examples. On the other hand, finding an exact expression for the AUC of this ideal observer is difficult, so we will not attempt to do that.

A. Example 6: Location Uncertainty with Normal Noise

We suppose that the tumor shape and size are known, but that the location of the tumor could be at any of the positions $\mathbf{r}_1, \ldots, \mathbf{r}_M$ in a noisy image, which is sampled at the same points described by the data vector $\mathbf{g}$. This gives a set of possible signal vectors whose components are

$$[\mathbf{s}_k]_m = s(\mathbf{r}_m - \mathbf{r}_k) = s_{km}$$

The function $s(\mathbf{r})$ is this expression describes the known tumor profile. If we let P_k be the prior probability that a tumor will be located at $\mathbf{r}_k$, and the noise is normally distributed with covariance $\mathbf{K}$, then the likelihood ratio is given by (34)

$$\Lambda(\mathbf{g}) = \sum_{k=1}^{M} P_k \exp\left[-\frac{1}{2}\mathbf{s}_k^T\mathbf{K}^{-1}\mathbf{s}_k\right]\exp[(\mathbf{g} - \mathbf{b})^T\mathbf{K}^{-1}\mathbf{s}_k]$$

If the noise is stationary, then the quantity in the first exponential is independent of k. With a constant prior probability on k and $\Delta\mathbf{g} = \mathbf{g} - \mathbf{b}$, we then have

$$\Lambda(\mathbf{g}) = \frac{1}{M}\exp\left[-\frac{1}{2}\mathbf{s}_1^T\mathbf{K}^{-1}\mathbf{s}_1\right]\sum_{k=1}^{M}\exp[\Delta\mathbf{g}^T\mathbf{K}^{-1}\mathbf{s}_k]$$

Statistical Decision Theory

In this equation, the quantity in the second exponential is the correlation of the prewhitened signal vector with the prewhitened $\Delta \mathbf{g}$ vector, evaluated at the shift corresponding to $\mathbf{r}_k$. This correlation output is then exponentiated and summed over k to get the likelihood ratio. If the noise is gaussian, so the covariance is a multiple of the identity, then an ordinary correlation is performed before exponentiating and summing. A common procedure is to leave out the prewhitening and exponentiating steps and simply sum the ordinary correlation between the signal and the data over all positions (35–37). We can see that this is not an optimal procedure even if the noise is gaussian.

B. Example 7: Location Uncertainty with laplacian Noise

If a tumor of known shape and size is located somewhere in a medical image that has been through a high-pass filter, then the laplacian noise model may be of interest. With the signal notation as in the previous example, the likelihood ratio is now given by

$$\Lambda(\mathbf{g}) = \sum_{k=1}^{M} P_k \prod_{m=1}^{M} \exp\left[-\frac{1}{c_m}|\Delta g_m - s_{km}| + \frac{1}{c_m}|\Delta g_m|\right]$$

When the pixel variances are all the same, we have $c_1 = \ldots = c_M = c$. If we define the total signal amplitude S by

$$\sum_{m=1}^{N} s_{km} = S$$

then an ideal observer calculates the quantity

$$\Lambda(\mathbf{g}) = \frac{1}{M}\exp\left[\frac{S}{c}\right]\exp\left[-\frac{2}{c}\sum_{m=1}^{M}\min\{\Delta g_m, 0\}\right]\sum_{k=1}^{M}\exp\left[\frac{2}{c}\sum_{m=1}^{M}\min\{\Delta g_m, s_{km}\}\right]$$

when all locations are equally likely. In this expression the quantity in the third set of square brackets is the morphological correlation of the net data vector $\Delta \mathbf{g}$ with the signal vector, evaluated at the shift corresponding to $\mathbf{r}_k$. The output of this operation is exponentiated and summed over k. The first exponential in $\Lambda(\mathbf{g})$ is also data dependent and affects the outcome of the calculation. The most common way to use morphological correlation, as with the ordinary correlation, is to simply sum over k, without exponentiating, and use the result for the decision statistic. As was the case with ordinary correlation in the previous example, this simplified procedure is not the optimal way to use the morphological correlation for tumor detection, at least with this noise model.

Because we have analytical expressions for the ideal observer in these examples, we could estimate the AUC by simulating a two-alternative forced-choice experiment with them. The fraction correct would then be a good approximation to the ideal-observer AUC if there are a large number of samples in the simulation. An appeal to the central limit theorem and the Hotelling observer may also be possible, as in the SKE case. Note, however, that the ideal observers in these two examples are highly nonlinear.

IX. NKE

NKE stands for nothing known exactly, which is quite often the situation in medical imaging. The background is not known exactly because of anatomical variation in the population, among other factors. The signal is not known exactly when some parameters of the tumor, such as size, shape, or location, are unknown. If we have prior probabilities for the background vectors **b** and parameter vectors **θ**, then, with the same assumption about how the signal affects the data as earlier, we may write a general expression for the data probability densities under the tumor-absent and tumor-present hypotheses:

$$pr(\mathbf{g} \mid H_0) = \int pr_n(\mathbf{g} \mid \mathbf{b}) pr_b(\mathbf{b}) d\mathbf{b}$$

$$pr(\mathbf{g} \mid H_1) = \int \left[\int pr_n(\mathbf{g} \mid \mathbf{b} + \mathbf{s}(\boldsymbol{\theta})) pr_\theta(\boldsymbol{\theta}) d\boldsymbol{\theta} \right] pr_b(\mathbf{b}) d\mathbf{b}$$

$$= \int \left[\int pr_n(\mathbf{g} \mid \mathbf{b}) pr_b(\mathbf{b} - \mathbf{s}(\boldsymbol{\theta})) d\mathbf{b} \right] pr_\theta(\boldsymbol{\theta}) d\boldsymbol{\theta}$$

In principle, with a noise model incorporated into $pr_n(\mathbf{g} \mid \mathbf{b})$, these quantities could be computed and the likelihood ratio formed by their quotient. In practice the high-dimensional integrals make this difficult. Current research is focusing on other ways to compute $\Lambda(\mathbf{g})$, or some equivalent statistic, and AUC_Λ, which does not involve explicit evaluation of these integrals.

We could, of course, retreat to linear observers again and find the appropriate expression for the Hotelling observer. From the examples we have seen so far, though, we suspect that the ideal observer in this kind of real world task is not linear. This makes numerical searches for the ideal observer more complicated, because parametrizing a general nonlinear observer is more difficult than it is for a general linear observer. With the increasing size and speed of computers, however, this kind of computation is becoming more and more feasible.

X. SUMMARY

We have shown how the ideal observer and Hotelling observer compute a test statistic for the task of tumor detection in digital imaging data. The ideal observer is optimal by several criteria, including minimizing the Bayes risk and maximizing the AUC. The Hotelling observer maximizes the SNR among all linear observers. We have provided exact and approximate formulas for computing the AUC of an ideal observer, which can be used as a figure of merit for the imaging system itself on a particular tumor detection task.

For SKE/BKE tumor detection tasks, we have given some examples of analytical expressions for the ideal observer and the exact and approximate AUC values for this observer. In these examples, the $G(0)$ approximation to the ideal-observer AUC was generally better than the well-known approximation using the SNR of the log-likelihood. For SKE tumor detection tasks, we have outlined the general procedure for computing the likelihood ratio and shown how the AUC for a linear observer may be estimated. For BKE tumor detection, we have shown analytically that common procedures, such as computing the correlation or morphological correlation, are used by the ideal observer in certain circumstances. These operations must be used correctly, though, to yield optimum performance. Finally, in the NKE situation, we have provided a general formula for the likelihood ratio and have indicated the difficulties involved in computing the AUC for the ideal observer in this most general setting.

REFERENCES

1. MP Eckstein, CK Abbey, JS Whiting. Proc SPIE 3340:16–26, 1998.
2. HH Barrett, CK Abbey, B Gallas. Proc SPIE 3340:27–43, 1998.
3. HH Barrett, JP Rolland, RF Wagner, KJ Myers. Proc SPIE 1090:176–182, 1989.
4. AE Burgess. J Opt Soc Am 16:694–703, 1999.
5. CK Abbey, MP Eckstein. Proc SPIE 3981:70–77, 2000.
6. FO Bochud, CK Abbey, MP Eckstein. Proc SPIE 3663:273–281, 1999.
7. JP Rolland, A Goon, E Clarkson, L Yu. Proc SPIE 3340:85–90, 1998.
8. HH Barrett. J Opt Soc Am A 7:1266–1278, 1995.
9. HH Barrett, JL Denny, RF Wagner, KJ Myers. J Opt Soc Am A 12:834–852, 1995.
10. RD Fiete, HH Barrett. Optics Lett 12:643–645, 1987.
11. RD Fiete, HH Barrett, WE Smith, KJ Myers. J Opt Soc Am A 4:945–953, 1987.
12. MP Eckstein, CK Abbey, FO Bochud. Proc SPIE 3663:243–252, 1999.
13. CK Abbey, MP Eckstein, FO Bochud. Proc SPIE 3663:284–295, 1999.
14. MP Eckstein, CK Abbey, JL Bartroff. Proc SPIE 3981:106–115, 2000.
15. X Pan, CE Metz. Stat Radiol 4:380–389, 1997.
16. CA Roe, CE Metz. Stat Radiol 4:587–600, 1997.
17. EJ Halpern, M Albert, AM Krieger, CE Metz, AD Maidment. Stat Radiol 3:245–253, 1996.
18. CE Metz. Semin Nucl Med 8:283–298, 1978.
19. JA Swets. Invest Radiol 14:109–121, 1979.
20. CE Metz. Invest Radiol 21:720–733, 1986.
21. JA Swets. Science 240:1285–1293, 1988.
22. RF Wagner, KJ Myers, MJ Tapiovaara, DG Brown, AE Burgess. Proc SPIE 1231:195–204, 1990.

23. HH Barrett, CK Abbey, E Clarkson. J Opt Soc Am A 15:1520–1535, 1998.
24. DM Green, JA Swets. Signal Detection Theory and Psycophysics. New York: Wiley, 1966.
25. HH Barrett, CK Abbey, E Clarkson. Proc SPIE 3340:65–77, 1998.
26. E Clarkson, HH Barrett. Appl Optics 39:1783–1793, 2000.
27. RF Wagner, SW Smith, JM Sandrik, H Lopez. IEEE Trans Sonics Ultrason 30:156–163, 1983.
28. RF Wagner, MF Insana, DG Brown. J Opt Soc Am A 4:910–922, 1987.
29. RF Wagner, MF Insana, SW Smith. IEEE Trans Ultrason Ferroelec Freq Control 35:34–44, 1988.
30. SW Smith, RF Wagner, JM Sandrik, H Lopez. IEEE Trans Sonics Ultrason 30:164–173, 1983.
31. HH Barrett, W Swindell. Radiological Imaging: The Theory of Image Formation, Detection and Processing. New York: Academic Press, 1981.
32. JJ Heine, SR Deans, LP Clarke. J Opt Soc Am A 16:6–16, 1999.
33. JJ Heine, SR Deans, DK Cullers, R Stauduhar, LP Clarke. J Opt Soc Am A 15:1048–1058, 1998.
34. HH Barrett, CK Abbey. In: J Duncan and G Gindi, eds. Lecture Notes in Computer Science 1230: Information Processing in Medical Imaging. New York: Springer, 1997, pp 155–166.
35. D Casasent, D Psaltis. Appl Optics 15:1795–1799, 1976.
36. D Casasent, D Psaltis. In: E Wolf, ed. Progress in Optics. Amsterdam: North Holland, 1978, pp 289–356.
37. DO Siegmund, KJ Worsley. Ann Stat 23:608–639, 1995.

5
Display, Including Enhancement, of Two-Dimensional Images

Stephen M. Pizer,
Bradley M. Hemminger and
R. Eugene Johnston
University of North Carolina, Chapel Hill, North Carolina

In this chapter the recorded image is assumed to have the form of a single intensity value at each point in a two-dimensional (2D) array of image points. Sec. I will face the question of what representation of displayed intensity should be used and how the displayed intensity should change as we move across the display scale. Sec. II will then address the question of how to assign display scale values to the recorded intensities at each image position.

I. DISPLAY SCALES

A. Quantitative and Classification Display: Discrete Scales

In classification display the viewer's job is to distinguish the class of each pixel corresponding to its recorded intensity. Quantitative display, while providing an interval scale, can be viewed as a nominal scale in which individual numeric recorded intensities or recorded intensity ranges form the classes. Probably the most effective form of classification display is interrogative—the viewer is given a pointing device, and the display systems responds with the class name or the quantitative value corresponding to the pixel or region to which the viewer has pointed. However, if such interaction is inconvenient, it may be useful to produce a single image to communicate the classes associated with pixels.

The class boundaries are assumed to be sharp, and thus the locations in one class should be perceptually distinguishable from those in another. To do this, we can effectively take advantage of the object-forming functions of the visual system. From this we see that adjacent ranges of recorded intensities corresponding to different classes should have discontinuously distinct luminances. Hue and saturation can nicely be used to label the classes as well, with the caveat that the perceived color depends on the spatial pattern and that many viewers will be to some degree color blind, at least between red and green.

B. Qualitative Display: Perceptually Continuous Scales

In qualitative display the viewer's job is to discern patterns of anatomy or physiology from the measurements of a scalar recorded intensity that can in principle vary over a continuous range at each pixel. Because the human visual system is especially sensitive to local, considerable changes in intensity, using them as boundary measurements to form objects, it is important that unimportant changes in recorded intensity not be represented as considerable changes in displayed intensity. Thus, at least the mapping from recorded intensity to displayed intensity should be smooth.

The objective of qualitative display is to optimize the transmission of information about pattern properties in the recorded image. Because the job that we are discussing is display and not image restoration, let us assume that the image has been processed to show the patterns in question with an optimal tradeoff of resolution, noise, and object contrast. More strongly, let us assume that our job in display is to present information as to patterns in the recorded image. Any detail in the image should be assumed to be of potential interest, even though in fact it might have come from noise of imaging. If it is not of interest, it is because the information is not relevant to the task of the viewer, not because the information is not relevant to the scene to be viewed.

Fig. 1 shows the sequence of stages for 2D display, from the point of view of intensity transformations. The middle stage is the display device itself, which includes analog hardware for turning analog intensities into luminances, colors, heights, or other perceivable features preceded by either hardware or software for doing the lookup that turns the numeric displayable intensities into analog intensities that drive the analog display hardware. From the point of view of intensity transformations, the display device is characterized by a display scale; the device takes numeric values indicating displayable intensities at each image point and produces displayed intensities on the display scale. In the final stage these displayed intensities are transformed by a viewer into a perceived image. At the beginning of the process the recorded image's intensities must be assigned to intensities on the scale of displayable intensities. This assignment is intended to optimize the contrast of important objects, and it is specified by a function from the recorded intensities to the ideal scale given by the displayable intensities.

Display of Two-Dimensional Images

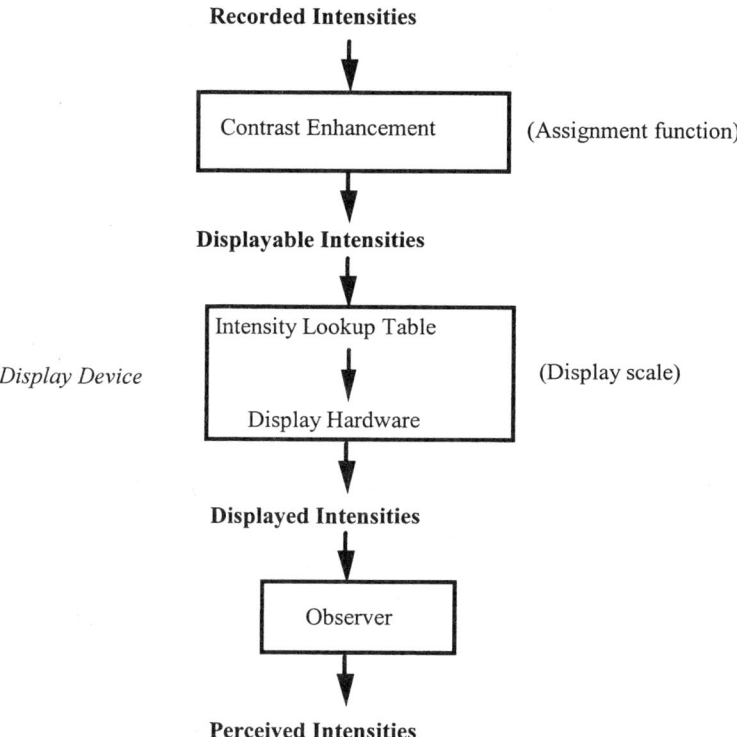

Fig. 1 Two-dimensional display sequence.

To give a feeling for the range of possible display scales, here are a few possibilities (see Fig. 2 for illustrations):

1. A gray scale, beginning at black and going through white, with the property that for all intensities on the scale the luminance that is at fraction ϕ along the scale is a fixed multiple of the luminance that is at fraction $\phi - 1/n$ along the scale, for some step parameter n.
2. A gray scale, beginning at black and going through white, with the property that for all intensities on the scale the luminance that is at fraction ϕ along the scale is a fixed *increment* over the luminance that is at fraction $\phi - 1/n$ along the scale, for some step parameter n.
3. A gray scale, beginning at white and going through black, which is the reverse of black to white scale number 1.
4. A gray scale, beginning at dark gray and going through light gray and comprising the middle half of scale number 1.

5. A color scale, beginning at black and going through white, with the hue following some specified path through red, orange, and yellow, the saturation following some specified path, and the luminance following the rule in scale 1.
6. A height scale, in which the intensity is displayed as a surface height proportional to its value, and the resulting surface is written onto a screen using three-dimensional (3D) display techniques that transfer a height into a shading and a stereo disparity.
7. A height scale as in scale 6, but in which the surface is painted with a combination of hue and saturation that is a function of the height, with the hue and saturation following some specified path in the space of hue, saturation possibilities.

These examples suggest that to specify a display scale, one must specify

1. The display parameter(s), which are to represent the displayable intensity (e.g., luminance, or color—luminance, hue, saturation), or height. Let us use the symbol f to stand for this collection of features.

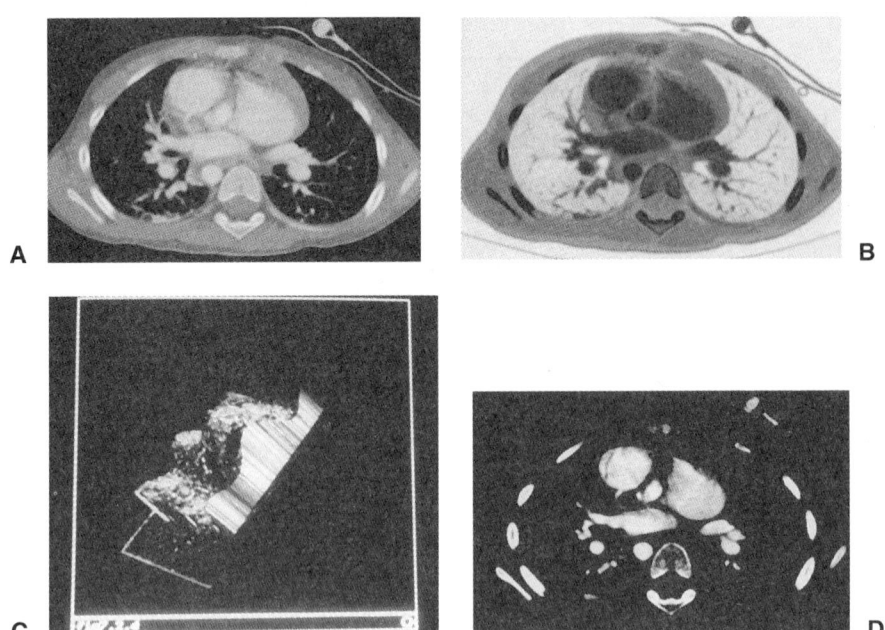

Fig. 2 A chest computed tomography (CT) medical image displayed with four different display scales. (a) standard intensity windowed for soft tissues view, (b) inverted grayscale view, (c) bone intensity window view, and (d) height (topography) scale.

Display of Two-Dimensional Images

2. The path that these parameters must follow. In the case of a single parameter the beginning and the end of the path specify the path (e.g., black to white, white to black, or 0 cm to 5 cm of altitude). With multiple parameters, a curve through the multidimensional parameter space must be specified (e.g., a path through the double-cone representation of color space).
3. The speed at which the path is traversed, as a function of position on the path. Scales 1 and 2, for example, differ only in this parameter. For these different scales the luminance corresponding, for example, to the middle of the scale is quite different.

For single parameter display the basis of comparison of different scales is the discrimination sensitivity that the scale provides. In early work at the University of North Carolina (1), we attempted to define a number, called *perceived dynamic range (pdr)*, which measures this property. The idea is that a perceptual unit called the *just noticeable difference (jnd)* is defined, and the pdr gives the number of jnd's that the scale provides. The difficulty in doing so is that the jnd depends on the spatial size and structure of the target and background, so the hope to measure pdr's of two scales, even relative to others, in a fully image-independent fashion is unfulfillable. Nevertheless, practice and visual experiments have suggested that it is reasonable to measure jnd's and thus pdr's with a particular, reasonably selected family of targets and backgrounds and that scale choices made on this basis will roughly accord with choices made with other families.

Intuitively, if the displayed intensity $i + j$ is just noticeable from a reference displayed intensity i, we call j the jnd for that reference intensity. To define the jnd more strictly, we strictly need to specify target and background structures, the viewing environment, a criterion true-positive rate of detection, and a criterion false-positive rate of detection. That is, a jnd is a change required by a viewer operating at a certain degree of conservatism to correctly detect the change at a specified (true positive) rate of correct calls. The jnd thus corresponds to receiver operating curve passing through a specified (true-positive rate, false-positive rate) point. The jnd may be a different value for every reference displayed intensity i, so it is given by a function $j(i)$.

Jnd's provide the units for perceived intensity. If $P(i)$ is the perceived intensity corresponding to a displayed intensity i, it can be shown (1) that

$$P(i) = \int_{i_{min}}^{i} \frac{j'(i)}{j(i) \log(1 + j'(i))} di$$

where i_{min} is displayed intensity on the bottom of the display scale. The perceived intensity corresponding to $i = i_{min}$ is zero. The perceived dynamic range of a display scale is simply the number of jnd's from the bottom of the display scale to the top: pdr $= P(i_{max})$.

For display scales that are smooth, one way to increase the pdr is to cycle many times up and back along a particular display scale. But despite increasing the pdr, this does not improve the displayed images, because the perceived patterns formed from regions crossing more than one cycle do not correspond to patterns in the recorded image. Similarly, color scales that are not monotonic in luminance produce such misleading patterns despite having large pdr's, because visual object formation in 2D images seems to be largely controlled by the luminance cue. It is therefore recommended to restrict color and gray display scales to those that are monotonic in luminance. Similarly, scales based on altitude (depth) should be monotonic in this parameter. With such a restriction comparisons on the basis of the pdr seem useful.

The greater the pdr of a scale, the more sensitively it can show intensity differences. Intuitively, sensitivity is a desirable feature, but it has been questioned whether it might not be the case that sensitive display of detail that is irrelevant to the task might not be distracting. That is, might it be the case that if image detail, such as that coming from imaging noise, has an amplitude less than signal contrast, then lowering the sensitivity with which image intensity changes are shown would decrease the visibility of distracting noise while leaving signal contrast adequately visible? Klymenko (2) has shown experimentally that this is not the case, at least in the situations he measured. In his studies, increasing the pdr never decreased the ability of the observer to perform his task of determining the orientation of a small Pacman-shaped object. Thus, of available display scales that are monotonic in luminance, it is always beneficial to use the display scale with the largest pdr.

Results (3) from psychophysical experiments from nearby but separated square targets in a uniform background on 100 Cd/m^2 (30 ftL) monitors with 8-bit DACs demonstrated the pdr for a gray scale as 90 jnd's and for a heated object pseudocolor scale as 120 jnd's. The pdr for a continuous gray scale over any luminance range can be derived from the Rose–de Vries and Weber's laws. These laws state, respectively, that in the scotopic or low-luminance range the jnd is proportional to the square root of the luminance of the reference intensity; in the photopic or high-luminance range the jnd is proportional to the reference intensity; and in a luminance range separating these two ranges there is a transition between these two rules. Roughly the Rose–de Vries range goes up to 5×10^{-3} Cd/m^2, and the Weber range begins about 1 Cd/m^2. Barten (4) and Daly (5) give models of these composite jnd functions. Using these new composite visual models, with the most sensitive targets as parameters, calculated for the luminance range of current high-brightness cathode ray tube (CRT) displays suggests significantly higher maximum pdrs, around 500 for high-brightness (340 Cd/m^2) CRTs, and around 1000 for 3425 Cd/m^2 lightboxes (6). Recent experimental work using 10 bit DACs suggests similar experimental results for video monitors (an estimated 300–600 JNDs for 340 Cd/m^2) and similar experimental results for lightboxes (es-

Display of Two-Dimensional Images

timated 500–700 JNDs, lower than the predicted 1000 JNDs because inaccuracies in reproduction of contrast signal when producing film images limit detection by human observers) (7).

The constants of proportionality between luminance or its square root and the jnd depend on many factors, including target shape, the spatial scale and intensity of confusing detail (e.g., image noise), the spatial structure of the background, and the time of exposure. These can cause the pdr to vary by up to a factor of 10. Hemminger (8) suggests that display scale choices depend on the lower envelope of all these jnd curves. Specifically, they analyzed the family of curves resulting from varying the parameters of the visual models across what is commonly found in medical imaging, and after finding similarity in the shape of these curves, they proposed using the jnd from the combination of parameters to the Barten visual model that gives the smallest jnd (the most sensitive discrimination of intensities). Very similar parameters to the Barten model were proposed by Blume (6). The Blume and Hemminger proposed parameters were incorporated into the Standard Display Function defined by DICOM for medical imaging for the purpose of display standardization. In the following, reference to the jnd curve will be taken to be to the DICOM GreyScale Standard Display Function (9).

Given a display with a given sequence of the features f mediating intensity, the speed at which we should move along this sequence at each point in the sequence has yet to be specified. Any display scale with the rates specified can be given by a function $f(i)$ from displayable intensity i to displayed intensity f. For any fully specified scale $f(i)$, each monotonic onto function g on displayable intensities on the range $[i_{min}, i_{max}]$ will correspond to a different fully specified scale $f(g(i))$ with the same sequence. Two separate objectives seem affected by the choice of the traversal speed modification function g. The first objective is the optimization of the effectiveness of image information transmission with respect to the viewing task (i.e., contrast enhancement). As the display scale traversal speed changes along the display scale, the perceived contrast for a fixed distance in displayable intensity changes, and this affects how the image looks. The second objective is the standardization across display systems. It seems desirable that the same image presented on two different displays with the same pdr communicate the same information.

Matters of display system standardization have to apply over all images that will be displayed on the system and all viewing tasks that will be accomplished with it. On the other hand, matters of effectiveness of information transmission are deeply tied up with the particular image and the particular viewing task. Therefore, it seems desirable to separate the standardization objective from the contrast enhancement objective. It is for this reason that Fig. 1 has separate boxes for contrast enhancement and for intensity lookup. The latter is intended to accomplish the standardization task. The contrast enhancement is intended to produce in the displayable image those contrasts that allow the viewing task to be best accomplished.

A fixed perceptual property needs to be chosen to specify the scale traversal speed modification function g, given a basic scale sequence $f(i)$. At the University of North Carolina much effort has been spent working on perceptual linearization (i.e., arranging the relation between displayable intensity and perceived intensity so that it would be linear). Given the convention that the minimum displayable intensity is called zero, perceptual linearization corresponds to arranging the perceived intensity corresponding to displayable intensity i $c \times i$ for a constant c given by the ratio of the pdr of the display scale and the number range of displayable intensities. Figure 3 shows that to accomplish this, we simply need to realize that the display device and observer together apply the intensity transformation P, so we need to precede them by a multiplication by c and an application of the function inverse to P. This fixed function can be applied by means of lookup, assuming that intensity sampling in the displayable intensity is fine enough (see later). The resulting scale will have a constant jnd function vs displayable intensity. Implementation of this lookup correction using discrete values on computer systems has pitfalls, with the result that a careful correction may reduce the available number of contrasts levels. This is discussed further in the next section.

The difficulty in the preceding argument has already been stated: the perceived intensity function P is not independent of the image and the task. To the extent that the changes caused by image and task are linear, the lookup table will not be changed, because c and P^{-1} will change in reciprocal fashion. However, further work is necessary to determine in which circumstances this change in P caused by image and task is linear. To the extent that there is a nonlinear dependence of P on image and task, the separation between contrast enhancement and standardization may seem misguided. However, for practical purposes, it is very advantageous to be able to standardize across display devices. Without this, adopted standards for medical image communication, like DICOM, would be meaningless. Furthermore, once a standard has been decided on, even if it is not perfect, it is well defined and provides a perceptually approximately linear re-

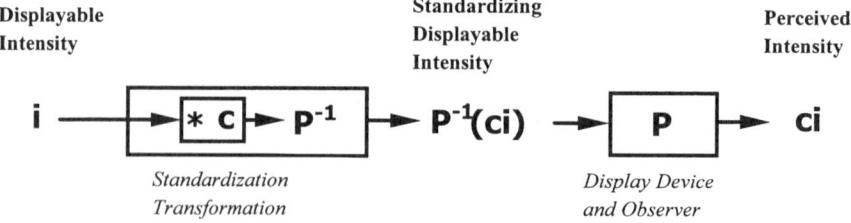

Fig. 3 Perceptual intensity standardization.

Display of Two-Dimensional Images

sponse for the display system, so that contrast-enhancement algorithms can be applied with the knowledge that a known expected perceptual linear response transfer function will approximately occur on the display system. As a result, the medical imaging community is currently adopting in practice this separation of standardization and contrast enhancement.

C. Gray and Color Scales for Image Presentation

The gray scale going from the darkest luminance producible by the display device to the brightest is the obvious first choice for a single parameter scale for 2D display. Such a display, when viewed in a room with ambient light, can be thought of as having a scale going from the ambient light level to the maximum screen luminance. This yields an approximate pdr, because factors such as screen glare, phosphor nonuniformities, CRT noise, etc. all affect the actual pdr.

A common assumption is that for a gray-scale image, reversal of the image can sometimes improve, or at least change, the visibility of objects in the image. If a display system is perceptually linearized, the pdr is independent of which direction the scale is presented. By definition of perceptual linearization, a just noticeable difference is the same whether it runs from black to white or from white to black.

Many display designers have suggested that the pdr could be strikingly increased by the use of a color scale. In that case the display scale will involve a track through the 3D color space. There are many coordinate systems for this space, including red-green-blue (the intensity of each of these light primaries for CRT's) and hue-saturation-intensity (normally shown on a color double-cone). It has been suggested that a path should cover as many hues as possible to optimize the pdr. But many commonly used scales, including scales passing through the colors of the rainbow, have failed to accept the aforementioned restriction that luminance should be monotonic, and these scales are guaranteed to produce artifacts for qualitative display. Moreover, because perceived chromanence varies strongly with the form and location of object boundaries and the chromanence of the objects and surrounds, such display scales cannot be counted on to be seen in a way that is close to the presenter's intentions, and jnd and other experiments based on test patterns cannot be expected to be usable to predict the behavior or the scale with real images. Display designers and users are thus strongly warned against so-called pseudocolor display, the use of single parameter qualitative display scales going over many hues.

A few pseudocolor scales in which the hue change is slow and the luminance is monotonic have been found to have some benefit of increase of pdr without obvious artifacts. One of these with among the highest pdrs is the so-called heated object scale. Also called the hot body scale and the temperature scale, it approximates the colors taken by a black body as it is heated: black-red-orange-yellow-white. It can be produced by monotonically modulating the three color beams in a color CRT. However, this scale increases the pdr over a CRT gray scale by at most one-third, according to the kind of test pattern jnd experiments described earlier. This is a modest increase for the extra cost.

Several authors, including ourselves, have investigated pseudocolor scales other than gray scale as alternatives for increasing the pdr. However, the evidence to date suggests that observers perform as well, or better, using gray scales for clinical tasks (10). Furthermore, radiologists generally indicate they are much more comfortable using the gray scales. Until experimental evidence shows a substantial increase in performance as a result of using a different pseudocolor scale, gray scale display seems indicated for single parameter qualitative 2D display. Furthermore, for these same reasons, the DICOM standards for medical image presentation are currently limited to gray scale presentation.

D. Sampling Issues for Digital (Discrete) Displays

Until now, all of the discussions on display scales have assumed that the scale was continuous. This is essentially true for analog displays such as analog filmscreen films displayed on a lightbox. However, many modern display systems, including laser printed films, video monitors, and reflective paper hardcopy are digital and thus have discrete intensity scales. The question of how a continuous scale should be sampled to produce a discrete scale and the number of samples that are necessary must therefore be addressed.

Recall the need for qualitative display scales to be perceptually continuous. From this it can be concluded that successive discrete intensities on a scale must be distinctly unnoticeable when they are in adjacent regions, even when the boundary of these regions is smooth and long. That is, using such a test pattern for jnd experiments, the intensity differences between successive scale intensities should be around a half of one jnd. Finer sampling will not increase perceptibility of displayed objects, and coarser sampling brings with it the jeopardy of artifactual object boundaries. Thus, a perceptually linear scale should be sampled equally, with the number of samples being approximately double the pdr. For a gray scale if we assume under the best circumstances the human observer could see approximately 500 jnds (9 bits), then this would result in the display device needing to provide 10 bits of standardized response.

This is likely an overestimate of what is required. To date, little work has been done to quantify how much contrast resolution is required for different clinical protocols. Sezan (11) found that 8 bits standardized film presentations was sufficient to avoid contouring on a general collection of x-ray protocols. Similarly, Hemminger found 7 bits on standardized film and video presentations sufficient to avoid contouring artifacts on mammograms (7). Thus, it is likely that between 8 and 10 bits will be required on the display system DAC.

Unfortunately, many scales are far from perceptually linear. An example is the raw scale of many digital gray scale devices; the bottom 15% and the top 10% are frequently far from perceptually linear. If in this case the voltages driving the scales are to be uniformly sampled, the number of samples will need to be small enough so that the smallest intersample perceptual difference is a fraction of a jnd. Hemminger studied existing video and laser printed film displays and found that in general a resampling of the characteristic curve of the display system to closely approximate the perceptual linear DICOM Standard Display Function required reducing the contrast resolution by a factor of 2 (8). Thus, for instance, to accurately achieve 8 bits of contrast on a display system, it required starting with 9 bits of contrast in the display system.

II. ASSIGNMENT OF DISPLAY SCALE INTENSITIES TO RECORDED INTENSITIES*

Given a display scale and a 2D recorded image of a single parameter, the remaining step in the display process is the rule by which the recorded intensities of the original image are mapped to the display scale intensities (see Fig. 1). When performed explicitly, this step is called contrast enhancement. This name suggests that it is an optional step, that an unenhanced displayed image exists. In fact, this step is not optional. To produce an image that a viewer can look at, the assignment must be done. The issue is simply whether we will do it better or worse.

Confusion has arisen from medical imaging systems in which the display is entangled with the acquisition. For example, in ordinary (analog) radiography, the film is exposed by light scintillations generated directly from the transmitted x-rays, and to determine properties of the display the viewer only has the choice of film type, development procedure, and lightbox intensity. But even these choices give different images, (i.e., different contrast enhancements). With digitally acquired images the choice of contrast enhancements is simply more flexible.

After the contrast-enhancement mapping is performed, the image undergoes further transformations, first within the display system and then in the human visual system. The effective design of contrast enhancement mappings requires a thorough understanding of these transformations. It would be ideal if the display device/observer combination could be made linear, so that equal differences in display scale intensity would be perceived as equally different. Methods for attempting to achieve this linearity given an appropriate model of luminance per-

---

* Based on Edge-Affected Context for Adaptive Contrast Enhancement by R. Cromartie and Stephen Pizer, Department of Computer Science, University of North Carolina. In: Information Processin in Medical Imaging (IPMI XII), Lecture notes in Computer Science, ACF Colchester, DJ Hawkes, eds, Vol. 511, New York: Springer-Verlag, 1991, pp 474–485.

ception and difficulties in doing so have been discussed in the previous section. However, ultimately, the step of standardizing the display scale and assigning intensities to it both depend on the spatial structure of the image (the target and its context) and of human visual perception, so it makes limited sense to separate the display scale rate and contrast enhancement determinations. Thus, the contrast-enhancement step needs to concern itself with mapping to an arbitrary well-constructed display scale.

In this chapter we first present a survey of contrast-enhancement techniques, concentrating on locally adaptive methods. Classical adaptive methods have centered on the calculation of various statistics of the local intensity distribution and the use of these to amplify local contrasts. More recently, methods have been developed that attempt to take explicit account of local image structure in terms of objects, especially object edges. These methods are based on advances in our understanding of human visual perception.

The notation used here is that i is the recorded intensity to be assigned and I is the displayable intensity that is the result of the contrast enhancement.

A. Global (Stationary) Contrast Enhancement

A global or stationary enhancement mapping is an intensity transformation based solely on the intensity of each pixel: $I(x, y) = f(i(x, y))$. The goal is to find a function that best uses the full range of display gray levels. Among these methods are intensity windowing, histogram equalization, and histogram hyperbolization.

If we identify a subrange of image gray levels corresponding to features of interest, this subrange can be expanded linearly to fill the full range of intensities (see Fig. 4). This technique is called intensity windowing. Pixels whose values fall outside the selected range are mapped to the minimum or maximum level. This technique is commonly used in the presentation of computed tomography (CT) images. For example, in chest CT images, a "lung window" and a "mediastinum window" are chosen and applied, producing two images. These two images are then viewed side-by-side by the radiologist. This method has the advantage of being easily computed and can be made interactive by an implementation that directly manipulates the lookup table of the display device. One difficulty is that objects occupying widely separated areas of the intensity range cannot be well presented in a single image. A perhaps more serious difficulty is that the perception of object boundary locations can depend critically on window selection (Fig. 5).

Although fixed intensity window choices are appropriate for CT images in which the pixel values are Hounsfeld units and represent physical 3D locations, in standard x-rays in which the pixels represent projections from 3D to 2D, this type of relationship may not hold. Intensity windowing in such situations needs to be able to accomodate shifts or changes in the shape of the histogram caused by dif-

Display of Two-Dimensional Images

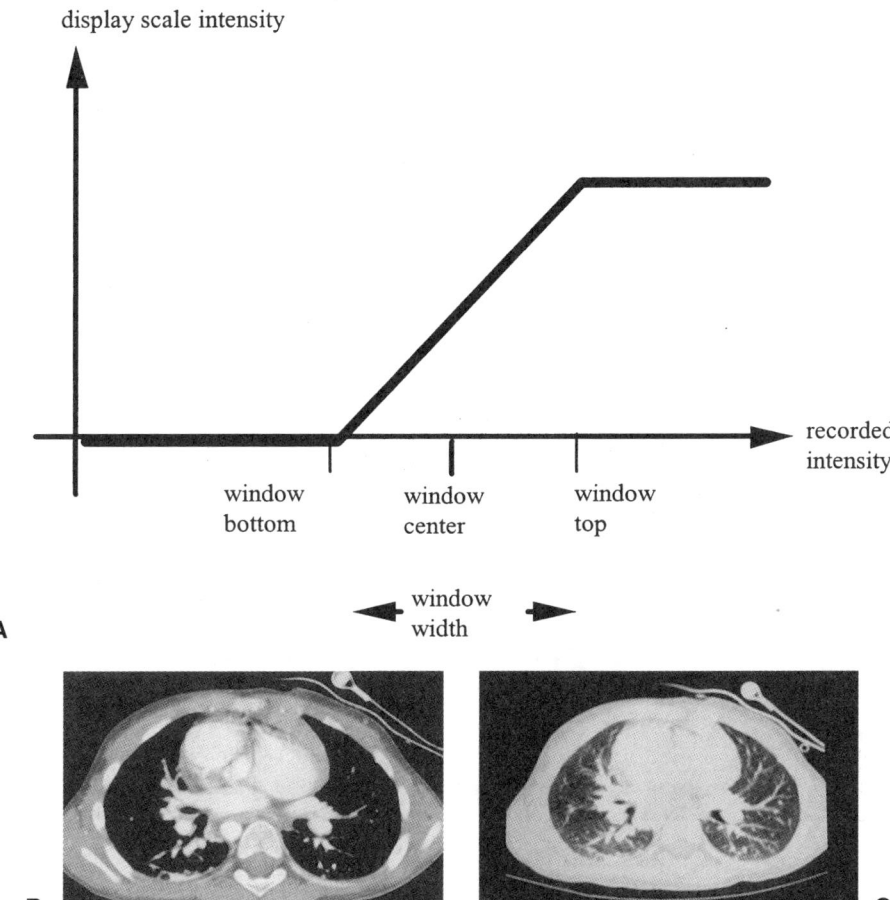

Fig. 4 The intensity windowing contrast enhancement mapping. The intensity window, giving the linear range of the mapping, is normally specified by either the window width and center or by the window bottom and top. (a) depicts the intensity windowing algorithm. (b) and (c) show the two common chest CT presentations, soft-tissue intensity windowed and lung intensity windowed.

ferences in acquisition parameters and projection angles. The most common technique for dealing with this is histogram-based intensity windowing techniques, which attempt to recognize the shape and location of the histogram to localize the intensity window to the appropriate range of contrast values for each individual image. Such techniques are becoming more common with the advent of digital scanners (computed x-ray, direct digital mammography, etc). An example depict-

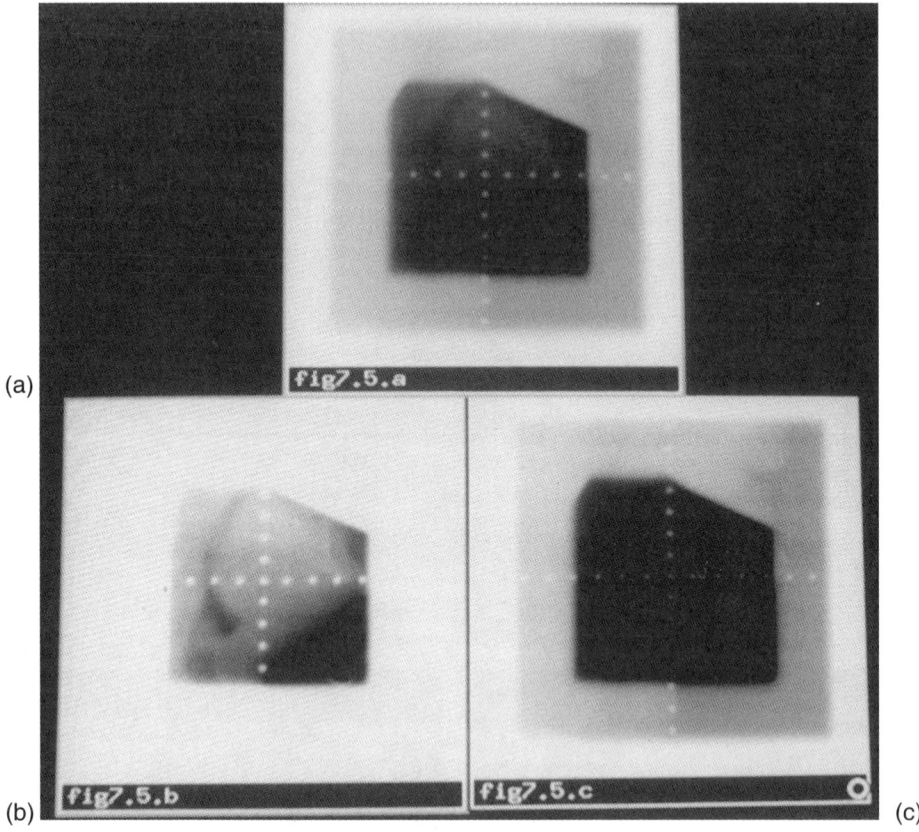

Fig. 5 A radiotherapy portal verification film. (a) The original image. (b) intensity windowed to show contrast in the center of the image. (c) intensity windowed to show contrast in the outer portion of the image.

ing histogram-based recognition of the breast tissue in a mammogram is shown in Fig. 6. Taking this approach a step further, another related method is to recognize the individual components of the histogram to more accurately choose the intensity windowing based on specific components. For instance, a general histogram-based intensity windowing technique may accurately recognize an appropriate window for "overall" breast tissue, whereas a technique that recognized the individual components of the breast (background, uncompressed fat, fat, dense, muscle) would be able to provide intensity windows tuned specifically to dense areas of the breast or to combinations of components (for instance fatty and dense areas of the breast). An example of this approach using mixture modeling (12) to intensity window the dense part of the breast is shown in Fig. 7.

Display of Two-Dimensional Images

Cormack (13) argued that the display intensity napping f should be chosen to maximally transmit information as to scene intensity values. In the case of noise-free, high-resolution imaging and display, the probability of a display scale intensity $p(f(i))$ is equal to the histogram of displayable intensities. Assuming that intensities equally far apart on the display scale are equally discernible (the display scale is linearized), the information increase by looking at (coming to know the value of) an image intensity is maximized by maximizing the average displayed intensity uncertainty before viewing, a property that occurs when $p(f(i))$ is flat (i.e., a constant function of displayable intensity) $f(i)$. Thus, on the assumption that intensities that are adjacent on the display scale are separated by a fixed number of jnd's and on the (very poor) assumption that intensity values are uncorrelated, so that what is right for coming to know the value of a single pixel is right for the collection of pixels, it follows from the preceding that flattening of displayed intensity histogram optimizes the image information increase to the viewer.

This flattening of the histogram of intensities in the whole image is called *global histogram equalization.* In this method, a pixel's gray level is mapped to its rank in the intensity histogram of the entire image, scaled so that the output image fills the full range of intensities. The enhancement mapping is thus proportional to the cumulative distribution function of the recorded image intensities. The result is that intensity values having greater numbers of pixels will be allo-

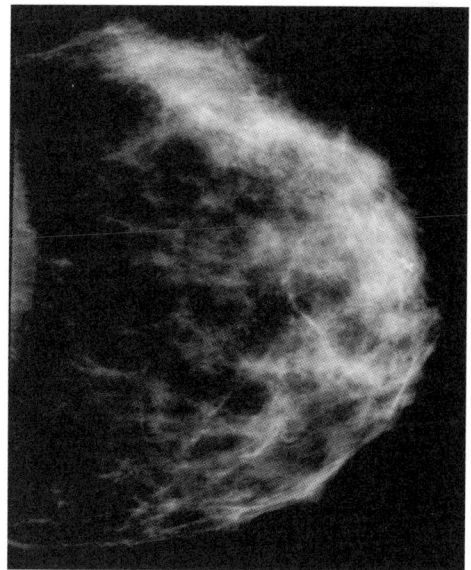

Fig. 6 Histogram based intensity windowed mammogram image. The parameters are chosen for best overall visualization of fatty and dense breast tissue.

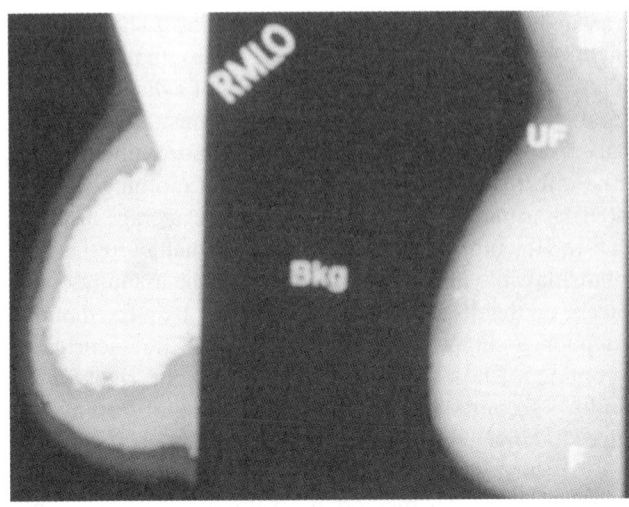

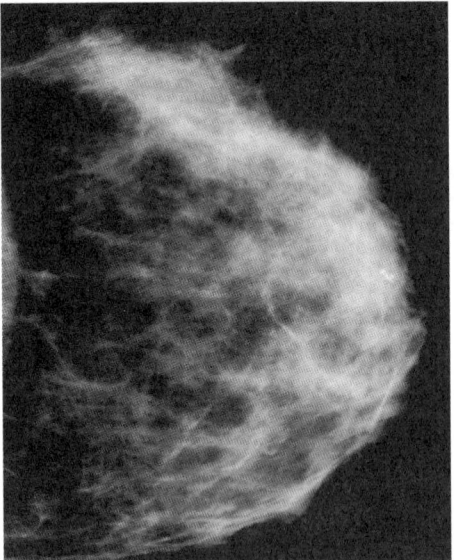

Fig. 7 Mixture-modeling based intensity window (MMIW) approach. (a) On the right panel: an example mammogram labeled with different breast tissue components (Bkg = Background, UF ultra fatty, F = fatty, M = muscle, D = dense). (a) On the left panel: the segmentation calculated by MMIW from this mammogram. (b) shows MMIW applied to the same mammogram of Fig. 6.

Display of Two-Dimensional Images

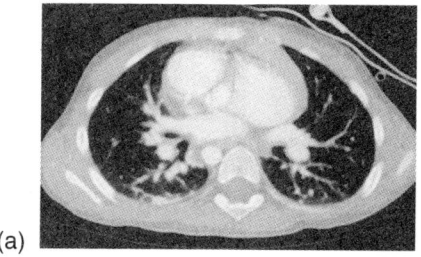
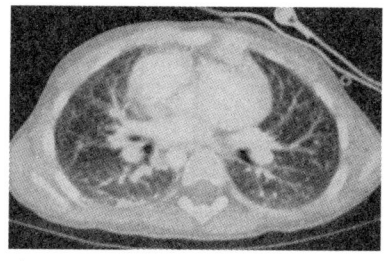

(a)   (b)

Fig. 8 (a) Original chest CT scan and (b) same CT scan processed using global histogram equalization.

cated a greater number of display levels, and the resulting histogram will be as flat as possible. Intensities that occur less frequently in the global histogram can combine with adjacent intensities into a single displayed intensity, resulting in a loss of contrast for the less frequently occurring intensities, but according to the preceding theory, this loss is more than compensated for by the greater sensitivity to changes in the other parts of the recorded intensity range (Fig. 8). Limitations of the flattening caused by discrete recorded and displayable intensities can cause some difficulties of overcompression of the infrequently appearing intensities, but these problems can be limited by adjustments of the algorithm.

In histogram hyperbolization (14), a transformation of intensities is sought that results in a flat histogram of *perceived* intensities. Because the luminance response of the first stage of the human visual system is approximately logarithmic, Frei argued that the shape of the histogram of displayed intensities should be approximately hyperbolic. Essentially, what is sought is histogram equalization after the effect of retinal processing. Thus a histogram-equalized image presented on a perceptually linearized display should result in perceived brightnesses very close to those of a histogram-hyperbolized image displayed without linearization. This approach assumes a display device the luminance output of which is linear in displayable intensity, not a common occurrence. Its main weakness is the strong dependence of our visual system on local object structure; brightness (perceived luminance) is not a logarithmic function of luminance.

B. Adaptive Contrast Enhancement

An adaptive contrast-enhancement mapping is one in which the new intensity value for a pixel is calculated from its original value and some further information derived from local image properties:

$$I(x,y) = f(i(x,y), D_N(x,y)) = f_N(i(x,y))$$

where $N(x,y)$, the *contextual region,* is some spatial neighborhood of (x,y) in the image that includes the pixel of interest (see Fig. 9) and $D_N(x,y)$ is some collection

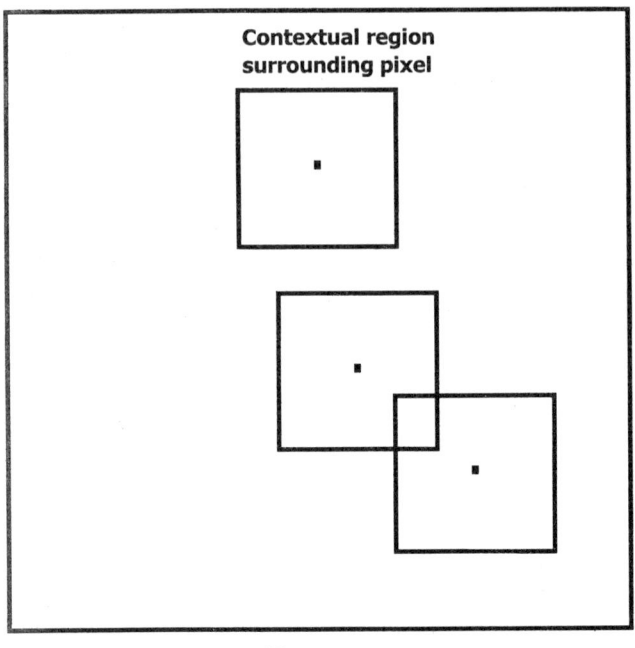

Fig. 9 Three pixels and their contextual regions for AHE processing.

of measurements over $N(x,y)$. For computational efficiency, it is most usual for N to be a square region centered on (x,y), but as we shall see, this need not be the case. Furthermore, the size and shape of the contextual region may itself vary throughout the image, based on either local statistics or local structural information.

The reason for contrast enhancement being adaptive is that the visual system perceives an object according to the shape of the object, its contrast with its local background, the structure of that local background, and variations of intensity within the object. To maximize perceivability of all changes, it is desirable to bring all contrasts within and in the vicinity of the object to a high value while making these local contrasts monotonic with the information they transmit. At the same time, there is no benefit to concerning oneself with global interluminance relationships because of the weak abilities of the visual system to perceive such relationships. The dependence of perception on local contrasts means that specifying the display contrast between local objects and distant objects does not change what will be perceived as objects. Although there is some ability to compare absolute intensities at a distance, and these relationships will be disturbed by arbitrary changes of the relation of intensities at a distance, the visual system cannot be trusted to determine absolute intensities, because the object structure strongly

Display of Two-Dimensional Images

affects perceived brightnesses. It follows that one should not even insist that for two spatially distant positions the order of the values of the recorded intensities be maintained into the display scale intensities under contrast enhancement. Rather, only appropriate local relationships should be optimized, as discussed earlier.

Any adaptive contrast-enhancement method with a fixed sized contextual region will produce a sort of shadowing artifact at sharp high-contrast boundaries. As the pixel moves toward the boundary, the contextual region passes across the boundary, and within the contextual region there is an exchange of pixels on one side of the boundary for those on the other side. That is, the average intensity of the context gets sharply lighter and lighter (darker and darker) as the center pixel on the dark (light) side of the boundary is moved toward the boundary. Thus, relative to its context, the center pixel will get darker and darker (lighter and lighter) as that pixel on the dark (light) side of the boundary is moved toward the boundary, so the result of the adaptive mapping will have the same behavior. Fig. 10 shows the general shape of the so-called edge-shadowing behavior that results.

Original image

Intensity on horizontal cross-section

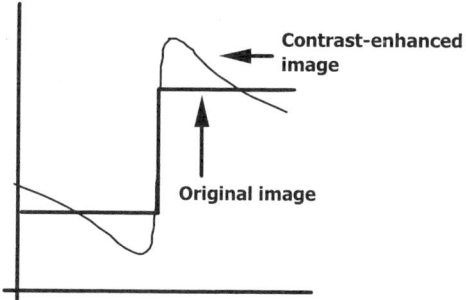

Fig. 10 Edge-shadowing intensity behavior near a sharp high-contrast edge.

This problem is common to all algorithm methods based on a contextual region including a sharp edge. This leads to a display mapping that can change too quickly with image position. Chan (15) has suggested a method of explicitly controlling this rate of change of the mapping with image position.

Many adaptive contrast-enhancement methods can be viewed as some variation of detail amplification (high-pass filtering). The oldest and most widely used of these is *unsharp masking*. Known in its photographic form for at least 60 years, unsharp masking has also been applied to digital images. It is defined as

$$I(x,y) = \gamma(i(x,y) - i_N^*(x,y)) + i_N^*(x,y)$$
$$= \gamma i(x,y) + (1 - \gamma) i_N^*(x,y)$$

where $i_N^*(x,y)$ is a positively weighted average of intensities over the contextual region and γ is a constant gain factor. $i_N^*(x,y)$ is referred to as the *background image*, because it represents the smooth background to the image detail. The term $(i(x,y) - i_N^*(x,y))$ is a high-frequency component referred to as the *detail image*. A γ between 0 and 1 results in a smoothing of the image, and the values of γ greater than 1 that are normally used in contrast enhancement result in emphasis of the detail image. Unsharp masking has been applied and tested with varying but frequently good success on a wide range of medical images (16,17). It has a noticeable contrast-enhancing effect on edges, but when the gain factor is high enough to present very small details well, ringing (edge-shadowing) artifacts are introduced across strong edges and breakup of image objects can occur (Fig. 11).

Note that although unsharp masking is frequently viewed as a shift-invariant linear filtering process, when viewed as a contrast enhancement it is

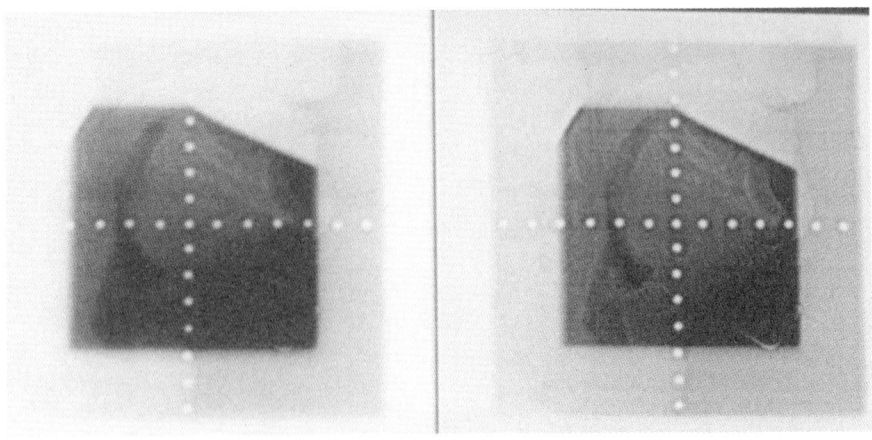

Fig. 11 Unsharp masking applied to the same portal image as in Fig. 5 with two different gain factors- $\gamma=4$ (a) and $\gamma=10$ (b).

Display of Two-Dimensional Images

adaptive (i.e., context-sensitive). It needs to be understood that sharpening (filtering) and contrast enhancement are two complementary ways of looking at the same process. In the former there is a focus on the spatial relations between pixels, and the intensity relations come along for the ride, whereas in the latter there is a focus on the intensity relations between pixels, and the spatial relations are secondary.

Unsharp masking can be generalized in a number of ways. One way is to replace the constant gain with separate weights for the background and detail terms:

$$I(x,y) = A(i(x,y) - i_N^*(x,y)) + B(i_N^*(x,y))$$

An example of a method using this formulation is the statistical difference filter (18,19). In this method, A is chosen so that the variance within the contextual region is made as nearly constant as possible, subject to a preset maximum gain to avoid overenhancement of areas of very small standard deviation. B is a constant that serves to restore part of the background component. The method has been shown to produce objectionable artifacts, and finding suitable values for the weighting factors, the maximum gain and the window size proves difficult.

Multiscale Image Contrast Amplification (MUSICA™) (20) is an algorithm based on a multiresolution representation of the original image. The image is decomposed into a weighted sum of smooth, localized, 2D basis functions at multiple scales. Each transform coefficient represents the amount of local detail at some specific scale and at a specific position in the image. Detail contrast is enhanced by nonlinear amplification of the transform coefficients. An inverse transform is then applied to the modified coefficients. This yields a uniformly contrast-enhanced image without apparent artifacts (see Fig. 12 for an example).

Another well-accepted adaptive method generalizes histogram equalization to local context. In *adaptive histogram equalization* (AHE) (21,22), the histogram is calculated for the contextual region of a pixel, and the transformation is that which equalizes this local histogram. Its development is logical both from the point of view of optimization of information, the basis for histogram equalization, and of the local sensitivity of the human visual system. It gives each pixel an intensity that is proportional to its rank in the intensity histogram of the contextual region centered at that pixel. AHE provides a single displayed image in which contrasts in all parts of the range-recorded intensities can be sensitively perceived. AHE has demonstrated its effectiveness in the display of images from a wide range of imaging modalities, including CT, magnetic resonance imaging (MRI), and radiotherapy portal fims.

The size of the contextual region used is a parameter of the method. Generally, the contextual region should be proportional to the size of the objects or object details to be visualized from the image. For 512 × 512 CT or MR or radiographic images, contextual regions of between 32 × 32 and 64 × 64 have been found to be the best for clinical use.

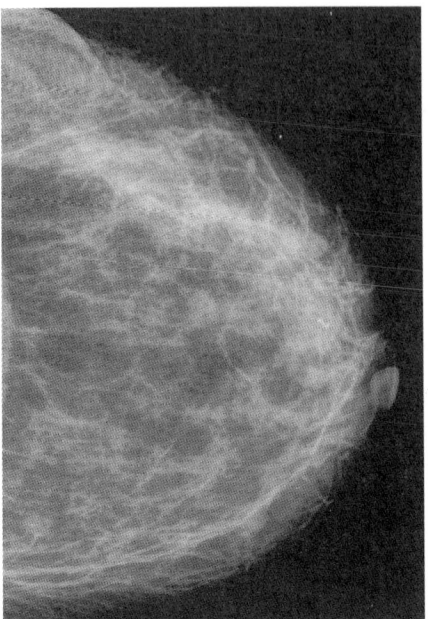

Fig. 12 The same mammogram processed with MUSICA. See Fig. 6 and 7 for comparison with MMIW and HIW methods.

AHE as it stands requires the computationally expensive process of computing a histogram for every pixel. Algorithms have been developed for streamlining this process while not changing the result (23,24), and for fitting this process on parallel processors (25,26), with only minor effects on the results. A great speedup on sequential machines has been achieved by interpolative AHE, in which the histogram and thus the local function f_N is computed for only a sample of pixels, and the value $I(x,y)$ is bilinearly interpolated from the results of f_N ($i(x,y)$) for each of the f_N appropriate for the nearest pixels in the sample (24). However, interpolative AHE has been shown to produce certain artifacts that are in some cases damaging, so full AHE is to be preferred if the time or the parallel machine it requires can be accepted.

While providing excellent enhancement of the signal component of the image, AHE also enhances noise, as it should if the perceptual task is to view all recorded image information. In addition, as with all adaptive methods with a fixed contextual region, shadowing of strong edges can occur in certain types of images. *Contrast-limited adaptive histogram equalization* (CLAHE) (24) was designed to lessen these behaviors in those cases in which the perceptual task leads to the desire to ignore salt-and-pepper noise. CLAHE proceeds from the realization that

Display of Two-Dimensional Images

overenhancement of noise occurs when the recorded intensity is approximately uniform in the contextual region. This nearly constant intensity reflects itself in a large peak in the contextual region's histogram, and this in turn leads to a high slope in the cumulative histogram. Because the slope of a normalized version of the cumulative histogram gives the degree of contrast amplification, that amplification is great when the contextual region has nearly constant intensity. Moreover, the main contrast to be amplified there is that caused by noise. This reasoning suggests that the enhancement calculation be modified by imposing a user-specified maximum on the height of the local histogram, and thus on the slope of the cumulative histogram that defines the contrast amplification in that region (see Fig. 13). This is exactly what CLAHE does, except that an additional normalizing transformation must be done, as discussed in the next paragraph. The enhancement is thereby reduced in very uniform areas of the image, which prevents overenhancement of

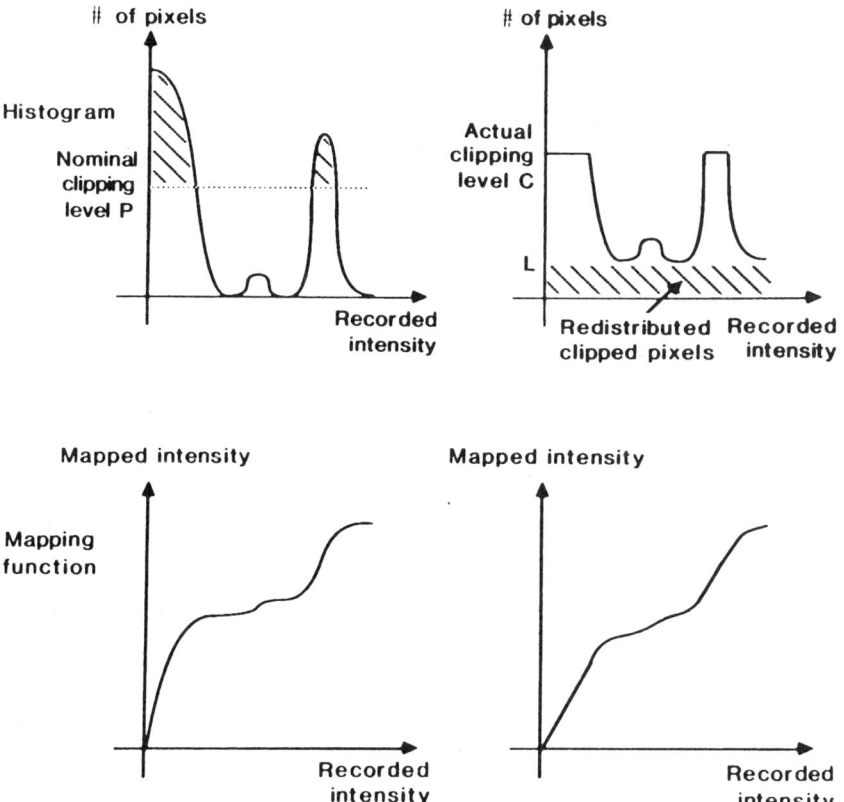

Fig. 13 Histogram clipping and renormalization and its effect on the intensity mapping.

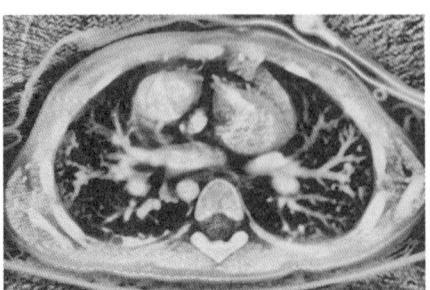 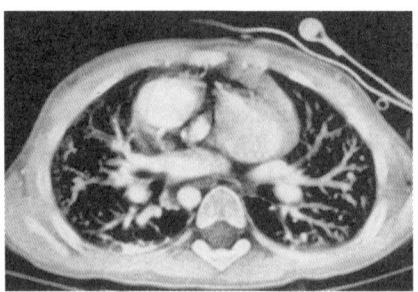

Fig. 14 (a) The original CT image shown in Fig. 8 processed by AHE and (b) CLAHE.

noise. At the same time lowering the contrast amplification reduces the edge-shadowing effect of unlimited AHE (see Fig. 14). More about this will be said later.

For any contrast-enhancement function f_N that maps the full range of i (in the contextual region) to the range of displayable intensities, the modification of by limiting its slopes will lead to a function that does not map to the full range of displayable intensities. Some renormalization is necessary to achieve a mapping to the full range. Basically, what needs to be done is to replace parts of the histogram that have been clipped off by the limitation in contrast amplification. The renormalization that produces a minimum change in the maximal contrast amplification caused by the renormalization is achieved by adding a constant level to the histogram so that its area is returned to its value before the clipping or, equivalently, by adding a constant to the slope of the cumulative histogram, which for histogram equalization is proportional to f_N. The result of adding a constant to the slope of the mapping is equivalent to adding a multiple of the original image into the image mapped by the unrenormalized cumulative histogram. In fact, it is best for this constant to be added only to histogram bins that have a nonzero content to make the method insensitive to pixels with strongly outlying intensities.

Another method for limiting the shadowing problem was discovered by Rehm (27) in the context of high-resolution digital chest radiographs. Her solution is a variant on unsharp masking. Instead of amplifying the detail image by multiplying it by a constant before adding it back to the background image, she applied CLAHE to (only) the detail image before adding a multiple of the result back. The limited excursions in intensity in the detail image and the limited edge-shadowing of CLAHE with heavy histogram height limitation led to limited edge shadowing in the final result.

C. Methods Incorporating Object Structure

The local image structure in terms of object geometry plays a crucial role in our perception of contrast. Enhancement techniques that incorporate local object geometry are a logical result. There are two ways in which the preceding methods may be extended to include object information. One is to change the enhancement calculation itself; the other is to change the contextual region over which the calculations are done. Examples of each of these approaches are presented in the following.

An interesting extension of the two-coefficient generalization of unsharp masking (28) chooses the coefficients to produce a local contrast modification based on the detection of edges within the contextual region. In essence, the recorded intensity of a pixel is weighted by the local edge strength at that pixel as computed by the Sobel, Laplacian, or other edge operator. These edge-weighted values are then used in the calculation of the local f_N. This method has an edge-enhancing effect.

Several ways have been proposed of adjusting the contextual region over which the contrast enhancement is calculated. The idea is to adaptively restrict the local context to that which is relevant to perception of the pixel under consideration. Exactly what constitutes relevance in this sense depends to a large extent on the visual model that is used, but it is certain that perceived object boundaries are important in defining relevant context.

Gordon's version of two-coefficient generalization of unsharp masking (29) has been extended by introducing a limited set of different window sizes and choosing the appropriate size on a pixel-by-pixel basis throughout the image. This is done by analyzing how the contrast function changes across these different window sizes. As the window size increases, the contrast of a central object will increase until the inner window just covers the object. This window is then used to calculate the enhancement. Even by restricting the available windows to a few possible sizes, the computational burden is large. Moreover, the use of square windows limits the ability to adapt to actual image structure.

Kim and Yaroslavskii (30) propose analyzing the local histogram to define a subset of the contextual region and determining the enhancement mappings from the histogram of this subset only. One method uses only that portion of the histogram of the contextual region that falls within a certain intensity range surrounding the value of the center pixel. To the extent that nearness in the histogram or nearness in absolute intensity corresponds to closeness within the image, this has the effect of restricting the calculations to within-object boundaries. The method unfortunately may result in a contextual region of disconnected pixels. Moreover, although the contextual region does indeed change across the image, the overall window size remains fixed. To be entirely satisfactory, an adaptive neighborhood must both have some mechanism for responding to object boundaries and also not be limited by an imposed overall shape. Two methods that meet both these criteria are now examined.

In designing an effective variable contextual region calculation, we seek some way of determining the relevant context. The context is the local object and its near background. The very variable conductance diffusion (VCD) that produces object formation in certain models of human vision also gives a measure of relevance of one pixel to another, thus offering a way of producing truly object-sensitive contextual regions.

One way of using VCD is called *sharpened histogram equalization* (SHAHE) (31), the background image of an unsharp masking is formed using VCD, and the resultant unsharp masking is followed by CLAHE.

The form of VCD used diffuses intensity according to a conductance determined by the rate of change of intensity. That is, conductance is lower in regions with high rate of change of intensity (near edges) than in those where intensity is more homogeneous. The scale at which intensity change should be measured at the beginning part of the diffusion determines what spatial degree of edge coherence is necessary for the location to form a significant degree of insulation.

SHAHE is a somewhat ad hoc combination of the ideas of object-sensitive contrast enhancement, but it frequently produces good results. It is unusual by having been proven to make a clinically significant difference, namely on radiotherapy portal films (32). The method consists of an unsharp masking based on smoothing by means of variable conductance diffusion, followed by CLAHE. VCD is used to define the background region in unsharp masking. The standard unsharp masking formula $I(x,y) = \gamma i(x,y) + (1 - \gamma) i_N^*(x,y)$, is used, but the background $i_N^*(x,y)$ is produced using a variable rather than fixed contextual region. The background thus reflects a relatively small blurring of high contrast, sharp edges while keeping a relatively large blurring of low-sharpness or low-contrast edges. This means that the detail image shows a strong sharpening of the weak edges while maintaining the sharpness but decreasing the sharpness of the strong edges. The step amplifying the detail image and adding back the background thus results in a relative increase in the enhancement of small details while producing no overshoot or even an undershoot along the edges. This is exactly what is needed to counteract the shadowing effect of CLAHE. Thus, when CLAHE with a significant contrast-enhancement limitation is applied (thus itself resulting in low shadowing) to the result of the unsharp masking, a high-contrast result without much edge shadowing is produced (Fig. 15).

D. Quality of Contrast-Enhancement Methods

The ultimate test of any contrast-enhancement method designed for use with medical images is whether it provides increased diagnostic accuracy or efficiency in a clinical setting. In choosing among contrast-enhancement methods, we must generally be content with some approximation to this test. Most frequently, enhanced images are judged purely subjectively. Unfortunately, there is a lack of correlation between performance as an observer executing a viewing task and subjective rating of image quality. Thus, observer experiments comparing different enhancement techniques have become an important part of the field. Enhancement meth-

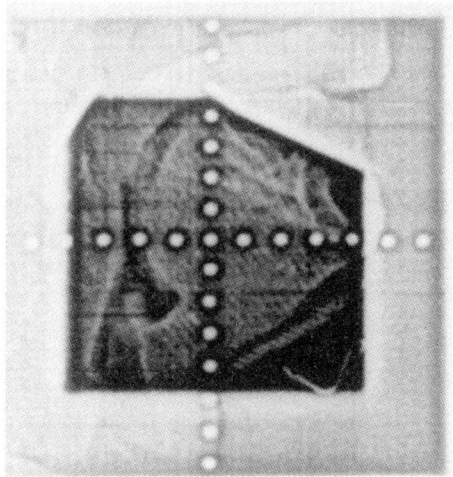

Fig. 15 Results of applying SHAHE algorithm to the portal image shown in Fig. 5.

ods are often compared on the basis of their ability to increase detectability of either standard test patterns or very subtle artificially produced lesions imposed on real medical images. This detection task is certainly important for many imaging modalities but may not be the most important in every case. Boundary localization, shape characterization and comparison of absolute luminances are some viewing tasks that may be of importance. It may take a considerable amount of training for the clinician to effectively use images processed by means of these enhancements.

Another task-related matter is how noise is treated. Noise is unwanted image detail, so its definition depends on what detail is wanted, as well as what is known about the properties of the image-formation process. With such a decision, the contrast enhancement must be chosen not simply to convey signal differences but to convey them relative to noise.

If one does not understand the effect of the display system, one cannot design contrast-enhancement mappings that best present the information of the recorded image to the human observer. We cannot control the processing that takes place inside the human visual system; indeed, we design our contrast-enhancement methods to best match this processing as we understand it. But nonlinearities in the display system can confound the most carefully designed enhancement mapping, and these effects can and must be controlled. Standardization of display systems is absolutely critical, especially when comparing different contrast-enhancement ideas.

We have discussed these techniques without paying particular attention to the cost of computing them. Certainly, for a method to be usable in the real world, the implementation must be relatively fast, even real-time. Many of the methods discussed previously, particularly the adaptive ones, have in the past been too computationally expensive to be clinically valuable. However, many algorithms are approaching real-time computation speeds as general purpose computers become more powerful. Furthermore, in most cases specialized hardware optimized for a specific method would be capable of real-time computation of that method.

We have presented a survey of recent advances in contrast-enhancement techniques and tried to give some indication of the importance of an accurate visual model in the development of these techniques. As better models of human visual perception are formulated, we will be able to design contrast-enhancement methods that more effectively complement our perceptual capabilities.

REFERENCES

1. SM Pizer. Intensity mappings to linearize display devices. Computer Graphics Image Processing 17:262–268, 1981.
2. V Klymenko, RE Johnston, SM Pizer. Visual increment and decrement threshold curves as a function of luminance range and noise in simulated computed tomographic scans. Invest Radiol 27(8):598–604, 1992.
3. SM Pizer, RE Johnston, JB Zimmerman, FH Chan. Contrast perception with video displays. SPIE 318 (part 1) Picture Archiving and Communication Sustems (PACS) for Medical Applications. 1982, pp 223–230.
4. PGJ Barten. Physical model for the contrast sensitivity of the human eye. Proceedings Human Vision, Visual Processing, and Digital Display III, SPIE 1666, 1992, pp 57–72.
5. S Daly. The visible differences predictor: an algorithm for the assessment of image fidelity, Proceedings Human Vision, Visual Processing, and Digital Display III, SPIE 1666, 1992, pp 2–15.
6. H Blume, S Daly, E Muka. Presentation of Medical Images on CRT displays A Renewed Proposal for a Display standard. Preceeding of Medical Imaging: Image Capture, Formatting and display. SPIE 1897, 1993, pp 215–231.
7. BM Hemminger, Panel on Image Display Quality. SPIE Medical Imaging: Image Perception Conference. Vol 3340, San Diego, CA, Feb. 1998.
8. BM Hemminger, RE Johnston, JP Rolland, KE Muller. Perceptual linearization of video display monitors for medical image presentation. SPIE Medical Imaging '94: Image Capture, Formatting, and Display, 2164, 1994, pp 222–240.
9. H Blume, BM Hemminger, et al. The ACR/NEMA Proposal for a Gray-Scale Display Function Standard. Proceedings of Medical Imaging 1996: Image Display, SPIE Vol 2707-35, 1996, pp 344–356.
10. H Leikowitz, GT Herman. Color Scales for Image Data. IEEE Computer Graphics and Applications 12:72–80, 1992.
11. MI Sezan, KL Yip, SJ Daly. Uniform perceptual quantization: applications to digital radiography. IEEE Trans on Man, Machine and Cybernetics, vol SMC-17:(4), pp 622–634, 1987.

12. GJ McLachlan, KE Basford. Mixture Models. Inc., New York: Marcel Dekker, 1988.
13. J Cormackand, BF Hutton. Quantitation and optimization of digitized scintigraphic display characteristics using information theory. Medical Image Processing: Proceedings of the VIIth International Meeting on Information Processing in Medical Imaging, Stanford University, 1981, pp 240–263.
14. W Frei. Image enhancement by histogram hyperbolization. Computer Graphics Image Processing 6:286–294, 1977.
15. H Zhu, FHY Chan, FK Lam. Image contrast by constrained local histogram equalization. Computer Vision and Image Understanding 73(2):281–290, 1999.
16. LD Loo, K Doi, C Metz. Investigation of basic imaging properties in digital radiography 4. Effect of unsharp masking on the detectability of simple patterns. Med Physics 12:209–214, 1985.
17. J Sorenson, CR Mitchell, JD Armstrong, H Mann, DG Bragg, FA Mann, IB Tocina, MM Wojtowycz. Effects of improved contrast on lung-nodule detection: A clinical ROC study. Invest Radiol 22:772–780, 1987.
18. R Wallis. An approach to the space variant restoration and enhancement of images. Proceedings of the Symposium on Current Mathematical Problems in Image Science, Monterey, California, Naval Postgraduate School, 1976.
19. JL Harris, Jr. Constant variance enhancement: a digital processing technique. Appl Optics 16:1268–1271, 1977.
20. P Vuylsteke, E Schoeters. Multiscale image contrast amplification (MUSICA™). SPIE 2167, Medical Imaging: Image Processing. 1994, pp 551–560.
21. SM Pizer. An automatic intensity mapping for the display of CT scans and other images. Medical Image Processing: Proceedings of the VIIth International Meeting on Information Processing in Medical Imaging, Stanford University, 1981, 276–309.
22. JB Zimmerman. Effectiveness of adaptive contrast enhancement. PhD dissertation, Department of Computer Science, The University of North Carolina at Chapel Hill, 1985.
23. K Zuiderveld. Contrast limited adaptive histogram equilization. In: T Heckbert, ed. Graphic Gems IV. Boston: Academic Press, 1994, pp 474–485.
24. SM Pizer, EP Amburn, JD Austin, R Cromartie, A Geselowitz, B ter Haar Romeny, JB Zimmerman, K Zuiderveld. Adaptive histogram equalization and its variations. Computer Vision, Graphics, and Image Processing 39:355–368, 1987.
25. JP Ericksen, JD Austin, SM Pizer. "MAHEM: A multiprocessor engine for fast contrast-limited adaptive histogram equalization. Medical Imaging IV, SPIE Proc 1233:322–333, 1990.
26. A Ramsisaria. University of North Carolina, Chapel Hill Department of Computer Science internal report. 1991.
27. K Rehm, GW Seely, WJ Dallas, TW Ovitt, JF Seeger. Design and testing of artifact-suppressed adaptive histogram equalization: A contrast-enhancement technique for the display of digital chest radiographs. J Thoracic Imaging 5(1):85–91, 1990.
28. A Beghdadi, A Le Negrate. Contrast enhancement technique based on local detection of edges. Comput Vision, Graphics, Image Processing 46:162–174, 1989.
29. R Gordon. Enhancement of mammographic features by optimal neighborhood image processing. IEEE Trans Medical Imaging MI-5 No. 1:8–15, 1986.

30. V Kim, L Yaroslavskii. Rank algorithms for picture processing. Comput Vision, Graphics, Image Processing 35:234–258, 1986.
31. R Cromartie, SM Pizer. Edge-effected context for adaptive contrast enhancement. In: ACF Colchester, DG Hawkes, eds. International Proceedings in Medical Imaging: Lecture Notes in Computer Science. Vol. 511. Berlin: Springer-Verlag, 1991, pp 477–485.
32. JG Rosenman, CA Roe, R Cromartie, KE Muller, SM Pizer. Portal film enhancement: technique and clinical utility. Int J Radiat Oncol Biol Physics 25:333–338, 1992.

6
Detection of Microcalcifications

Robert M. Nishikawa
The University of Chicago, Chicago, Illinois

I. INTRODUCTION

Breast cancer is one of the few diseases that uses asymptomatic screening as a method for controlling the disease. Several countries in the world have national screening programs, and many others have recommendations for regular mammographic screening for asymptomatic women. Consequently, mammography is becoming a high-volume subspecialty. Furthermore, it is becoming one of the most common areas for radiological malpractice suits in the United States (1). Radiologists read screening mammograms in batches, sometimes 100 or more at a sitting. Because only about 0.5% of these cases will have breast cancer, it can be difficult to be ever vigilant to find the often subtle indications of malignancy on the mammogram. Consequently, between 5% and 30% of women, who have breast cancer and have a mammogram, are diagnosed as normal. Computerized detection of breast lesions can be used by radiologists as a "second opinion" and thereby reduce the chances that a cancer is missed. Therefore, automated analysis of mammograms is the most active area in computer-aided diagnosis research.

Microcalcifications appear grouped on a mammogram—typically, at least 5 microcalcifications per square centimeter are required to be considered a cluster, but three suspicious microcalcifications could be enough to prompt a biopsy. Because isolated calcifications are not clinically relevant, the detection of clustered microcalcifications is somewhat unique. Multiple individual microcalcifications compose the target lesion: a cluster of microcalcifications. Therefore, it is not necessary to detect every calcification to detect the cluster. In theory, a detection scheme could have low sensitivity for the detection of microcalcifications, while having high sensitivity for the detection of a cluster of microcalcifications.

Calcifications are a result of either a benign or a malignant process that causes the epithelial cells lining the ducts of the breast to secrete calcium salts into the duct lumen. As a result, what appears mammographically as a calcification is a concretion of varying size composed of calcium phosphates, mainly hydroxyapatite, or calcium oxalate crystals. Thus, the calcifications themselves are neither benign nor malignant but are the result of cells that have undergone a benign or malignant transformation. Although it appears mammographically as a single entity, a calcification is actually composed of multiple crystals. Because these crystals can adhere in multiple ways, the size and shape of the calcification can vary greatly—from 10 μm up to several millimeters in diameter and from spherical to elongated. Furthermore, the density of the calcifications can vary, depending on the amount of fluid trapped in the concretion. Consequently, the radiographic contrast of the calcifications can differ even for calcifications of the same size and shape. These factors add to the complexity of detecting calcifications on mammograms.

Mammographic screen-film systems are capable of imaging very high-contrast objects down to 25 μm or less. However, small calcifications are not high-contrast objects. Typically, the smallest calcifications that can be seen with conventional mammography are around 200 μm microns (2,3). This is because the detection of calcifications is limited by the calcification's signal/noise ratio (4). Smaller calcifications or better detail of larger calcifications can be obtained using geometric magnification techniques when producing the image because of improved signal/noise ratio (5,6). These special views may be done as part of a diagnostic mammogram workup but are not normally done in screening mammography.

Historically, the first report of automated detection of microcalcifications was by Spiesberger in 1979 (7). His technique examined the mammogram in sections, using a 25 μm pixel size. For each point in the image, the local maximum pixel value was found. For each candidate, the contrast was calculated and compared with two times the standard deviation in pixel values of the boundary pixels. Finally, compactness was computed, and only compact candidates were kept. Modest performance was obtained using 132 regions of interest (ROIs) of 512 × 512 pixels: 68% sensitivity at a false-positive rate of 1% and a false-negative rate of 31%. A number of other published reports followed over the next few years, none showing conclusively a technique that was accurate enough to be used clinically.

The turning point in the field occurred in 1990, when Chan and colleagues showed that an automated detection scheme could improve radiologists' ability to find clustered microcalcifications on mammograms (8). In this carefully controlled observer study, seven attending radiologists and eight radiology residents each read 60 images. Half the images contained a cluster of calcifications, and the other half did not. The readers used a five-category rating scale to give their confidence that a cluster was present. The data were analyzed using the receiver operating characteristic (ROC) method (9,10). The computer scheme had a sensitivity of 87% with an average of four false clusters per image. The area under the ROC curve increased from 0.924 to 0.953 when the observers used the computer aid. This increase was statistically significant at the $p < 0.001$ level. On average, the readers' sensitivity increased by 10% at a constant specificity. This study was in fact the first computer-assisted diagnosis (CAD) algorithm of any kind shown to be a beneficial aid to radiologists. It has spurred CAD research in mammography and in other organs and other imaging modalities.

There are probably 100 or more groups developing an automated detection method for clustered microcalcifications on mammograms. It is not possible to describe them all. There is, however, commonality between most approaches. Nearly all methods can be described generically, as outlined in Fig. 1, as consisting of three steps: preprocessing, segmentation of candidate microcalcifications, and feature analysis to remove false-positive detections.

Almost all techniques developed to date have relied on digitized screen-film mammograms as a source of image data. The quality of the digitized mammogram

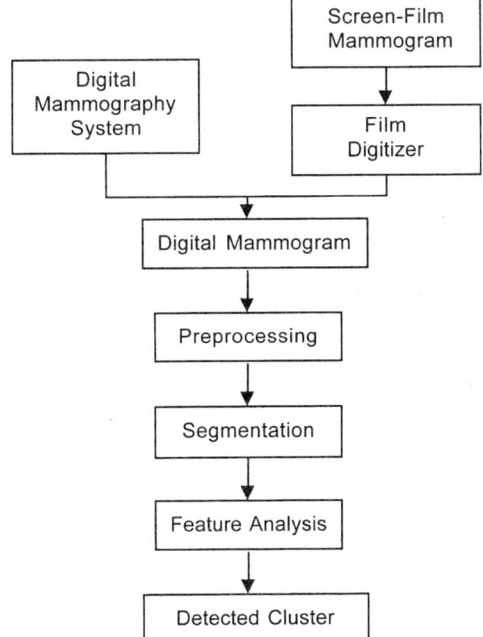

Fig. 1 Flowchart of a generic scheme for the detection of clustered microcalcifications. Most approaches reported in the literature follow this paradigm.

will depend on the characteristics of the digitizer used: pixel size, gray-scale resolution, noise properties, and artifacts. Because microcalcifications are small—microcalcifications as small as 200 μm can be reliably seen mammographically—the choice of pixel size is critical and is a current point of controversy (11–16). Chan et al. have examined the performance of their automated detection scheme on mammograms digitized with different pixel size and gray-scale resolution (14). They found that the performance of their scheme for detecting microcalcifications decreased when the pixel size was 70 μm or larger (compared with 35 μm). Note that this result is for the detection of *individual* microcalcifications and not for the detection of *clusters* of microcalcifications. It is possible to detect a cluster of pleomorphic calcifications by detecting the larger calcifications while missing the smaller, subtler ones. Most algorithms are currently being developed using images digitized at 100 μm. Table 1 is a surrey of the pixel sizes used by different investigators.

Another limitation of using digitized film mammograms is the high amount of noise in dark regions of the image. When the film optical density is high, light transmission through the film is low and, consequently, few photons are measured by the digitizer. Under such conditions, the electronic noise of the digitizer will be a significant fraction of the measured signal, resulting in poor signal-to-noise characteristics. This can lead to false-positive detections if one is not careful in designing a technique. This situation is exacerbated, because the newer screen-film systems have maximum optical densities greater than 4.0 (17), which is beyond what most digitizers can accurately measure.

The remainder of the chapter will describe techniques used to accomplish the three different parts of a detection scheme; this will not be a comprehensive listing, but rather a survey. There are a number of different approaches to accomplishing these three tasks. Unfortunately, at present, it is not possible to compare

Table 1 A Survey of Pixel Sizes Used by Different Investigators

Pixel size μm	Number of investigators	Reference number
25	1	(54)
35	1	(93)
40	3	(31, 55, 65)
50 (8 bit)	4	(35, 45, 62, 68)
50 (≥10 bits)	7	(22, 30, 46, 49, 61, 73, 85)
80	1	(47)
100 (8 bit)	3	(57, 58, 94)
100 (≥10 bits)	23	(8, 23–25, 33, 34, 40, 44, 51, 53, 59, 60, 63, 64, 66, 74, 77, 80, 84, 95–98)

Microcalcifications

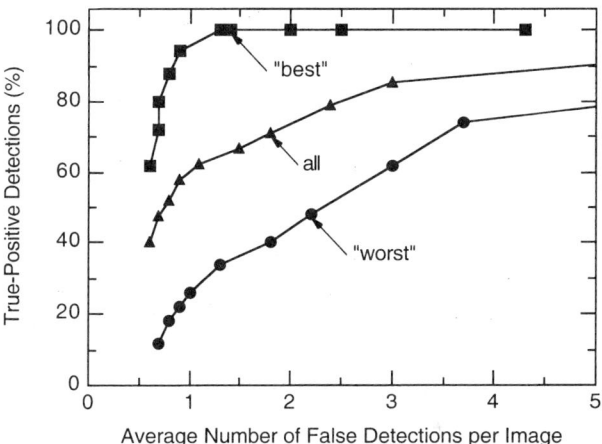

Fig. 2 The effect of a database on measured performance. Here, the performance of a detection scheme on a database of 90 mammograms (all) is compared with a subset of 50 mammograms that gives the best performance and a subset of 50 mammograms that give the worst result.

the different approaches in a meaningful way. This is principally because different images are used to evaluate performance of the different methods, and this can introduce great variations in measured performance (18). This is illustrated in Fig. 2, where selecting a subset of cases from a larger set of images can produce large variation in measured performance. Furthermore, the exact criterion used to score the computer detections can influence measured performance (19,20). Because no standard test set or scoring method exists, no attempt is made in this chapter to compare different techniques. Large databases are becoming available (21), and this should facilitate direct comparisons of techniques in the future.

II. PREPROCESSING

Preprocessing is used in an effort to reduce the effects of the normal anatomy of the breast, which acts as a camouflaging background to clustered microcalcifications. In addition, because the response of the screen-film system is nonlinear, the background optical density will affect the image contrast of the microcalcifications (see Appendix to this chapter). In bright or dark areas of the image, the contrast is reduced compared with regions that are optimally exposed. This reduces the effectiveness of pixel-value–based and contrast-dependent techniques.

One approach to preprocessing is to fit a polynomial to the background and subtract the fitted background from the original image. Cubic polynomials have been found to be useful by Bottema et al. (22). When analyzing smaller ROIs, background trend correction by polynomial fitting has been found to be useful (8,23,24).

Because microcalcifications contain relatively large amounts of high spatial frequency information, a high-pass filter would enhance the signals while reducing the background structure. Unsharp masking will accomplish this goal (25). However, a large component of the power in a mammogram at high spatial frequencies is noise, both quantum mottle and film granularity (4,26,27). Therefore, a band-pass filter would be more effective, because there is little information at the highest spatial frequencies in the image.

One strategy for enhancing calcifications is to subtract two processed images: one in which calcifications or high spatial frequencies have been enhanced and another in which the calcifications or high spatial frequencies have been removed or diminished. The first group to use this approach was Chan et al. (28,29). They applied two linear filters by means of convolution on images digitized at 100-μm pixel size. The template for the enhancing filter was a 3×3-pixel kernel, with the center pixel having a higher weighting factor than the surrounding pixels in a 4:3 ratio. The suppression filter used a 9×9 kernel, with the center 5×5 pixels having 0 weighting and the 2-pixel rim perimeter having a value of 1/56. This filter would enhance calcifications 500 μm and smaller. An example of applying such a technique is shown in Fig. 3.

Similar principles are used in applying a top hat operator. The top hat template includes components for enhancement of calcifications and suppression of background but uses mathematical morphological operators instead of convolution operations. Several groups have found this approach useful (30–32). An extension of the top hat transformation has been proposed by Kobatake et al., which multiple structuring elements, which are linear or curvilinear, are used. In one implementation, there are 16 structuring elements, each 5 pixels (100-μm pixel size), radiating from the same pixel out to a pixel on the perimeter of a 9×9 box. The termination points are every other perimeter pixel, starting it the pixel directly above the central pixel (33). This approach is less likely to have false detection because of ducts and ligaments that form part of the normal background structure in the mammogram.

A difference of gaussian band-pass filtering can also be used to create an enhanced image with reduced background structure. In this approach, an image is convolved by two gaussian functions, and the resulting filtered images are subtracted. Empirical data by Zheng et al. show that a 1.55 and 2.33 pixel full width at half-maximum intensity (100-μm pixel size) are effective sizes for the gaussian function (34). This corresponds to a kernel size of 5 and 7 pixels, respectively.

A directional recursive median filter with principal component analysis (PCA) has been developed by Cernadas et al., in which one-dimensional recursive median filters are applied at 12 different angles (35). The recursive median filter is

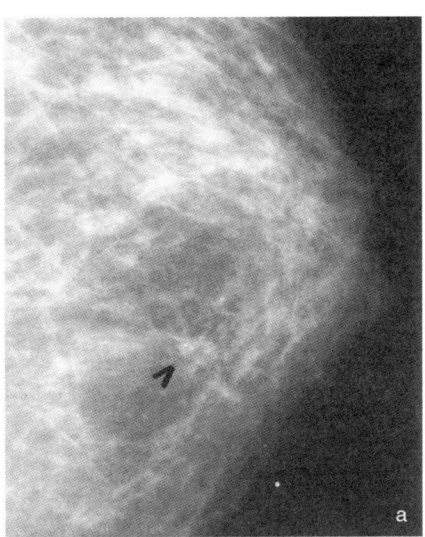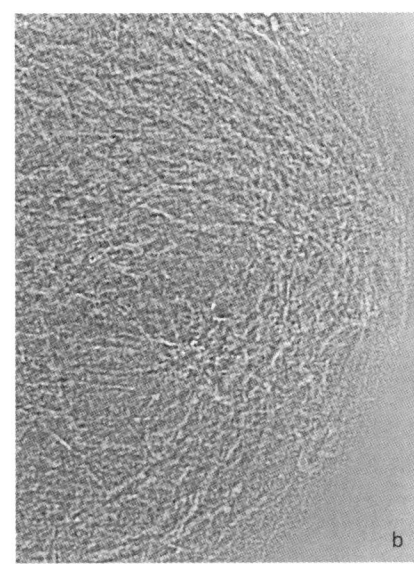

Fig. 3 A preprocessing technique, in which the normal breast structure shown in (a) is greatly suppressed in (b). A cluster of calcifications is marked in the unprocessed image. The suppressed image is presented with greatly enhanced contrast to show that the large-area variation in the background has been successfully suppressed.

a class of filters known as sieves (36) and is closely related to morphological operators. This allows a scale-orientation signature to be built for each pixel. In this signature, a column represents constant orientation, a row constant scale, and the values are the changes in gray level of the pixel with respect to the image filtered at the next smaller scale. PCA (Principle Component Analysis) is then applied to reduce the dimensionality of the signature. Typically, the first 80 components are used.

Wavelets are an effective method of preprocessing, because a multiple number of band-pass filters can be chosen on the basis of which daughter wavelet decomposition is used in reconstructing the image. The principle of applying wavelets to medical images is discussed in Chapter 6. In mammography, a weighted sum of the different levels in the wavelet domain is performed to enhance calcifications (37). Different approaches differ in their choice of wavelets and the selection of which levels to use in the reconstruction. A list of different wavelets used for processing microcalcifications on mammograms is given in Table 2.

Although most implementation of wavelets is decomposition and reconstruction of selected levels, Strickland and Hahn use wavelets as means of applying match filters to an image (38). Undecimated wavelet transforms are used to

Table 2 List of Different Mother Wavelets Used for Processing Mammograms Containing Microcalcifications

Lead investigator	Wavelet
Brown (61)	Undecimated spline
Chen (55)	Morlet
Lo (66)	Daubechies 8-tap
Strickland (38)	Biorthogonal B-spline
Wang (99)	Daubechies' 4- and 20- coefficient
Yoshida (95)	8-tap least asymmetric Daubechies

adjust the filter for the range in sizes of calcifications. To implement a match filter, in addition to the size and shape of the object, the power spectrum of the image noise needs to be known. To estimate the noise power spectrum a stochastic model is used (39), which consists of a stationary and nonstationary components. The two components are modeled as separable Markov process with autocorrelation of $r_{nn}(k,l) = \sigma_n^2 e^{-\alpha(|k|+|l|)}$, and a nonseparable Markov process with autocorrelation of $r_{nn}(k,l) = \sigma_n^2 e^{-\alpha \sqrt{k^2 + l^2}}$. The power spectrum can be computed from a weighted sum of the two Markov processes and by estimating the Markov correlation parameter, α, from the background texture.

A very sophisticated filter has been designed by Qian et al. (40). They have developed a tree-structured nonlinear filter coupled with wavelets. The front end of their method is a cascade of centrally weighted median filters that reduce the image noise while trying to maintain the structure of the calcifications. This is done, in part, by using eight different 5×5 linear or curved windows. A two-channel tree-structured wavelet transform that incorporates quadrature-mirror filter banks is then applied.

A different preprocessing technique has been developed by Karssemeijer (41). In his method, the gray level values are rebinned, so that each gray level contains the same amount of noise, as opposed to the same amount of signal. This eliminates the dependency of the noise on the gray-level value. To do this the number of bits in the image to be analyzed is reduced from 12 to 8. Because the noise properties of the image depend on the film's optical density (26,27), the transformation from 12 to 8 bits is nonlinear. The method estimates the standard deviation as:

$$\hat{s}(k) \propto \int_{c_{min}}^{c_{max}} c^2 \hat{f}(c \mid k) \, dc \tag{1}$$

where c is the radiographic contrast measured in pixel values [i.e., a constant times ΔD of Eq. (A5), assuming the digitizer is linear] calculated in a small region of interest, and $\hat{f}(c \mid k)$ is the estimated conditional probability density of the local contrast conditioned on the gray level value. Estimates of the local standard deviation can be made by using measurements from nonoverlapping bins (42).

In 1990, Caldwell et al. showed that the film optical density pattern on a mammogram could be used to determine a fractal dimension (43), implying that the distribution of tissue within the breast was fractal in nature. Two different investigators have used this fact to segment calcifications on a mammogram. The reasoning is that the presence of a calcification will change the fractal dimension of a local area. Li et al. have applied a fractal model to the normal background structure in a mammogram (44). Then by subtracting the model from the original image, an image of calcifications can be obtained. A threshold is also applied to the difference image to eliminate weak intensities caused by noise. Lefebvre et al. (45) plotted the logarithm of the surface area as a function of the logarithm of the elementary ruler area for small 16×16-pixel ROIs (50-µm pixel size). The slope of this plot is related to the fractal dimension, because, for a true fractal, this plot is a straight line. When a calcification is present, the plot becomes concave, and the maximum deviation from the theoretical straight line is determined. ROIs with the highest deviation are kept as containing possible calcifications.

Another approach for preprocessing that uses fractals is by Sari-Sarref et al. (46). Instead of filtering the image, they select ROIs that are unlike other regions in the given mammogram. That is, a region that is dissimilar to all other regions in an image is likely to contain an abnormality. Determining dissimilarity is done by partitioning the image into regions, initially 256×256 pixels (50-µm pixel size). Then two classes of regions are created: range and domain. If a given region in the domain pool cannot be mapped to any region in the range pool, then that domain region is partitioned into smaller subregions. The partitioning continues until a match from the range pool is found or the region is subdivided down to 8×8-pixel subregions. Subregions that do match are considered to be suspicious and are kept. All matched subregions are eliminated. In this way, the amount of the image that needs further analysis is greatly reduced, by approximately 80%.

Guillemet et al. use a texture model based on noisy fractional brownian motion to eliminate regions on the mammogram that are too regular to contain microcalcifications (47). The model assumes that image texture is caused by fractional brownian motion and an independent gaussian white noise source. There are three parameters in the model: signal dynamic, signal fractal dimension, and noise level. Details of the method are given elsewhere (48).

III. SEGMENTATION

Because calcifications have higher mass attenuation coefficients than any other structure in the breast, they appear as bright areas in the mammogram. This makes gray-level thresholding a potentially useful method for segmentation. Unfortunately, a mammogram is a two-dimensional projection of a three-dimensional object, so that summation of overlapping tissues can produce areas in the mammogram that are brighter than calcifications. Furthermore, the appearance of the calcification depends on the type and amount of tissue surrounding it, in addition to the tissue that is directly above and below it. As can be seen in Fig. 4, a calcification can have a low optical density or a relatively high optical density, depend-

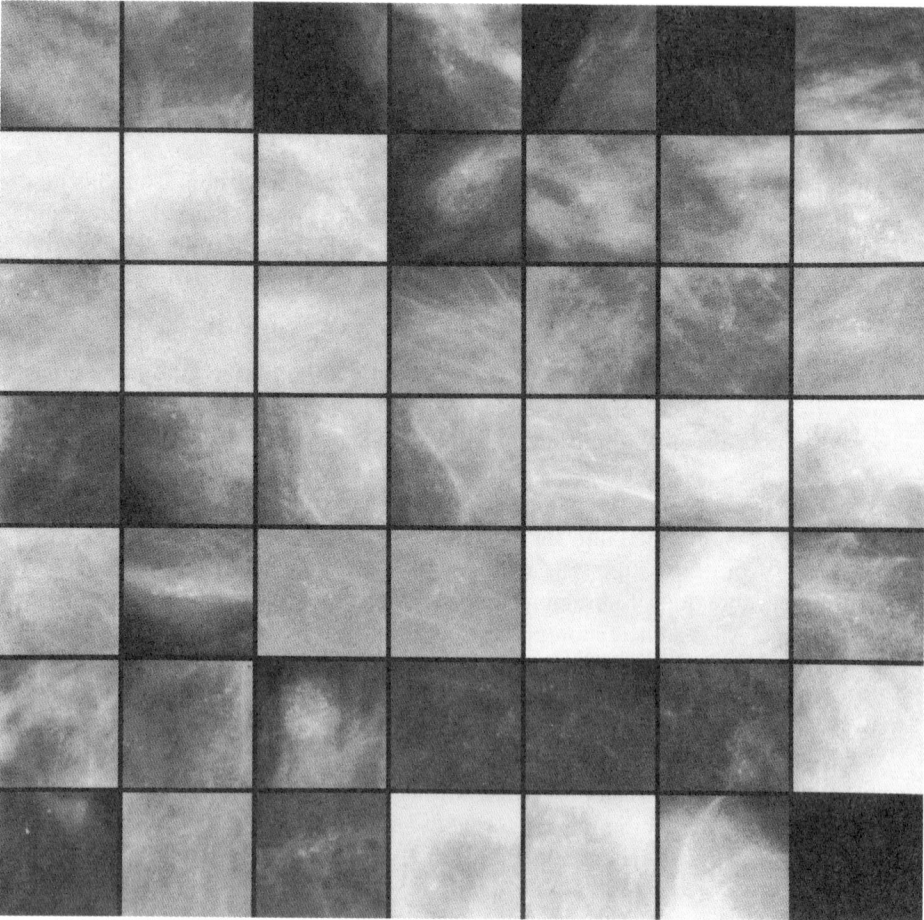

Fig. 4 A collage of regions of interest, each 1.28- × 1.28-cm in size. There are microcalcifications centered on the middle of each ROI. Although the microcalcifications may not be visible in all ROIs, one can see the range in contrast and background film density for clustered microcalcifications on mammograms. The bottom right ROI is empty.

ing on its surrounding tissue. Therefore, keeping a small fraction of the brightest pixels will be effective in identifying calcifications, but it also will include other noncalcification objects in the image. In a small ROI, however, calcifications should again be the brightest objects present. This may also be true for images that have been preprocessed appropriately. The problem then becomes one of signal/noise ratio. That is, small calcifications will have relatively low contrast and tend to be masked by image noise. Therefore, to segment the most subtle calcifications on the basis of gray-level thresholding will result in the inclusion of pixels caused by image noise. After thresholding, region growing is used to identify connected pixels as individual calcifications.

The global thresholding can be refined by applying a local threshold. The local threshold is determined as the mean plus a multiple of the standard deviation of pixel values in a small region of interest, for example 5 × 5-mm square, as done by Chan et al. (29). In this way, the local statistics (i.e., noise) of the region around the calcification influence the threshold.

Shen et al. have developed a variation on local thresholding. They compare the seed pixel value to the average of the maximum and minimum pixel value of the four connected neighbors (49). If the pixel value is within plus or minus a percentage of the average, then that pixel is grown as part of the signal.

Zheng et al. implemented segmentation using the quantity (34):

$$a = \frac{(I_1 - I_2)}{(I_1 + I_2)/2} \qquad (2)$$

where I_1 and I_2 are pixel values of the object and its background (a 5 × 5-mm square region). A 2% threshold is then applied, so only those signals with a >0.02 are kept. This is combined with a local minimum search ring, in which each pixel in the thresholded image is compared with 16 pixels that form a circle of radius 3 pixels.

Note that several investigators use the preceding definition in Eq. (2) for contrast. For digitized screen-film mammograms, however, the contrast is just the difference in pixel value, not the difference divided by the mean. This is shown in the Appendix to this chapter.

Jiang et al. (50) and Veldkamp and Karssemeijer (51) have independently developed a segmentation technique based on background-trend correction and signal-dependent thresholding. In these two approaches, corrections for the non-linear response and the blurring of the calcification by the screen-film system and film digitizer are performed. At low and high x-ray exposures to the screen, the contrast, which is proportional to the slope of the characteristic curve, is reduced [see Eq. (A5) and Fig. 5]. That is, the inherent contrast of the calcifications [i.e., radiation contrast, given by Eq. (A1)] is reduced when recorded by the screen-film system. This can be seen in Fig. 4. Therefore, the image or radiographic contrast [given by Eq. (A5)], will depend on the background intensity. If a correction is not

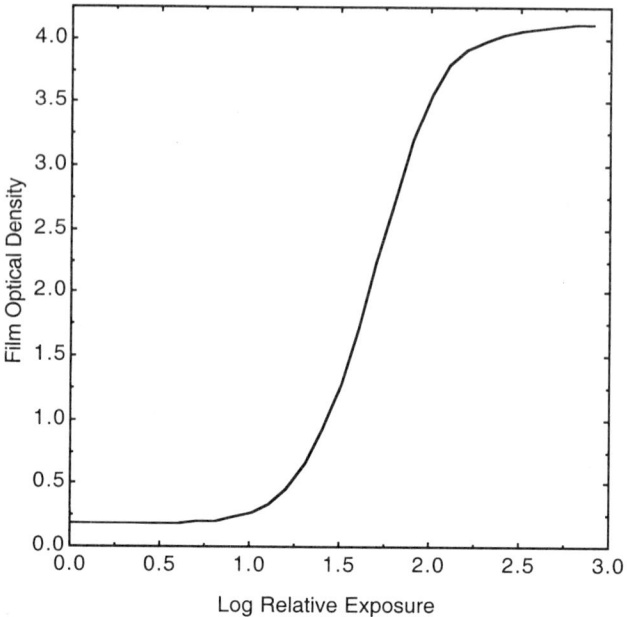

Fig. 5 A typical characteristic curve for a mammographic screen-film system.

made for nonlinearity, then it becomes extremely difficult to segment accurately calcifications in dense and fatty regions of the image simultaneously with calcifications in other regions of the breast. Similarly, the smaller the calcification, the more that its contrast is reduced because of blurring. This can be corrected based on the modulation transfer function of the screen-film system (52).

Gürcan et al. use a two-dimensional adaptive filtering method, which is based on the assumption that the prediction error has a gaussian distribution if no calcifications are present (53). The prediction error is the difference between the actual pixel value and the weighted sum of the eight nearest neighbor pixels. Next, a gaussianity test is applied in which the moments of the prediction error for a 30 × 30-mm squared area are computed. Then the moments are combined as:

$$h = M_3 - 3M_1(M_2 - M_1^2) - M_1^3 \qquad (3)$$

M_1, M_2, and M_3 are the first, second, and third moments, respectively. If the prediction error follows a gaussian distribution, then h goes to zero as the size of the ROI goes to infinity. A threshold of approximately 5 is applied to segment the calcifications.

Bankman et al. have developed a method that operates without threshold or window selection or parametric data models (54). Given a local maximum pixel value at (x_0,y_0), then an edge pixel is given by the value of (x,y) that maximizes the difference in pixel value between pixels at (x,y) and (x_0,y_0) divided by the euclidean distance between the two pixels. In this way edge pixels from 16 different lines equally spaced radiating from (x_0,y_0) are determined. All pixels that lie within the contour defined by the edge pixels are then determined on the basis of the radial angle from (x_0,y_0). This technique works well when the object consists of many pixels. In their work, images with 25-μm pixel size were used, resulting in each calcification being at least 100 pixels in size. If images of 100-μm pixel size were used, then the calcification could consist of only 6 pixels. It is unclear how effective the Bankman technique would then be.

Stochastic approaches have also been used to segment calcifications, in particular, a Markov random field model (41,55). Karssemeijer et al. use the Markov random field to model pixels in the image as belonging to one of four classes: background, calcification, lines/edge, and film emulsion errors (42). Three different features are used in the model: local contrast at two different spatial resolutions and the output of a line/edge detector. The line/edge detector resembles a Hough transform analysis (41).

IV. FEATURE ANALYSIS

To reduce the number of false detections, features are extracted and are used to differentiate true calcifications from false detections. A large number of different features are being used by different investigators. A large, but not complete, list is given in Table 3. The drawback of having a large number of features to choose from is that the selection of the optimum set of features is difficult to do, unless a very large number of images are available for feature selection (56). This is in addition to images needed for training and images needed for testing the technique.

Most of the features listed in Table 3 use standard techniques for determining their value. One feature, effective thickness of the calcification developed by Jiang et al., is calculated using a model of image formation (50). That is, what thickness of calcification will give rise to a given measured contrast in the digital image. To do this, corrections for the blurring of the digitizer and the screen-film system are performed, along with corrections for the characteristic curves of the digitizer and the screen-film system. The assumption is that, in general, calcifications are compact, so their diameter and thickness should be comparable. Film artifact, such as dust on the screen, will have a very high thickness value compared with its size and, therefore, can be eliminated. Similarly, detections that are thin compared with their area are likely to be false positives because of image noise.

Most features are extracted from either the original image or a processed image that has sought to preserve the shape and contrast of the calcifications in

Table 3 List of Different Features Used for Distinguishing Actual Calcifications from False Detections

Pixel-value based	Morphology based	Derivative based	Other
Contrast (7, 28, 45, 60, 68, 83)	Area (28, 45, 60, 100, 101)	Mean edge gradient (25, 33, 57–60, 66, 68, 83)	Number of signals per cluster (45, 93, 101)
Average pixel value (7, 49)	Area/maximum linear dimension (57)	Standard deviation of gradient (58)	Density of signals in cluster (45, 100, 101)
Maximum value (22, 66)	Average radius (22)	Gradient direction (25)	Distance to nearest neighbor (93)
Moments of gray-level histogram (67)	Maximum dimension (58)	Second derivative (68)	Distance to skin line (93)
Mean background value (66)	Aspect ratio (93)		Mean distance between signals (101)
Standard deviation in background (66, 83, 100)	Linearity (59)		First moment of power spectrum (8)
	Circularity (22, 60, 101)		Effective thickness (50)
	Compactness (7, 57, 68)		Peak contrast/area (22)
	Sphericity (contrast is the third dimension) (22)		

the original image. Zheng et al. have used a series of topographical layers ($n = 3$) as a basis for their feature extraction. The layers are generated by applying a 1%, 1.5%, and 2% threshold using Eq. (2). This allows for features related to differences between layers (e.g., shape factor in layer 2 and shape factor in layer 3) and changes between layers (e.g., growth factor between layers 1 and 2) to be used.

Once a set of features has been identified, a classifier is used to reduce the number of false detections, while retaining most of the actual calcifications that were detected. Several different classifiers are being used: simple thresholds (7,29,33,34,45,57–60), artificial neural networks (61–64), nearest neighbor methods (32,60,65), fuzzy logic (66,67), linear discriminant analysis (35), quadratic classifier (61), bayesian classifier (68), genetic algorithms (69), and multiobjective genetic algorithms (70).

Once individual signals have been identified, they need to be grouped or clustered, because only clustered microcalcifications have clinical significance.

Microcalcifications

This usually is done based on the spacing between detected signals (58,71,72). Not only will this eliminate isolated detections, but false signals that are in close proximity to each other (i.e., a false-positive cluster) can be eliminated (71).

V. ALTERNATIVES TO FEATURE EXTRACTION

In lieu of feature extraction, several investigators have used the image data as input to a neural network. The difficulty with this approach is that the networks are usually quite complex (several thousand connections). Therefore, to properly train the network and to determine the optimum architecture of the network requires a very large database of images.

Stafford et al., after application of a high-pass filter and normalization, used 16×16-pixel ROIs (50-μm pixel size) as input to a feed-forward neural network (73). They use 16 neurons in the hidden layer and a single neuron at the output. They repeated this structure three times to create a parallel network. The inputs to the other two subnetworks are the original image reduced by 4 and 16 times in size by pixel averaging. In this way, the network using the unreduced image is "tuned" for calcifications in the 100–500-μm size range, once-reduced-image network 200–1000 μm, and the twice-reduce-image network 400–2000 μm. The three outputs are then subjected to a winner-take-all filter, in which the output from the network with the largest value is kept.

Rosen et al. used a bayesian artificial neural network to examine the image using 7×7-pixel ROIs (100-μm pixel size) (74). Their network had a single hidden layer with nine hidden units and one output unit. They found that the weights from the inputs to one of the hidden units resembled a Mexican hat filter—a peak at the center decreasing to negative value in the surround.

These and similar approaches are limited, because extremely high performance is needed to avoid having a high false-positive rate. Most mammograms are normal, and most of the area of mammograms that are abnormal do not contain calcifications. Mammographically, the average breast is approximately 100 cm^2 in area. For a 50-μm pixel, there will be 4 million pixels to be analyzed. If there are 13 calcifications of 500 μm in diameter, then only 0.01% of pixels will belong to a calcification. Therefore, a specificity of 99.9% will give rise to 10 false ROIs per image.

Wu et al. used a feed-forward neural network to examine regions that contained potential calcifications as specified by a detection scheme (75). This reduces the number of ROIs that need to be examined and thus reduces the demand for extremely high specificity. They used 32×32-pixel ROIs (100-μm pixel size) that have background trends removed using a third-degree polynomial. These ROIs are then subjected to a fast fourier transform. The resulting values are then scaled logarithmically between 0 and 1 and are used as input values. The network had 15 hidden units and one output unit.

Zhang et al. (23,76) and Hasegawa et al. (77) have developed a shift-invariant or convolution artificial neural network to further refine suspicious areas detected by a computer scheme. This network is a simplified version of the neocognitron (78) and is a multilayer, back-propagation neural network with local, shift-invariant interconnections. The advantage of this network is that its output is not dependent on the location of a calcification in the input layer. Zhang et al. (23) have shown that this network outperforms the network developed by Wu et al.

Sajda et al. have developed a hierarchical/pyramid artificial neural network (HPNN) to detect calcifications (24). The advantage of their technique is that the network automatically learns context information relevant to calcifications. In their technique, illustrated schematically in Fig. 6, the input to the neural networks come from an integrated feature pyramid (IFP) (79). The IFP is composed of fea-

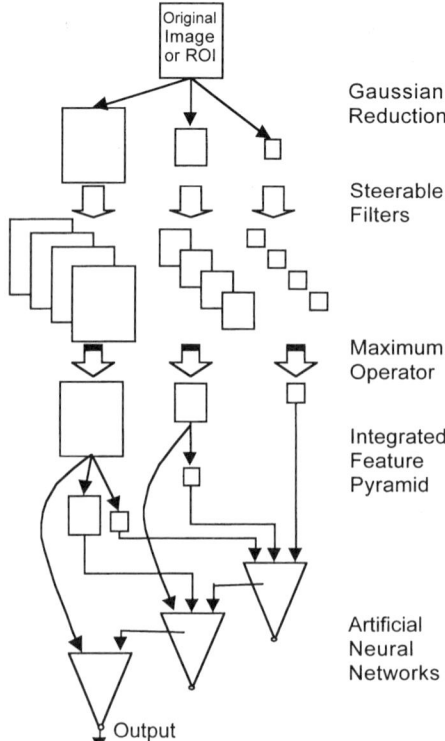

Fig. 6 Schematic diagram of the hierarchical/pyramid artificial neural network to detect calcifications (24). This is an example of a technique that inputs the image data, in this case preprocessed, to a neural network, as opposed to feature values extracted from the image.

Microcalcifications

tures constructed at several scales, generated using gaussian reduction. At each scale, steerable filters are used to produce four orientation-invariant features at each pixel. The filtered images are then squared to compute the energy. Then, for each pixel, the orientation that produced the maximum energy is kept. In this way, the resulting image is invariant to orientation. From these images, images at different scales are produced and are then input to a series of multilayer perceptrons with connections between the hidden units at low resolution and the input to the next level network. In this way, the network takes advantage of coarse-to-fine search.

VI. COMPUTATION TIMES

The computation times are not often stated by most investigators, perhaps under the belief that this is not an important factor, because computers will always get faster. In general, times range from 20 seconds (80) up to several tens of minutes (inferred by this author from description of the technique), depending on the platform and pixel size of the image. For any of the techniques to be used clinically, they must be able to process images at a rate that is useful clinically. For "real-time" analysis, such as for diagnostic mammography, there is approximately one patient approximately every 20 minutes per x-ray machine. This means there is 5 minutes available per film, including the time to digitize the film. However, many clinics have several mammography units, with large centers having four or more. In this situation, computation times of about a minute per film may be necessary. This also assumes that only one detection scheme is run. Most likely, at least one other algorithm, for the detection of masses, will be implemented, cutting the available time for computation in half.

In most centers, screening mammograms are not read until the next day. This allows for processing overnight, and computation time becomes less critical, but still important. To analyze 20 cases (80 films) in 15 hours (overnight) is 11 minutes per film for at least two different algorithms. For a higher volume center (40 cases), this gives less than 3 minutes for each algorithm. Computation time is not a trivial matter.

VII. DIGITAL MAMMOGRAMS

Developing in parallel to CAD is the development of digital detectors for mammography. Small-field digital detectors for stereotactic needle biopsy systems are commonly used clinically. So-called full-field digital mammography systems are being developed by several companies (81). Digital acquisition of the mammogram overcomes several limitations of screen-film systems (82). The resulting images should have higher signal/noise ratios, and thus detection algorithms should have higher performance when analyzing these images (81).

Because digital mammography is a new modality, cases for developing, training, and testing detection schemes are not readily available, especially in the United States. In Japan, computed radiography (CR) systems have been in use at several hospitals, including the largest cancer hospital in the country. At the cancer center, a large number of cases have been performed. Kobatake et al. have used this large database (953 patients) to develop a detection scheme (83). McLeod et al. have begun a preliminary study using wavelets to detect calcifications again on CR images (84). Their database had 248 images from 62 patients. These studies, however, do not allow a comparison of digitized film versus digital mammograms. Further studies on other digital mammography systems need to be performed, because the different systems have different imaging characteristics (e.g., pixel size).

VIII. CONCLUSION

In about 20 years, the automated detection of clustered calcifications has gone from a crude tool in the research laboratory to a commercial system being sold and used clinically. The performance obtained on a large, consecutive set of cancer cases can be as high as 98.3% sensitivity at a false-positive rate of 0.3 clusters per image (85). This extremely high level of performance indicates that such a system should be beneficial clinically. Clinical trials to prove this hypothesis are now ongoing.

Although a high level of performance has been achieved, there are still a number of areas that need to be addressed, such as:

1. Defining a standard test set (18).
2. Defining a standard scoring methodology (19,20).
3. How to deal with finite size databases (86–88).
4. Comprehensive comparison of different classifiers (89).
5. Clinical trials (90).
6. Understanding the relationship between the computer's performance (false-positive and true-positive rates) and clinical efficacy, which includes, but is not limited to, reduction in mortality and morbidity, cost-effectiveness, acceptance by radiologists, and improvement in radiologists' performance.
7. Should a detection algorithm identify calcifications associated with benign breast disease or only identify cancers, and how does this affect radiologists' ability to use the computer aid (91)?

IX. APPENDIX

In this Appendix, the relationship between radiographic contrast measured on the film and the inherent contrast of the object (radiation contrast) is shown. The contrast, in terms of differences in number of x-ray quanta, is given as (92):

$$c = \frac{(N_1 - N_2)}{(N_1 + N_2)/2} = \frac{\Delta N}{N} \tag{A1}$$

The contrast given by Eq. (A1) is called the radiation contrast. Film optical density (D) is related to the incident x-ray exposure (E) by the characteristic curve of the screen-film system (see Fig. 5). The contrast, as recorded by the film (i.e., radiographic contrast), is given by:

$$D_1 - D_2 = G(\log E_1 - \log E_2) \tag{A2}$$

where G is the slope of the characteristic curve. Now, for a given x-ray beam, E is related to N by a constant, k, so that Eq. (A2) becomes:

$$\Delta D = G \, \Delta(\log kN) \tag{A3}$$

Given that:

$$\Delta(\log kN) = (\log_{10}e)\Delta(\ln kN)$$

$$= (\log_{10}e)\frac{\Delta N}{N} \tag{A4}$$

then, by Eq. (A1), Eq. (A3) becomes:

$$\Delta D = GC \log_{10}e \tag{A5}$$

That is, contrast measured on the film is the difference in measured film optical density, and this is related to the radiation contrast (difference divided by the mean) by a constant and the slope of the characteristic curve. So at x-ray exposures corresponding to dense breast tissue or fatty tissue (low and high exposures), the contrast of a calcification will be reduced compared with its contrast if it were in the "average" part of the breast, where the slope of the characteristic curve is maximum. This is illustrated in Fig. 4. The contrast measured on a digitized mammogram is directly proportional to the ΔD, because digitizers are generally have a linear relationship between pixel value and film density.

REFERENCES

1. RJ Brenner. AJR 156:719–723, 1991.
2. EA Sickles. AJR 139:913–918, 1982.

3. SL Olson, BW Fam, PF Winter, FJ Scholz, AK Lee, SE Gordon. Radiology 169:329–332, 1988.
4. RM Nishikawa, MJ Yaffe. Med Phys 12:32–39, 1985.
5. K Doi, H Imhof. Radiology 122:479–487, 1977.
6. EA Sickles, K Doi, HK Genant. Radiology 125:69–76, 1977.
7. W Spiesberger. IEEE Trans Biomed Eng 26:213–219, 1979.
8. H-P Chan, K Doi, CJ Vyborny, RA Schmidt, CE Metz, KL Lam, T Ogura, Y Wu, H MacMahon. Invest Radiol 25:1102–1110, 1990.
9. CE Metz. Invest Radiol 21:720–733, 1986.
10. CE Metz. Invest Radiol 24:234–245, 1989.
11. Y Higashida, N Moribe, K Morita, N Katsuda, M Hatemura, T Takada, M Takahashi, J Yamashita. Radiology 183:483–486, 1992.
12. N Karssemeijer, JT Frieling, JH Hendriks. Invest Radiol 28:413–319, 1993.
13. DS Brettle, SC Ward, GJS Parkin, AR Cowen, H Sumsion. Br J Radiol 1994.
14. H-P Chan, LT Niklason, DM Ikeda, KL Lam, DD Adler. Med Phys 21:1203–1211, 1994.
15. H-P Chan, B Sahiner, N Petrick, KL Lam, MA Helvie. Proc SPIE 2710:30–41, 1996.
16. AR Cowen, JH Launders, M Jadav, DS Brettle. Phys Med Biol 42:1533–1548, 1997.
17. PC Bunch. Proc SPIE 3659:120–130, 1999.
18. RM Nishikawa, ML Giger, K Doi, CE Metz, F-F Yin, CJ Vyborny, RA Schmidt. Med Phys 21:265–269, 1994.
19. RM Nishikawa, LM Yarusso. Proc SPIE 3338:840–844, 1998.
20. M Kallergi. Med Phys 26:267–275, 1999.
21. RM Nishikawa. Breast Disease 10:137–150, 1998.
22. MJ Bottema, JP Slavotinek. In: N Karssemeijer, M Thijssen, J Hendriks, L van Erning, eds. Digital Mammography Nijmegen 98. Amsterdam: Kluwer Academic Publishers, 1998, pp 209–212.
23. W Zhang, K Doi, ML Giger, RM Nishikawa, Y Wu. Med Phys 21:517–524, 1994.
24. P Sajda, CD Spence, JC Pearson, RM Nishikawa. Proc SPIE 2710:733–742, 1996.
25. H Fujita, T Endo, T Matsubara, K Hirako, T Hara, H Ueda, Y Torisu, N Riyahi-Alam, K Horita, C Kido, T Ishigaki. Proc SPIE 2434:682, 1995.
26. GT Barnes, DP Chakraborty. Radiology 145:815–821, 1982.
27. PC Bunch, KE Huff, R Van Metter. Proc SPIE 626:63–71, 1986.
28. H-P Chan, K Doi, CJ Vyborny, KL Lam, RA Schmidt. Invest Radiol 23:664–671, 1988.
29. H-P Chan, K Doi, S Galhotra, CJ Vyborny, H MacMahon, PM Jokich. Med Phys 14:538–548, 1987.
30. SM Astley, CJ Taylor. Proceedings of the 1st British Machine Vision Conference, 1990.
31. D Betal, N Roberts, GH Whitehouse. Br J Radiol 70:902–917, 1997.
32. SA Hojjatoleslami, J Kittler. In: K Doi, ML Giger, RM Nishikawa, RA Schmidt, eds. Digital Mammography '96. Amsterdam: Elsevier Science, 1996, pp 267–272.
33. H Kobatake, H-R Jin, Y Yoshinaga, S Nawano. In: H Lemke, K Inamura, C Jaffe, R Felix, eds. Computer Assisted Radiology. Berlin: Springer-Verlag, 1993, pp 624–629.

34. B Zheng, Y-H Chang, M Staiger, W Good, D Gur. Academic Radiology 2:655–662, 1995.
35. E Cernadas, R Zwiggelaar, W Veldkamp, T Parr, S Astley, C Taylor, C Boggis. In: N Karssemeijer, M Thijssen, J Hendriks, L van Erning, ed. Digital Mammography Nijmegen 98. Amsterdam: Kluwer Academic Publishers, 1998, pp 205–208.
36. JA Bangham, TG Campbell, RV Aldridge. Signal Processing 38:387–415, 1994.
37. W Zhang, H Yoshida, RM Nishikawa, K Doi. Med Phys 25:949–956, 1998.
38. RN Strickland, H Hahn. IEEE Trans Med Imaging 15:218–229, 1996.
39. BR Hunt, TM Cannon. IEEE Trans Systems, Man Cybernetics 6:876–882, 1976.
40. W Qian, LP Clarke, M Kallergi, RA Clark. IEEE Trans Med Imaging 13:25–36, 1994.
41. N Karssemeijer. Int J Pattern Recognition Artif Intell 7:1357–1376, 1993.
42. WJH Veldkamp, N Karssemeijer. In: N Karssemeijer, M Thijssen, J Hendriks, L van Erning, ed. Digital Mammography Nijmegen 98. Amsterdam: Kluwer Academic Publishers, 1998, pp 160–176.
43. CB Caldwell, SJ Stapleton, DW Holdsworth, MJ Yaffe. Phys Med Biol 35:235–247, 1990.
44. H Li, KJ Liu, SC Lo. IEEE Transaction on Medical Imaging 16:785–798, 1997.
45. F Lefebvre, H Benali, R Gilles, E Kahn, R Di Paola. Med Phys 22:381–390, 1995.
46. H Sari-Sarref, S Gleason, RM Nishikawa. Proc SPIE 3059:1535–1543, 1999.
47. H Guillemet, H Benali, E Kahn, R Di Paola. In: K Doi, ML Giger, RM Nishikawa, RA Schmidt, eds. Digital Mammography '96. Amsterdam: Elsevier Science, 1996, pp 225–230.
48. H Guillemet, H Benali, F Préteux, R Di Paola. Proc SPIE 2823:40–53, 1996.
49. L Shen, RM Rangayyan, JEL Desautels. Int J Pattern Recognition Artif Intell 7:1403–1416, 1993.
50. Y Jiang, RM Nishikawa, ML Giger, K Doi, CJ Vyborny, RA Schmidt. Proc SPIE 1778:28–36, 1992.
51. WJ Veldkamp, N Karssemeijer. Med Phys 25:1102–1110, 1998.
52. GT Barnes. Med Phys 9:656–667, 1982.
53. MN Gürcan, Y Yardimci, E Cetin. In: N Karssemeijer, M Thijssen, J Hendriks, L van Erning, ed. Digital Mammography Nijmegen 98. Amsterdam: Kluwer Academic Publishers, 1998, pp 157–164.
54. IN Bankman, T Nizialek, I Simon, OB Gatewood, IN Weinberg, WR Brody. IEEE Trans Infor Tech Biomed 1:141–149, 1997.
55. CH Chen, GG Lee. Graphical Models Image Processing 59:349–364, 1997.
56. M Kupinski, ML Giger. Med Phys 26:2176–2182, 1999.
57. DH Davies, DR Dance. Phys Med Biol 35:1111–1118, 1990.
58. BW Fam, SL Olson, PF Winter, FJ Scholz. Radiology 169:333–337, 1988.
59. T Ema, K Doi, RM Nishikawa, Y Jiang, J Papaioannou. Med Phys 22:161–169, 1995.
60. CS Carman, G Eliot. In: K Doi, ML Giger, RM Nishikawa, RA Schmidt, eds. Digital Mammography '96. Amsterdam: Elsevier Science, 1996, pp 253–255.
61. S Brown, R Li, L Brandt, L Wilson, G Kossoff, M Kossoff. In: N Karssemeijer, M Thijssen, J Hendriks, L van Erning, eds. Digital Mammography Nijmegen 98. Amsterdam: Kluwer Academic Publishers, 1998, pp. 189–196.

62. JG Diahi, A Giron, D Brahmi, C Frouge, B Fertil. In: N Karssemeijer, M Thijssen, J Hendriks, L van Erning, eds. Digital Mammography Nijmegen 98. Amsterdam: Kluwer Academic Publishers, 1998, pp. 151–156.
63. RH Nagel, RM Nishikawa, K Doi. Med Phys 25:1502–1506, 1998.
64. FYM Lure, RS Gaborski, TF Pawlicki. Proc SPIE 2710:16–23, 1996.
65. DH Davies, DR Dance. Phys Med Biol 37:1385–1390, 1992.
66. S-CB Lo, H Li, J-S Lin, A Hasegawa, O Tsujii, MT Freedman, SK Mun. Proc SPIE 2710:8–15, 1996.
67. H-D Cheng, YM Lui, RI Freimanis. IEEE Trans Med Imaging 17:442–450, 1998.
68. IN Bankman, WA Christens-Barry, DW Kim, IN Weinberg, OB Gatewood, WR Brody. Proc SPIE 1905:731–738, 1993.
69. MA Anastasio, H Yoshida, R Nagel, RM Nishikawa, K Doi. Med Phys 25:1613–1620, 1998.
70. MA Anastasio, MA Kupinski, RM Nishikawa. IEEE Trans Med Imaging 17: 1089–1093, 1998.
71. RM Nishikawa, ML Giger, K Doi, CJ Vyborny, RA Schmidt. Med Phys 20:1661–1666, 1993.
72. N Karssemeijer, L van Earning. Proc SPIE 1444:166–177, 1991.
73. RG Stafford, J Beutel, DJ Mickewich. Proc SPIE 1898:1993.
74. D Rosen, B Martin, M Monheit, G Wolff, M Stanton. In: K Doi, ML Giger, RM Nishikawa, RA Schmidt, eds. Digital Mammography '96. Amsterdam: Elsevier Science, 1996, pp. 277–282.
75. Y Wu, K Doi, ML Giger, RM Nishikawa. Med Phys 19:555–560, 1992.
76. W Zhang, K Doi, ML Giger, RM Nishikawa, RA Schmidt. Med Phys 23:595–601, 1996.
77. A Hasegawa, YC Wu, MT Freedman, SK Mun. Proc SPIE 2434:557–562, 1995.
78. K Fukushima, S Miyake, T Ito. IEEE Syst Man Cybern SMC-13:826–843, 1983.
79. P Burt. Proc IEEE 76:1006–1015, 1988.
80. RM Nishikawa, ML Giger, K Doi, CJ Vyborny, RA Schmidt. Med Biol Engin Computing 33:174–178, 1995.
81. SA Feig, MJ Yaffe. RadioGraphics 18:893–901, 1998.
82. RM Nishikawa, GE Mawdsley, A Fenster, MJ Yaffe. Med Phys 14:717–727, 1987.
83. H Kobatake, H Takeo, S Nawano. In: N Karssemeijer, M Thijssen, J Hendriks, L van Erning, ed. Digital Mammography Nijmegen 98. Amsterdam: Kluwer Academic Publishers, 1998, pp 201–204.
84. G McLeod, GJS Parkin, AR Cowen. In: K Doi, ML Giger, RM Nishikawa, RA Schmidt, eds. Digital Mammography '96. Amsterdam: Elsevier Science, 1996, pp 311–316.
85. J Roehrig, T Doi, A Hasegawa, B Hunt, J Marshall, H Romsdahl, A Schneider, R Sharbaugh, W Zhang. In: N Karssemeijer, M Thijssen, J Hendriks, L van Erning, ed. Digital Mammography Nijmegen 98. Amsterdam: Kluwer Academic Publishers, 1998, pp 395–400.
86. K Fukunaga, RR Hayes. IEEE Trans Pattern Anal Machine Intell 11:873–885, 1989.
87. HP Chan, B Sahiner, RF Wagner, N Petrick. Proc SPIE 3338:846–858, 1998.
88. RF Wagner, HP Chan, JT Mossoba, B Sahiner, N Petrick. Proc SPIE 3338:859–875, 1998.

89. KS Woods, JL Solka, CE Priebe, CC Doss, WW Bowyer, LP Clarke. Proc SPIE 1905:841–852, 1993.
90. RM Nishikawa, ML Giger, DE Wolverton, RA Schmidt, CE Comstock, J Papaioannou, SA Collins, K Doi. In: N Karssemeijer, M Thijssen, J Hendriks, L van Erning, ed. Digital Mammography Nijmegen 98. Amsterdam: Kluwer Academic Publishers, 1998, pp 401–406.
91. A Hume, P Thanisch, M Harwwood, R Procter. In: K Doi, ML Giger, RM Nishikawa, RA Schmidt, ed. Digital Mammography '96. Amsterdam: Elsevier Science, 1996, pp 273–276.
92. K Doi, PC Bunch, G Holje, M Pfeiler, RF Wagner. Modulation transfer function of screen-film systems. ICRU Report 41. Bethesda, MD: International Commission on Radiation Units and Measurements, 1986.
93. LN Mascio, JM Hernandez, CM Logan. Proc SPIE 1898:472–479, 1993.
94. J Dengler, S Behrens, JF Desaga. IEEE Trans Med Imaging 12:634–642, 1993.
95. H Yoshida, K Doi, RM Nishikawa, ML Giger, RA Schmidt. Acad Radiol 3: 621–627, 1996.
96. N Karssemeijer. Proc SPIE 1905:776–786, 1993.
97. AR Al-Hinnawi, PE Undrill, G Needham. In: N Karssemeijer, M Thijssen, J Hendriks, L van Erning, ed. Digital Mammography Nijmegen 98. Amsterdam: Kluwer Academic Publishers, 1998, pp. 481–482.
98. D Meersman, P Scheunders, D Van Dyck. In: K Doi, ML Giger, RM Nishikawa, RA Schmidt, ed. Digital Mammography '96. Amsterdam: Elsevier Science, 1996, pp. 287–290.
99. TC Wang, NB Karayiannis. IEEE Trans Med Imaging 17:498–509, 1998.
100. D Zhao, M Shridhar, DG Daut. Proc SPIE 1905:702–715, 1993.
101. D Fukuoka, S Kasai, H Fujita, T Hara, M Kato, T Endo, H Yoshimura. In: N Karssemeijer, M Thijssen, J Hendriks, L van Erning, ed. Digital Mammography Nijmegen 98. Amsterdam: Kluwer Academic Publishers, 1998, pp. 197–200.

7
Evaluation of a Multiscale Enhancement Protocol for Digital Mammography

Ralf Mekle
Columbia University, New York, New York

Andrew F. Laine and Suzanne J. Smith
Columbia-Presbyterian Medical Center, New York, New York

I. INTRODUCTION

We have carried out a receiver operating characteristics (ROC) study for the enhancement of mammographic features in digitized mammograms. The study evaluated the benefits of multiscale enhancement methods in terms of diagnostic performance of radiologists. The enhancement protocol relied on multiscale expansions and nonlinear enhancement functions. Dyadic spline wavelet functions (first derivative of a cubic spline) were used together with a sigmoidal nonlinear enhancement function (1,2). We designed a computer interface on a softcopy display and performed an ROC study with three radiologists, who specialized in mammography. Clinical cases were obtained from a national mammography database of digitized radiographs prepared by the University of South Florida (USF) and Harvard Medical School.

Our study focused on dense mammograms [i.e., mammograms of density 3 and 4 on the American College of Radiology (ACR) breast density rating], which are the most difficult cases in screening. To compare the performance of radiologists with and without using multiscale enhancement, two groups of 30 cases each were diagnosed. Each group contained 15 cases of cancerous and 15 cases of normal mammograms. Conventional ROC analysis was applied, and the resulting

ROC curves indicated improved diagnostic performance when radiologists used multiscale nonlinear enhancement.

Recently, research has focused on the development of digital displays and softcopy workstations for digital mammography. Limited spatial resolution, luminance, and dynamic range cannot be solved simply by hardware improvements or computer programming alone. A possible solution to these problems is the application of multiscale contrast-enhancement techniques derived from nonlinear models.

Radiologists are mostly familiar with films in which the Modulation Transfer Function (MTF) is approximately equal to 2^8 gray levels of contrast resolution. However, images acquired with digital detectors can record at least 2^{12} different gray levels of intensity and are now commercially available. The wealth of dynamic range within these digital acquisition systems provides strong evidence that the signal-to-noise-ratio (SNR) can be increased in digital mammography. For expert radiologists the human visual system can detect at most 2^7 shades of gray. These considerations motivate the need for judicious methods of processing digital radiographs that can optimize the bandwidth of the human visual system. We have designed enhancement software that is well adapted for this purpose and provides a "data mining" tool to map and make visible selected "quantum levels" of information living within the wide range of contrast resolution provided by digital detectors.

Medical imaging is a field in which quantitative accuracy and qualitative fidelity are paramount. In any image-enhancement process, distortion of the original image and artifacts are not affordable. Multidimensional feature enhancement by means of wavelet analysis has been previously demonstrated on mammograms (3–8) and is a powerful tool for processing digital medical images without artifacts. The enhancement process adjusts multiscale coefficients at some particular spatial-frequency scale by increasing, decreasing, or resetting their values. Each image is then reconstructed with modified coefficients. This simple enhancement technique relies on the idea that features of interest in a given radiograph are detectable at a particular scale and can be amplified, whereas noise and less clinically interesting features may live at other levels of analysis, whose visual appearance can be diminished or eliminated in a reconstructed image. Further results and detailed descriptions of these methods can be found in Refs. 9–15.

Surprisingly, there have been very few studies carried out to evaluate the benefits of multiscale enhancement methods in terms of diagnostic performance. Our study aimed at providing quantitative evidence of these benefits. ROC analysis (16) is most commonly used in medical imaging for such purposes, although alternative statistical approaches can be found as well (17). ROC curves have been compared to evaluate the visibility of malignancies (18), mass detection techniques (19), or algorithms for computer-aided diagnosis (CAD) that use neural networks (20).

Enhancement Protocol for Digital Mammography

The chapter is organized as follows. In Sec. II we describe a protocol for multiscale nonlinear contrast enhancement. After a short overview of the use of multiscale expansions for contrast enhancement, we discuss the dyadic spline wavelet selected, its implementation, and how a nonlinear enhancement function is applied to multiscale coefficients. Sec. III addresses the design of a graphical user interface (GUI) that was developed to carry out the ROC study, including high-performance displays and specialized hardware for softcopy display of digital mammograms. Next, the ROC study itself together with its results and subsequent data analysis is presented in Sec. IV. After a discussion of the results of the study, conclusions and possible directions of future research are presented in Sec. V.

II. ENHANCEMENT PROTOCOL

A. Contrast Enhancement by Means of Multiscale Expansions: A Short Overview

We summarize in the following, the advantages of the use of overcomplete multiscale representations for adaptive contrast enhancement of digital mammograms. Critically sampled multiscale representations are not suitable for detection and enhancement tasks because of aliasing effects introduced during downsampling of the analysis (21,22). However, overcomplete representations avoid such aliasing artifacts and have the desirable property of being shift invariant (23,24). Indeed, this property ensures that the spatial locations of any mammographic finding within an image are preserved across all scales. Thus, in our approach, the transform coefficient matrix size at each scale remains the same as the original spatial resolution of the digital mammogram, because there is no downsampling across each level of analysis.

Overcomplete multiscale analysis and reconstruction algorithms using dyadic scales previously developed in Refs. 25–27 were used as an initial choice of analysis function for our enhancement protocol. The implementation was carried out by the use of several low-pass and high-pass filters with localized frequency support. At each level of the multiscale expansion an input image is decomposed into a coarse approximation and detailed structures. The coarse approximation is the output from applying a low-pass filter, and the detailed structures are obtained from high-pass filtering. The approximation image corresponds to scaling coefficients, whereas the details extracted from the approximation are wavelet coefficients at a particular scale. This procedure is successively repeated on the approximation image to obtain multiple levels of analysis. The coarsest approximation is often referred to as the "dc-cap." A gain or enhancement function modifies the matrices of coefficients that have been isolated by the filters at each level and may boost coefficients at some scales and/or attenuate others. If the filters meet a perfect reconstruction condition, the image can be reconstructed from its wavelet representation of scaling and wavelet coefficients (28). The filter bank implementation of enhancement processing by an expansion-reconstruction algorithm for two levels of analysis is schematically illustrated in Fig. 1. Image reconstruction that is also accomplished by appropriate filtering operations is presented in a simplified manner in Fig. 1.

The modified matrices of coefficients are simply "plugged in" during reconstruction, producing a "focused" subband enhancement. As shown earlier, the enhancement function can be implemented independently of a particular set of filters and easily incorporated into a filter bank to provide the benefits of multiscale enhancement (1,29).

B. High-Speed Implementation to Support Interactive Processing

Similar to orthogonal and biorthogonal discrete wavelet transforms (30) the discrete dyadic wavelet transform can be implemented within a hierarchical filtering scheme. Let an input signal $x(n)$ be real, $x(n) \in l^1(Z)$, $n \in [0, N-1]$ (i.e., $x(n)$ is supported on the index interval $[0, N-1]$) and let $X(\omega)$ be its Fourier transform. Depending on the length of each filter impulse response, filtering an input signal may be computed either by multiplying $X(\omega)$ by the frequency response of a filter or by circularly convolving $x(n)$ with the impulse response of a filter. Of course, such a periodically extended signal may change abruptly at the boundaries and cause artifacts. A common remedy for such a problem is realized by constructing a mirror extended signal

$$x_{me}(n) = \begin{cases} x(-n-1), & \text{if } n \in [-N, -1] \\ x(n), & \text{if } n \in [0, N-1] \end{cases}$$

where we chose the signal $x_{me}(n)$ to be supported in $[-N, N-1]$. In Ref. 1 it is shown how a mirror extension is a particularly elegant solution in conjunction with symmetrical antisymmetrical filters, because a signal is of a particular type of symmetry at each stage of the filter bank. The optimized circular convolution described in Ref. 1 was implemented in native "ANSI C" to speed up performance for multiscale decomposition and image reconstruction. Parameters of this algorithm included number of levels of analysis, gain, and threshold. This algorithm was incorporated into a GUI developed during the preparation of the study.

As a further goal, we envision developing feature-specific enhancement protocols for each type of lesion. An enhancement protocol would consist of a multiscale expansion of a mammogram by a specific basis and an associated nonlinear enhancement function that is best matched to a specific type of lesion (e.g., microcalcifications). For the study under consideration, a dyadic spline wavelet function was used as the basis, and a nonlinear sigmoidal function was applied as the enhancement function. Both are described in greater detail next.

Enhancement Protocol for Digital Mammography

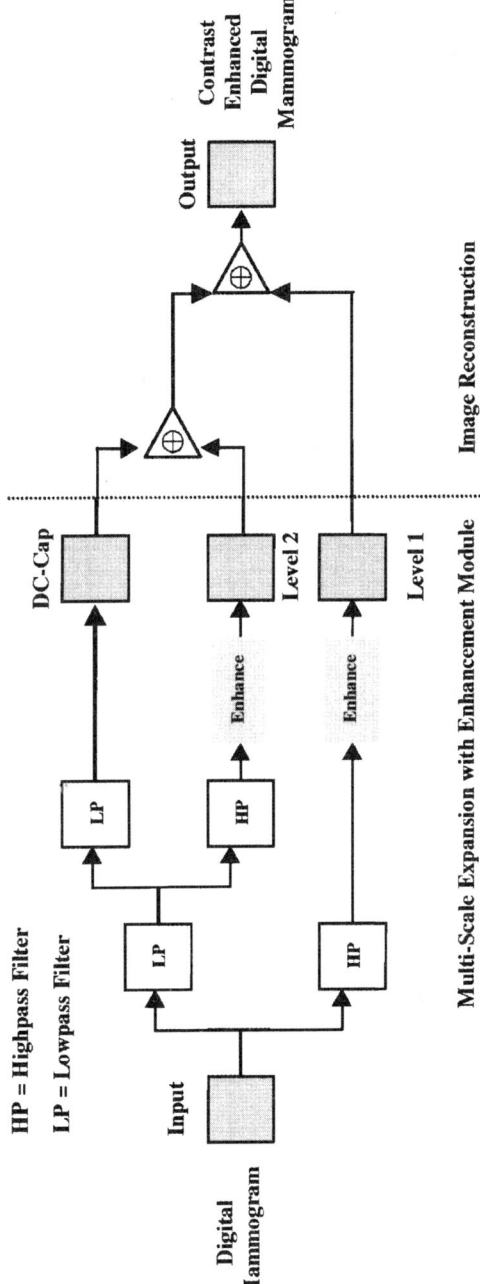

Fig. 1 Multiscale analysis with nonlinear contrast enhancement: Schematic of filter bank implementation. In the left part, multiscale expansion with enhancement for two levels of analysis is shown, and reconstruction is presented (in a simplified manner) in the right part.

C. Dyadic Spline Wavelet Algorithm

The wavelet transform of a signal $f(x)$ at scale s and position x is defined by $Wf(u,s) = f*\psi_{u,s} = \int_{-\infty}^{+\infty} f(x) \frac{1}{\sqrt{s}} \psi^* \left(\frac{x-u}{s} \right) dx$, where the function f is projected on a family of translated and dilated basis functions (wavelets) $\psi_{u,s}(x) = \frac{1}{\sqrt{s}} \psi \left(\frac{x-u}{s} \right)$. $\psi(x)$ is the mother wavelet of zero average. Both translation and dilation parameters u and s are continuous for the continuous wavelet transform. To allow fast numerical implementation of discrete wavelet transforms, Mallat and Zhong (31) introduced the dyadic wavelet transform, in which the scale parameter varies only along the dyadic sequence $\{2^j\}$, with $j \in Z$. Extending this approach to two dimensions by the use of a tensor product yields the two-dimensional (2-D) dyadic wavelet transform that partitions plane orientations into two bands. This means that there are two channels of analysis along orthogonal directions x and y. The wavelet transform of the 2-D signal $f(x,y)$ at the scale 2^j has two components defined by: $W_{2^j}^1 f(x,y) = f*\psi_{2^j}^1(x,y)$ and $W_{2^j}^2 f(x,y) = f*\psi_{2^j}^2(x,y)$, with $\psi_{2^j}^d(x,y) = \frac{1}{2^{2j}} \psi^d \left(\frac{x}{2^j}, \frac{y}{2^j} \right)$, $(d = 1,2)$. We used the quadratic spline wavelet function $\psi(x)$ defined by Mallat and Zhong in Ref. 31 of compact support and continuously differentiable. Its Fourier transform can be derived as $\hat{\psi}(\omega) = (j\omega) \left(\frac{\sin(\omega/4)}{\omega/4} \right)^4$. $\psi(x)$ is the first derivative of a cubic spline smoothing function $\theta(x)$, whose Fourier transform is $\hat{\theta}(\omega) = \left(\frac{\sin(\omega/4)}{\omega/4} \right)^4$ (1). These functions are displayed for the one-dimensional case in Fig. 2.

By use of a wavelet that is the derivative of a smoothing function, it can be shown that the wavelet transform $W_{2^j}^d f$ of the signal f is proportional to the deriva-

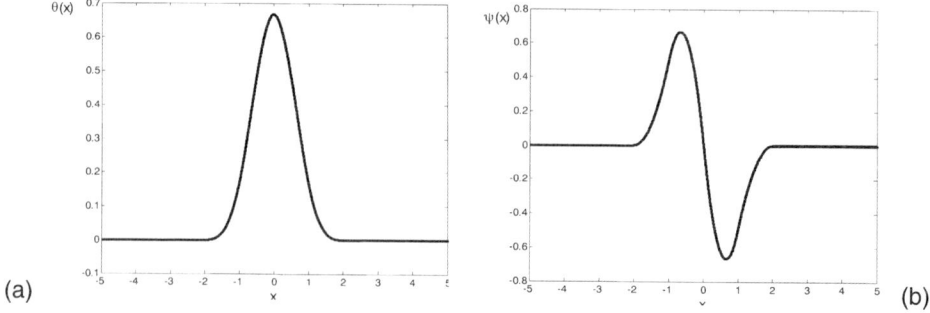

Fig. 2 (a) Cubic spline smoothing function $\theta(x)$. (b) Quadratic spline wavelet $\psi(x)$ of compact support defined as the first derivative of the smoothing function.

Enhancement Protocol for Digital Mammography

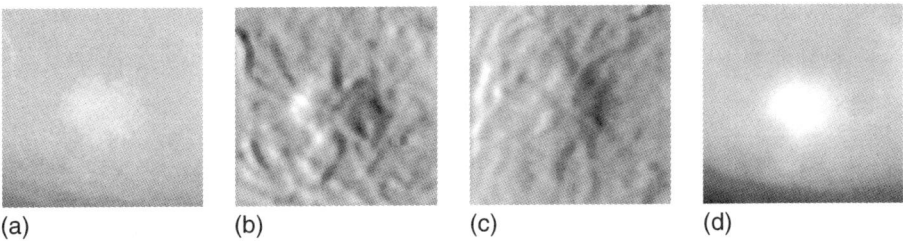

Fig. 3 Level 5 of an overcomplete dyadic wavelet expansion of a spiculated mass. (a) Original image. (b) Horizontal details. (c) Vertical details. (d) Approximation image.

tive of the signal smoothed at the scale 2^j (32). The coefficients of modulus maxima detection are then equivalent to an adaptive sampling that finds signal variation points in the two orthogonal directions x and y.

Because images represent finite energy signals measured at some finite resolution, we cannot compute the wavelet transform at scales below the limit set by this resolution. We applied this analysis at dyadic scales varying from 1 (original signal) to the limit imposed by acquisition (digitizer sampling rate). Fig. 3 shows an example for one level of an overcomplete wavelet expansion of a region of interest (ROI) with a spiculated mass at a dyadic scale, and in Fig. 4 wavelet coefficients of microcalcifications at the finest dyadic scale are presented.

D. Nonlinear Enhancement Function

Modification of selected analysis coefficients within a certain scale can make more obvious indiscernible or barely seen mammographic features (14). Contrast

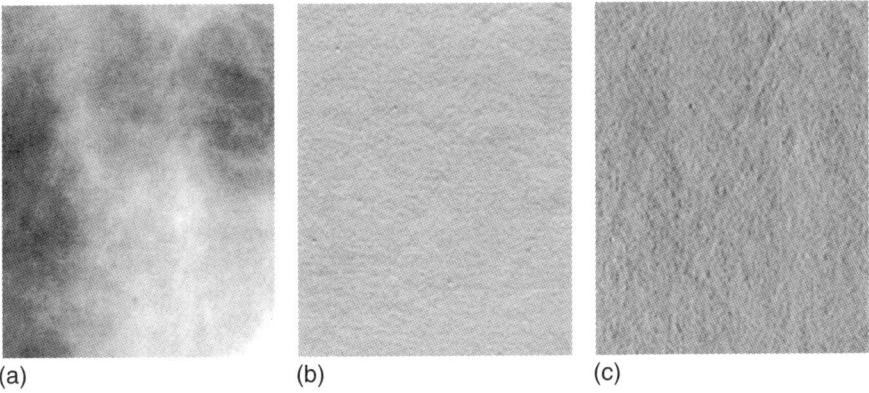

Fig. 4 (a) Original ROI with microcalcifications. (b) Horizontal and (c) vertical dyadic wavelet coefficients.

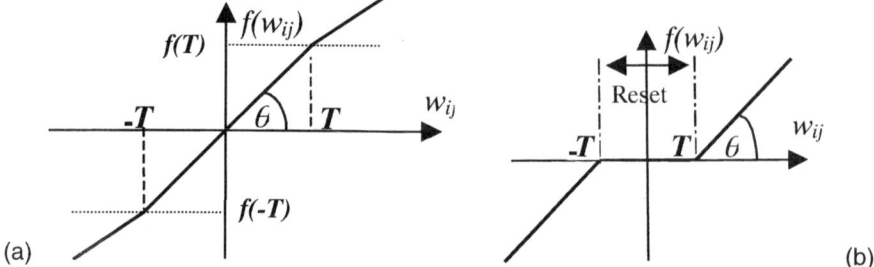

Fig. 5 (a) A simple piecewise linear enhancement function, (b) Hard-thresholding function.

enhancement was achieved by applying an enhancement function to transform coefficients at selected scales. This operation results in local attenuation or amplification of coefficients. Enhancement or gain functions must be cumulative and monotonically increasing to preserve the order of intensity information in the original image and to avoid artifacts (26). Fig. 5(a) provides a simple example of a piecewise linear enhancement function. Multiscale coefficients are denoted w_{ij}, which are modified by applying an enhancement function $f(w_{ij})$. T is the threshold of the function, and α the gain. The effect of the enhancement function depends on the value of the angle θ. For $\theta < 45$, there is an attenuation of the coefficients ($\alpha < 1$), at $\theta = 45$ we have the identity function ($\alpha = 1$), and for $\theta > 45$ there is a smooth amplification of the coefficients ($\alpha > 1$). The values of the two parameters, T and θ (or α), determine the final shape of the enhancement function. Fig. 5(b) displays a hard-thresholding function for denoising, in which coefficients with modulus $|w_{ij}| \leq T$ are set to zero. Unfortunately, these two particular functions have the disadvantage of being discontinuous at the threshold value $\pm T$. This could result in an abnormal distribution of coefficient values in the output and may create sharp peaks on both ends of the histogram of a particular output mapping. For this reason, smoother functions, like sigmoids, are preferable and were used in this study. Fig. 6 shows an example of such a function as described in Ref. 2.

The analytical formulation of the sigmoidal enhancement function as designed in Refs. 2 and 33 is the following:

$$f(w_{ij}) = a[sigm(c(w_{ij} - b)) - sigm(-c(w_{ij} + b))]$$

$$a = \frac{1}{sigm(c(1-b)) - sigm(-c(1+b))}, \quad 0 < b < 1 \tag{1}$$

$$sigm(y) = \frac{1}{1 + e^{-y}}$$

Parameters b and c control the threshold and the rate of enhancement (gain), respectively. This enhancement function is continuous, monotically increasing, and has a continuous first derivative. This ensures that the application of the function will not introduce any new discontinuities of coefficients in the transform domain.

From Fig. 6 we see that this enhancement function decreases the value of the coefficients around zero, which is equivalent to a denoising action, whereas it may increase values of the coefficients outside this range, equivalent to enhancement or amplification. This type of enhancement function, in "steps," offers a very rich and flexible paradigm to carry out nonlinear dynamic analysis of coefficients within a specific scale (34).

There are many criteria for the selection of the enhancement function applied to the coefficients of a particular level of analysis for contrast enhancement. One goal of the study described here was to develop a research tool for testing enhancement functions targeted for specific mammographic features. Because this process requires specialized expertise and a substantial time investment, no systematic study of the problem of associating enhancement functions with target features in mammograms has been reported in the literature.

In general, nonlinear estimators are signal dependent and behave differently for different realizations of each signal. In this context, Johnstone and Donoho have shown that by considering the signal as deterministic, thresholding of wavelet coefficients gives a nearly optimal estimation of piecewise smooth functions (35,36). More specifically, for a noisy signal of size N, thresholding of the wavelet coefficients with $T = \sigma \sqrt{2 \ln(N)}$, where σ is the standard deviation of the coefficients, provides an asymptotically optimal estimator of the original signal in

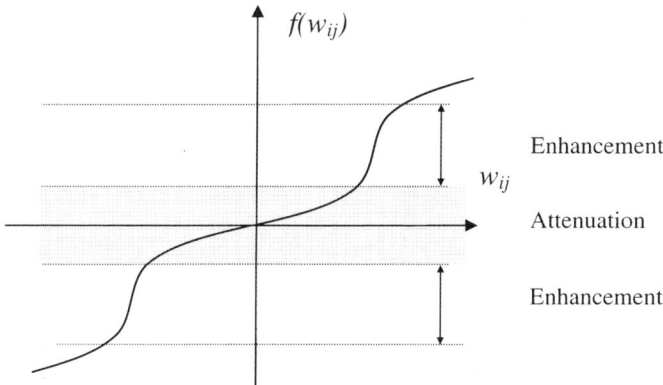

Fig. 6 A sigmoidal nonlinear enhancement function.

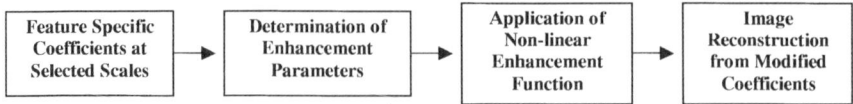

Fig. 7 Block diagram of modifying feature-specific coefficients at selected scales by applying a nonlinear enhancement function.

the mini-max sense (36). Thresholding of wavelet coefficients performs an adaptive smoothing of the image by averaging noisy areas and preserving or enhancing coefficients in areas of sharp transitions. Noise standard deviations can be estimated by determining the median wavelet coefficient value at the finest scale or with local discrete statistical estimation in the transform domain. The use of extremely local variances for the estimation of a threshold leads to a very aggressive posturing of the enhancement function and represents a high amount of intervention in adjusting the output, whereas global variance measurements are less noticeable. Superiority of either method depends on the screening protocol used by the radiologist and the kind of analysis to be performed. For example, fine microcalcifications represent high-frequency information of the image. We would expect the local variance for such a feature to be high within a selected ROI. Consequently, smooth amplification of coefficients within this particular spatial frequency range (in combination with possibly decreasing the information of other spatial frequencies) will enhance these features of interest. Similar analysis can be done to enhance low spatial frequency features such as masses. A block diagram of the enhancement process for coefficients at selected scales, which are chosen with respect to the particular mammographic feature to be enhanced, is shown in Fig. 7.

Because the computation of the enhancement parameters uses data-dependent information such as local or global coefficient variance, digital and digitized radiographs acquired under different imaging conditions are best processed independently to achieve optimal enhancement. Intrinsic properties of the radiograph are therefore incorporated in the setting of the parameters. In our work we used both coefficient variance computed with respect to a ROI and user input (see Sec. IIIB) to adapt the threshold and gain parameters.

III. DEVELOPMENT OF A GRAPHICAL USER INTERFACE

A. Motivation

Running such an enhancement algorithm in a batch mode might be sufficient for single experiments. However, adjustment of parameters tied to a data-dependent enhancement function is slow because of the repeated need to decompose and reconstruct from modified coefficients. A more desirable situation would be to observe the results of modified multiscale coefficients interactively and to continue the enhancement procedure until results are visually satisfactory or the decision is made that no further improvement can be achieved. In addition, with introducing fixed-enhancement protocols into a clinical screening paradigm, the algorithm must be simple, fast, and user-friendly (i.e., use of the algorithm should be familiar to the radiologist and intuitive). Because each radiologist may have preferences with respect to contrast in mammograms, it must be possible to adjust parameter settings to individual preferences. Thus, we designed a GUI to facilitate carrying out such a study and to create a softcopy display prototype, whose successors might find entrance into clinical screening. We call this application a "test bed" softcopy display tool. Its first version was used for the ROC study described in the next section.

B. Design and Implementation

The GUI developed for this study was written in Visual C++ 6.0. The code for the wavelet expansion and image reconstruction that was written in native "ANSI C" to speed up performance could be incorporated and executed in this environment without major modifications, thus shortening development time. Some of the guidelines and considerations for the design and implementation of the GUI are described next.

The prototype interface was primarily designed to process raw 16-bit data. Data were obtained from a national mammography database of digitized radiographs provided by the University of South Florida (USF, "Digital Database for Screening Mammography" (DDSM)). Our database of digitized mammograms (stored on 22 8-mm tapes) at the time of the study contained 586 selected cases of biopsy proven malignant lesions and 437 cases of normal breasts. More specifically, different types of lesions are represented in the following proportions: 100 round and oval malignant masses, 216 spicular lesions, and 248 microcalcifications. Five hundred fifty-nine cases of dense breasts (density of 3 and 4) with 266 normal and 293 cancerous, referred by radiologists as the most challenging cases, were included in the database.

Images from the mammography database were digitized from film at resolutions of 40 to 50 μm. Image line lengths (no. of columns) varied between 2000 and 3000 pixels, and number of rows from 4000 to 5900 pixels. Depending on the scanner used for digitization, the contrast resolution was either 12 bits or 16 bits per pixel, resulting in 15 to 50 megabytes per view. To handle this large amount of data and to provide the diagnosing radiologist as much information as possible, all four views (right and left mediolateral (RMLO, LMLO) and right and left craniocaudal (RCC, LCC) of a case were loaded into memory and displayed as downsampled images on display screen, which consisted of two high-resolution MegaScan monitors each with a screen size of 2048 by 2560 pixels. Specialized framebuffers allowed a display of 2^{10} gray levels (see Sec. IIIC). The four views were aligned to assist the radiologist to look for asymmetries. In addition, one view could be selected, and a viewport could display a selected ROI at full (original) resolution from a selected mammogram. The size of the viewport could be chosen as 512 by 512, 1014 by 1024, or even 2048 by 2048. The center of the ROI was determined through the mouse pointer in a chosen window. Thus, the original mammogram could also be examined through the viewport, if desired. More importantly, suspicious areas could be captured in the viewport and processed through enhancement by means of the multiscale expansion described in Sec. II. For the enhancement procedure, the user could adjust the number of subbands of the expansion as well. After selecting a ROI, the image was decomposed onto dyadic wavelet basis functions yielding wavelet coefficients. Coefficients were modified by a sigmoidal nonlinear enhancement function, and the image was reconstructed from these modified coefficients in nearly real time.

Fig. 8(a) shows Dr. Koenigsberg, one of three radiologists who participated in this investigation, during the ROC study, Fig. 8(b) depicts a typical screen display of the GUI showing additional viewports described earlier.

As mentioned in Sec. IID, the shape of the enhancement function can be changed through modification of the two parameters gain and threshold. Therefore, each parameter could be adjusted through sliders for each level (subband) of the multiscale expansion (see Fig. 9(b)). On release of the slider button, a reconstruction "event" was "triggered" and a resulting image presented in an output window. For example, reconstruction of a 512 by 512 matrix for five levels of decomposition

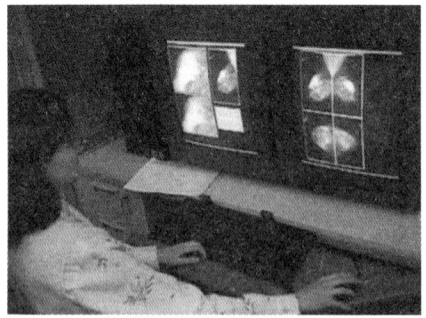
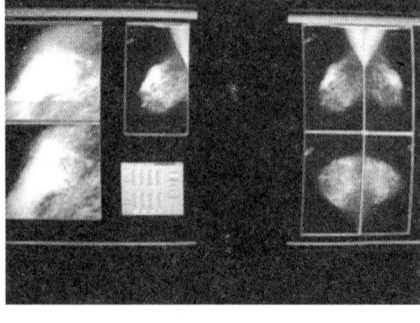

(a) (b)

Fig. 8 (a) Tova Koenigsberg, MD, using the GUI during the preliminary ROC study described earlier (b) Typical screen display used during the ROC study: four original digitized mammograms of one case on the right monitor, and a selected view, the GUI interface for parameter adjustments, original and enhanced ROI are shown on the left monitor.

Enhancement Protocol for Digital Mammography

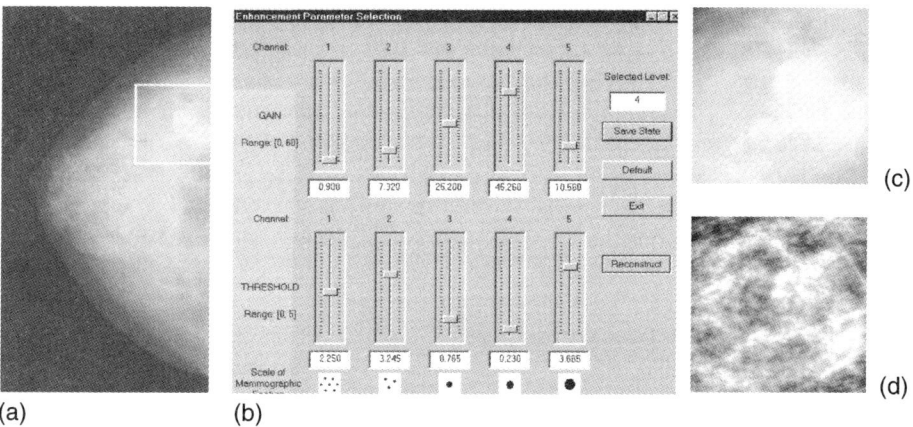

Fig. 9 (a) Original mammogram with selected ROI containing a mass, (b) Multi-Scale Contrast Enhancement (MSCE) GUI, (c) original ROI, and (d) enhanced ROI.

(five subbands) took 5 to 6 seconds. For four subbands reconstruction time shortened to 4 to 5 seconds. Reconstruction times t_{recon} for different sizes of the ROI and different number of levels of analysis are presented in Table 1. However, reconstruction time can certainly be improved to achieve true real-time performance by use of faster algorithms.

After processing, enhanced images could be saved together with information about the location of the ROI (the position of the ROI was marked in its corresponding downsampled view) to facilitate evaluation of a particular diagnosis for each case in comparison with the "ground truth" provided in the USF database. All suspicious areas in a case could be carefully examined by sequentially choosing different views and multiple ROIs.

Fig. 9(b) shows the test bed interface as an illustration. Interactive (real-time) enhancement was accomplished by means of sliders shown in the graphical user interface (GUI). The enhancement operation relied on the optimality of parameters derived from their nonlinear models and on the strategy used for the type

Table 1 Reconstruction Times T_{recon} for Two Different Levels of Analysis and Two Sizes of ROI

Size of region of interest (ROI)	T_{recon} for four levels of analysis	T_{recon} for five levels of analysis
512 × 512	4–5 sec	6–7 sec
1024 × 1024	19–20 sec	24–25 sec

of enhancement applied to each subband of coefficients (amplification, preservation, or diminution). Selected subband coefficients at a particular level could be strongly suppressed by choosing large thresholds (>2) and small gains (<1), which can be desirable for the elimination of (structured and acquisition) noise or normal benign anatomical (fibroglandular) structures.

Because the size of digital mammograms is quite large, an ROI (fixed at either 512 × 512 or 1024 × 1024) within the original image was chosen to avoid computing over regions that do not contain suspicious areas. This is also shown in Fig. 9, where Fig. 9(a) exhibits an original digitized mammogram with a 512 × 512 ROI that contains a possible mass. Fig. 9(c) and Fig. 9(d) display this ROI before and after enhancement by means of a nonlinear modification of multiscale coefficients, respectively.

C. Display and Hardware Settings

The enhancement protocol was executed on an IBM IntelliStation Z Pro Professional Workstation Type 6865. This machine had two Intel Pentium II Xeon microprocessors (450 MHz), 512 Mbytes of RAM, and was equipped with 36 Gbytes of hard disk space. Windows NT 4.0 with service pack 4 was the operating system.

To explore the richness of information quantized at 16-bit per pixel (bpp) gray scale data (65,536 shades of gray), the IBM IntelliStation workstation was equipped with two BARCOMed SMP1H Graphics controllers. These are high-resolution display subsystems for the PCI bus with a resolution of 2048 × 2560 pixels each, a digital-to-analog converter (DAC) capable of 1024 shades of gray and real-time window leveling. With the BARCO© framebuffers, an extended hardware palette of nearly 16,000 entries could be accessed through specialized "C" function calls that were part of a library provided to us as developers for BARCO/Metheus. By use of these library functions, the extended palette was loaded with a ramp of 4096 shades of gray corresponding to 12-bit resolution. Images stored in 16-bit per pixel format were rescaled to 12 bpp, if necessary (most of the mammograms were digitized at a resolution of 12 bpp), and then displayed at full resolution. Direct access to the video framebuffer also sped up the display process useful for updating and refreshing the different views on the screen.

Two high-resolution MegaScan monitors were attached to this workstation, providing dual-headed display on a single logical framebuffer or virtual desktop of 4000 × 2048 pixels, respectively, with Windows NT 4.0. To ensure the accurate depiction of the same image quality on both screens, a BARCO P1500 luminance photometer was used. It recognized the 1024 shades of gray displayed by a monitor and had a range of 0 to 450 ft-L. Both monitors were

Enhancement Protocol for Digital Mammography

calibrated to correct for nonlinearity of display properties through gamma correction.

Lighting conditions were controlled for the ROC study to model reading room conditions. The ambient light intensity was measured with the luminance photometer to be 12.802659 candelea/m^2. It is worthwhile to note that the optimality of enhancement parameters is independent of the cathode ray tube (CRT) display quality and the image acquisition quality. Because their computation is data driven, they are adapted to signal content and its characteristics. As our radiologists gave us feedback on the quality of the enhancement, we could adjust these initial default settings in future studies.

IV. DESCRIPTION OF THE RECEIVER OPERATING CHARACTERISTICS (ROC) STUDY

The first ROC study focused on overcomplete dyadic wavelets for enhancement of mammographic features in digitized mammograms. Specifically, dyadic spline wavelet functions were used together with a sigmoidal nonlinear enhancement function explicitly described in Sec. II. The ROC study included three radiologists specializing in mammography. The Director of the Breast Imaging Center at Columbia-Presbyterian Medical Center, Dr. Suzanne Smith, assisted in the selection of cases.

A. Selection of Cases

To measure the benefits of diagnosing digitized mammograms with enhancement through multiscale expansions, we focused on dense mammograms [i.e., mammograms of density 3 and 4 on the American College of Radiology (ACR) breast density rating], which are the most difficult cases in screening. In general, the enhancement protocol aimed at improving the detection and localization of mammographic features, such as microcalcifications, masses, and spicular lesions, without introducing "false positives."

To compare the performance of radiologists with and without the enhancement tool, two groups of 30 cases each were presented. Each group contained 15 cases of cancerous and 15 cases of normal mammograms. As mentioned earlier, a national mammography database of the USF provided "ground truth" (mostly through biopsy) for the selected cases. The selection was carried out very carefully under the guidance of a mammographer (Dr. Smith) to find rather challenging cases of similar difficulty for each group. Images showing metal markers ("bibis") to indicate suspicious regions of breast tissue were avoided, as well as obvious malignancies. Because of time constraints, the number of cases was limited for this initial study.

B. Paradigm of Diagnosis of Study

For each case presented to the radiologist, the enhancement procedure followed was the following:

1. Paradigm A: <u>Without Enhancement</u>

The radiologist made a diagnosis based only on the four original displays and the viewport. No processing of ROIs was allowed.

2. Paradigm B: <u>With Enhancement</u>

The radiologist selected an ROI in one of the views and could apply multiscale enhancement. Four levels of coefficients were computed. The radiologist then evaluated the quality of an enhanced ROI and adjusted the equalizer sliders of a channel to improve the visual quality of suspicious regions. Once he or she was satisfied with the visual result or if he or she judged that additional benefit could not be achieved, a diagnostic decision was made.

A diagnosis included specifying all lesions found and assigning a BI-RAD scale to each breast and the case. In addition, the radiologist was asked to choose a level of confidence (LOC) for each positive diagnosis (i.e., cancer is present) on an integer scale from 1 (definitely negative, i.e., total confidence that there are no malignant lesions) to 5 (definitely positive, i.e., total confidence that there is a malignant lesion). The value for the LOC was used in the analysis of data to decide whether a lesion was classified as malignant or benign (see discussion of LOC ratings in Sec. IVD).

C. ROC Data

Tables 2 and 3 summarize the data acquired during the study. Group 1 is composed of the set of cases in which the radiologists were allowed to take advantage of the enhancement protocol, whereas Group 2 contains those cases in which no processing could be applied. Each of the tables shows the case numbers, the case designation, and total number (#) of lesions for each case according to the mammography database (DB) and for each of the three mammographers the BI_RAD rating and level of confidence (LOC) values. The BI_RAD rating could be chosen from the standard categories 0–5 with 0 meaning that additional information for a more confident diagnosis was needed. In such cases, the radiologists were asked to also select a BI_RAD rating different from 0, if they were asked to make a diagnosis without any additional information. This number is shown in parentheses for such cases.

In each table, both groups are sorted into actually negative cases (normals with "0" lesions) and actually positive cases (cancers with at least "1" malignant lesion), because this is required for subsequent analysis of the data.

Enhancement Protocol for Digital Mammography

Table 2 ROC Data for Three Mammographers for Group 1 (i.e., with Enhancement Enabled)

Group 1 (With enhancement)

Case #	Database	DB total # of lesions	Mammographer 1		Mammographer 2		Mammographer 3	
			Bi Rad	Loc	Bi Rad	Loc	Bi Rad	Loc
2	A 0058	0	4	3	1	1	3	2
5	A 0069	0	1	2	1	1	1	1
6	A 0041	0	3	2	1	1	1	1
7	A 0077	0	3	2	2	1	2	1
9	A 0064	0	2	2	2	1	2	2
13	A 0067	0	0 (3)	2	1	1	0 (3)	3
15	A 0080	0	0 (3)	3	2	1	2	1
16	A 0089	0	3	3	1	1	1	2
19	A 0062	0	2	2	1	1	2	1
21	A 0057	0	2	2	1	1	0 (3)	3
24	A 0072	0	1	2	1	1	1	1
25	A 0070	0	1	2	0 (3)	2	1	2
26	A 0068	0	1	2	1	1	2	1
28	A 0039	0	3	2	1	1	0 (4)	3
30	A 0092	0	3	2	1	1	1	1
1	B 3044	1	4	4	4	4	4	3
3	B 3073	1	3	2	3	2	4	3
4	B 3006	1	5	5	5	5	5	5
8	B 3032	1	0 (3)	2	5	4	4	4
10	B 3107	1	5	4	4	4	5	4
11	C 0060	1	0 (3)	3	0	3	0 (4)	3
12	B 3057	1	4	4	5	4	4	4
14	B 3078	1	5	4	5	4	0 (4)	3
17	B 3033	1	0 (3)	2	0	2	0 (3)	3
18	B 3031	1	0 (4)	4	5	4	0 (3)	3
20	B 3076	1	0 (3)	3	0	3	0 (5)	4
22	B 3058	1	5	5	5	5	4	4
23	B 3079	1	2	2	1	1	1	1
27	B 3047	1	3	2	0 (4)	3	0 (4)	3
29	C 0008	1	0 (3)	3	3	3	0 (4)	3

D. ROC Analysis: General Principles

The most widely used method to objectively evaluate the performance of a diagnostic system or the difference in performance between two diagnostic systems is ROC analysis. It compares radiologists' image-based diagnoses with known states of disease and health. In ROC analysis, performance of a diagnostic system is de-

Table 3 ROC Data for Three Mammographers for Group 2 (i.e., without Enhancement)

Case #	Database	DB total # of lesions	Mammographer 1		Mammographer 2		Mammographer 3	
			Bi Rad	Loc	Bi Rad	Loc	Bi Rad	Loc
3	A 0015	0	2	2	1	1	1	1
4	A 0034	0	2	2	0 (3)	2	0 (3)	3
5	A 0112	0	2	1	1	1	0 (4)	3
8	A 0020	0	2	2	1	1	2	2
9	A 0003	0	3	2	1	1	1	1
13	A 0030	0	2	2	1	1	0 (3)	2
15	A 0009	0	2	2	1	1	2	2
16	A 0037	0	2	2	1	1	1	2
17	A 0099	0	0 (3)	2	1	1	2	1
18	A 0116	0	0 (3)	3	1	1	1	1
21	A 0035	0	0 (3)	2	0 (4)	3	0 (3)	3
23	A 0018	0	2	2	1	1	1	1
24	A 0022	0	2	2	1	1	0 (3)	3
27	A 0005	0	0 (3)	2	0 (3)	2	1	2
30	A 0016	0	2	2	1	1	1	2
1	B 3003	1	1	2	1	1	5	5
2	B 3389	1	2	2	1	1	1	1
6	B 3009	1	0 (4)	4	0 (3)	2	0 (4)	3
7	C 0309	1	4	4	1	1	0 (4)	3
10	C 0142	1	0 (3)	3	0 (3)	2	1	2
11	B 3016	1	0 (4)	4	0 (3)	2	4	4
12	B 3382	1	2	2	1	1	3	2
14	B 3134	1	5	4	4	4	5	5
19	B 3005	3	0 (3)	3	3	3	0 (4)	4
20	C 0127	1	0 (3)	3	0 (4)	3	0 (4)	4
22	C 0015	1	0 (4)	4	0 (4)	4	5	5
25	B 3007	1	3	3	4	3	4	4
26	B 3012	1	5	5	5	5	0 (4)	3
28	B 3380	1	0 (4)	4	4	4	0 (4)	4
29	C 0358	1	5	5	5	4	0 (4)	4

scribed by the indices of "sensitivity" and "specificity," in which "sensitivity" can be expressed as the true-positive fraction (TPF) and "specificity" by the true-negative fraction (TNF) of a diagnosis (16). In a complimentary way, the false-negative fraction (TNF) and the false-positive fraction (FPF) can be defined as FNF = 1-TPF and FPF = 1-TPF, respectively, with a similar interpretation. Because

Enhancement Protocol for Digital Mammography

of this dependence, it is only necessary to measure one pair of indices, and frequently TPF and FPF are used (as in our study).

The underlying model for ROC analysis is the use of probability density distributions of a radiologist's confidence in a positive diagnosis for a particular diagnostic task for true-positive and true-negative patients (16). It is currently accepted that based on a confidence threshold [i.e., a particular level of confidence (LOC) in a positive diagnosis], a diagnosis is considered to be positive if it exceeds this threshold, and a diagnosis is considered to be negative if it falls below the threshold. TPF and FPF are then calculated from the probability density distributions as areas under the curves delimited by the confidence threshold (see Fig. 10). If the confidence threshold is varied continuously, an ROC curve can be generated from the pair values for TPF and FPF. ROC curves that indicate better decision performance are positioned higher in the unit square spanned by FPF and TPF (higher TPF values for the same FPF values). The area under the ROC curve, A_z, provides a useful summary index for the inherent discrimination performance of a diagnostic system. Thus, A_z is the average value of sensitivity of a corresponding ROC curve, if the specificity of the system is selected randomly between 0.0 and 1.0. Conversely, it can be considered as the average value specificity of a corresponding ROC curve if the sensitivity of the system is selected randomly between 0.0 and 1.0 (16).

In practice, data for an ROC analysis are obtained by providing a set of rating categories to the radiologist. For a rating scale, we chose discrete values from 1 to 5 for the LOC in a positive diagnosis. The meaning of these values was as fol-

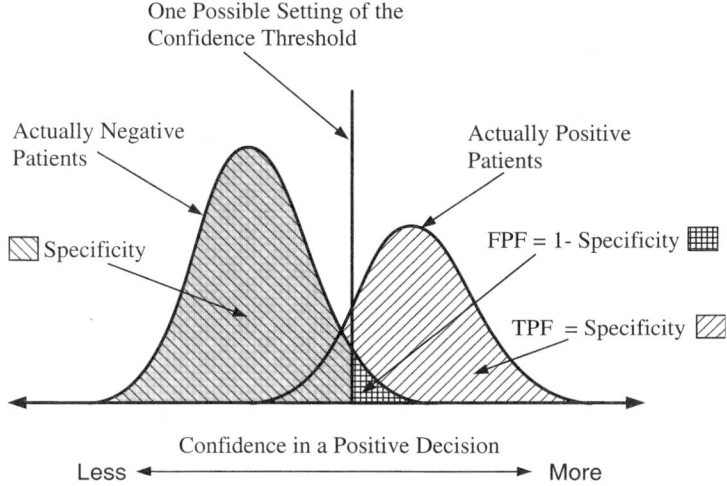

Fig. 10 Schematic example of the model that underlies ROC analysis. The bell-shaped curves represent probability density distributions of a radiologist's confidence in a positive diagnosis. A confidence threshold, represented by a vertical line, separates "positive" decisions from "negative" decisions.

lows: (a) definitely or almost definitely negative, (b) probably negative, (c) possibly positive, (d) probably positive, and (e) definitely or almost definitely positive. With this choice, the value for the LOC is similar to the standard BI_RAD rating scale used in screening.

To generate an ROC curve from discrete data requires assumptions about the functional form of the curve. The "binormal" model has been widely used in medical imaging. This model includes two adjustable parameters, and it is assumed that each conventional ROC curve has the same functional form as that implied by two "normal" (i.e., gaussian) decision-variable distributions with generally different means and standard deviations (37,38).

The two adjustable parameters of the binormal ROC curve can be taken to be the y intercept and the slope of the straight line that represents the ROC curve when it is plotted on normal-deviate axes. These two parameters, denoted as "a" and "b," can be interpreted as an effective pair of underlying gaussian distributions as the distance between the means of the two distributions and the standard deviation of the actually negative distribution, respectively, with both expressed in units of the standard deviation of the actually positive distribution (16). With the binormal model, a maximum-likelihood parameter estimation scheme is then used to generate an ROC curve that best represents the data.

If two different diagnostic systems are to be evaluated, the statistical difference of an apparent difference between measured ROC curves is of interest. Testing differences between ROC curves is well described in the literature (39,40).

E. Results from ROC Analysis

In our study, ROC analysis was possible, because the "ground truth" for each case was provided by the mammography database. In general, any enhancement protocol should increase sensitivity, [i.e., fraction of true positives (TPF)], without decreasing specificity, [i.e., essentially without increasing the fraction of false positives (FPF)] (41). An initial analysis of the data counted the number of false positives and true positives in each group of cases. Before a lesion was considered being diagnosed as malignant or benign, the LOC value was thresholded (16). The threshold value influences the shape of the ROC curve and its interpretation. For example, if the threshold for the level of confidence was chosen to be 3, meaning that lesions with a LOC greater or equal 3 were considered as malignant, then the average TPF was found to be 0.667 with enhancement, and TPF = 0.569 without enhancement. This observed increase in sensitivity is encouraging, although it was accompanied by a slight increase in the fraction of false positives (0.222 compared with 0.178). The latter is not too surprising, *because the applied enhancement protocol only used dyadic spline wavelets* with the nonlinear sigmoidal enhancement function, which is certainly not optimal for all types of lesions. We believe that dyadic spline wavelet expansions are best used to enhance microcalcifications. If the analysis of the data only focused on microcalcifications, then we observed TPF = 0.417 with enhancement compared with TPF = 0.222 without enhancement. No increase or decrease in FPF was noticed! The last finding supports the promise for future research to design specific enhancement protocols for each mammographic feature. Table 4 summarizes initial results of the ROC study using the single basis function described in Sec. IIC.

A more thorough analysis of the data was undertaken by using the *ROCKIT* software developed by a research group led by Charles Metz at the University of Chicago (42,43). This software package was written to analyze data from ROC studies and to generate corresponding ROC curves. More specifically, the purpose of *ROCKIT* is to calculate maximum-likelihood estimates of the parameters of a conventional "binormal" model for the input data, to calculate maximum-likelihood estimates of the parameters of a "bivariate binormal" model for data from two potentially correlated diagnostic tests, and, thus, to estimate the binormal ROC curves implied by those data and their correlation, and to calculate the statistical significance of the difference between two ROC curve estimates using any one of three distinct statistical tests:

1. The *bivariate test:* A bivariate chi-square test of the simultaneous differences between the "a" parameter and the "b" parameter of the two ROC curves. (*Null hypothesis:* the data sets arose from the same binormal ROC curve.)
2. The *area test:* A univariate z-score test of the difference between the areas under the two ROC curves. (*Null hypothesis:* the data sets arose from binormal ROC curves with equal areas beneath them.)

Table 4 Results of Preliminary ROC Study. TPF Refers to the Fraction of True-positives and FPF to the Fraction of False-positives

With enhancement (all types of lesions)		Without enhancement (all types of lesions)	
TPF	FPF	TPF	FPF
0.667	0.233	0.569	0.178
With enhancement (micros only)		Without enhancement (micros only)	
TPF	FPF	TPF	FPF
0.417	0.0	0.222	0.0

3. The ***TFP test:*** A univariate z-score test of the difference between the (TPFs on the two ROC curves at a selected FPF. (Null hypothesis: the data sets arose from binormal ROC curves having the same TPF at the selected FPF.)

Three types of input data are allowed for statistical testing of the differences between ROC curves:

1. Unpaired (uncorrelated) test results. The two "conditions" are applied to independent case samples—for example, from two different diagnostic tests performed on the different patients, from two different radiologists who make probability judgments concerning the presence of a specified disease in different images, etc.
2. Fully paired (correlated) test results, in which data from both of two conditions are available for each case in a single case sample. The two "conditions" in each test-result pair could correspond, for example, to two different diagnostic tests performed on the same patient, to two different radiologists who make probability judgments concerning the presence of a specified disease in the same image, etc.
3. Partially paired test results—for example, two different diagnostic tests performed on the same patient sample and on some additional patients who received only one of the diagnostic tests.

ROCKIT assumes that the population ROC curve for each condition plots as a straight line on "normal-deviate" axes, or equivalently, that the input data follow normal distributions after some unknown monotonic transformation (16) ROC curves measured in a broad variety of fields demonstrate this "binormal" form (44–46). The assumption may be satisfied even when the raw data have multimodal and/or skewed distributions (42,43).

With the *ROCKIT* software, the analysis was first applied independently to the datasets for Group 1 and Group 2 for each of the three radiologists. Unfortunately, this approach did not allow us to compare the diagnostic performance for the two diagnostic systems (softcopy display with and without enhancement). The reason for that was that the analysis for at least one group of cases could not be completed, because the data were found to be degenerate (41). In this case, the result of the ROC analysis would be a straight line with a constant value for TPF, and, therefore, the software aborts processing to avoid meaningless output. According to the authors of the software, a degenerate data distribution can be found if the number of samples is too small or in data sets with many tied values (43).

Because the number of cases could not be increased after conducting the study and to obtain more complete results, we decided to apply the analysis to the

Enhancement Protocol for Digital Mammography

union of data from all three radiologists. This was justified by the fact that all three radiologists came from the same population with a similar level of experience. Thus, their performance should be similar under the same conditions, and the data could be treated as independent samples (unpaired data). If the data did not have to be pooled, they would have been unpaired, because the two different conditions were applied to different sample cases. Nevertheless, we are well aware that the statistical significance of the results must be interpreted carefully. For future ROC studies, we plan to increase the number of cases to avoid such a problem. To check on our assumption of independent samples (unpaired data) and for completion, we also repeated the analysis with the input as paired data. These results are included in this chapter as well.

For the analysis, Group 1 (with enhancement) was set as Condition 1 and Group 2 (without enhancement) was considered as Condition 2. The resulting ROC curves for data analyzed as unpaired are shown in Fig. 11. Their corresponding values for FPF and TPF are given in Table 5. Finally, the most important results of ROC analysis, the binormal parameters a, b, and the area under the ROC curve A_z with their corresponding standard errors, 95% confidence intervals, and correlation of a and b are summarized for unpaired data in Table 6. Note that the 95% confidence intervals are symmetrical for the binormal parameters a and b, but asymmetric for the area index A_z. The corresponding results from the analysis as paired data follow directly afterwards. ROC curves are shown in Fig. 12, FPF and TPF values in Table 7, and parameters a, b, and A_z together with their corresponding standard errors, 95% confidence intervals, and correlation of a and b in Table 8.

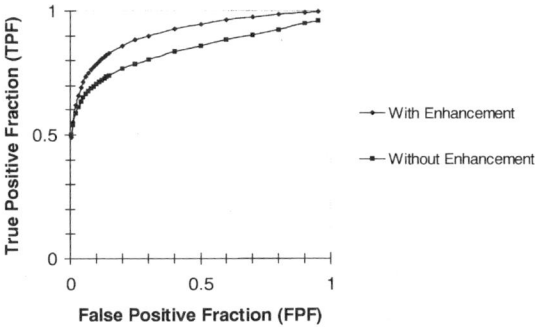

Fig. 11 ROC curves for data with Condition 1 (with enhancement) and Condition 2 (without enhancement) analyzed as unpaired data (independent analysis).

Table 5 Values for False-positive Fractions (FPF) and True-positive Fractions (TPF) for Condition 1 (with Enhancement, TPF 1) and Condition 2 (without Enhancement, TPF 2) Analyzed as Unpaired Data (Independent Analysis)

FPF	TPF 1	TPF 2	FPF	TPF 1	TPF 2
0.005	0.4886	0.4989	0.13	0.8155	0.7282
0.01	0.5521	0.5407	0.14	0.8232	0.7346
0.02	0.6199	0.5859	0.15	0.8304	0.7406
0.03	0.6612	0.614	0.2	0.86	0.7665
0.04	0.6911	0.6347	0.25	0.8825	0.7874
0.05	0.7145	0.6514	0.3	0.9003	0.8053
0.06	0.7338	0.6653	0.4	0.9274	0.8352
0.07	0.7501	0.6773	0.5	0.9472	0.8602
0.08	0.7642	0.6879	0.6	0.9625	0.8825
0.09	0.7767	0.6974	0.7	0.9746	0.9035
0.1	0.7878	0.7061	0.8	0.9845	0.9244
0.11	0.7979	0.714	0.9	0.9926	0.9475
0.12	0.8071	0.7213	0.95	0.9962	0.9619

F. Discussion

As seen from the analysis for unpaired data, the value for the area under the ROC curve A_z was 8.7% larger for Condition 1 (with enhancement) than it was for Condition 2 (without enhancement). In all cases the standard error for A_z was between 0.03 and 0.05, which was rather small. Although the 95% confidence intervals for A_z overlapped, there was a clear tendency that diagnostic performance improved *with enhancement* compared with diagnosis *without enhancement*. All ROC curves lay high in the unit square of FPF and TPF, which corresponded to accurate diagnostic performances in general, but the curve for Condition 1 was positioned slightly higher (see Fig. 11).

Similar results were generally obtained for the analysis as paired data. The increase in A_z for Condition 1 with respect to Condition 2 was 8.5%, but there was an overlap of the 95% confidence intervals for A_z as well. The ROC curve for Condition 1 was also positioned slightly higher than the one for Condition 2 (see Fig. 12). Values for *a, b,* and A_z were very similar for both types of analysis. Hence, the same tendency of improved diagnostic performance *with enhancement* compared with diagnosis without *enhancement* can be inferred.

The observed increase of the summary index A_z within statistical errors and the higher position of the ROC curve for diagnosis with enhancement encourage us to further pursue the application of enhancement protocols for mammographic screening. We are aware of the fact that there always are inherent sources of variability in the index A_z, such as a "case-sample" component caused

Enhancement Protocol for Digital Mammography

Table 6 Binormal Parameters a, b, Area Under ROC Curve A_z with their Corresponding Standard Errors, 95% Confidence Intervals, and Correlation (a, b) for Condition 1 (with Enhancement) and Condition 2 (without Enhancement) Analyzed as Unpaired Data (Independent Analysis)

Condition 1 (with enhancement)			Condition 2 (without enhancement)		
Binormal parameter a	Binormal parameter b	Area under ROC curve A_z	Binormal parameter a	Binormal parameter b	Area under ROC curve A_z
1.6183	0.6393	0.9136	1.0813	0.4208	0.8405
Standard error a	Standard error b	Standard error A_z	Standard error a	Standard error b	Standard error A_z
0.3162	0.2093	0.0325	0.2329	0.1307	0.0475
95% confidence interval for a	95% confidence interval for b	95% confidence interval for A_z	95% confidence interval for a	95% confidence interval for b	95% confidence interval for A_z
(0.9986, 2.2381)	(0.2291, 1.0495)	(0.8312, 0.9615)	(0.6247, 1.5379)	(0.1647, 0.6770)	(0.7301, 0.9162)
	Correlation (a, b)			Correlation (a, b)	
	0.6544			0.4989	

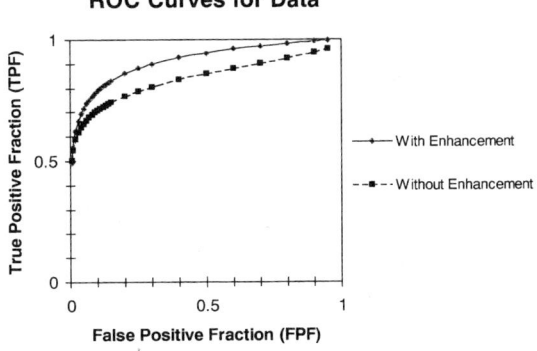

Fig. 12 ROC curves for data with Condition 1 (with enhancement) and Condition 2 (without enhancement) analyzed as paired data (correlated analysis).

Table 7 Values for False-positive Fractions (FPF) and True-positive Fractions (TPF) for Condition 1 (with Enhancement, TPF 1) and Condition 2 (without Enhancement, TPF 2) Analyzed as Paired Data (Correlated Analysis)

FPF	TPF 1	TPF 2	FPF	TPF 1	TPF 2
0.005	0.494	0.5036	0.13	0.8155	0.7304
0.01	0.5565	0.5451	0.14	0.8232	0.7367
0.02	0.6232	0.5898	0.15	0.8303	0.7426
0.03	0.6638	0.6176	0.2	0.8595	0.7682
0.04	0.6932	0.6381	0.25	0.8817	0.7889
0.05	0.7162	0.6545	0.3	0.8994	0.8066
0.06	0.7351	0.6683	0.4	0.9263	0.8361
0.07	0.7512	0.6801	0.5	0.9461	0.8608
0.08	0.7651	0.6906	0.6	0.9614	0.8829
0.09	0.7774	0.7	0.7	0.9737	0.9036
0.1	0.7883	0.7086	0.8	0.9838	0.9244
0.11	0.7982	0.7164	0.9	0.9922	0.9472
0.12	0.8073	0.7236	0.95	0.9959	0.9617

by random variations in the difficulty of the cases included in an ROC experiment, a "between-reader" component caused by random variations in the skills of the observers participating in the experiment, and a "within-reader" component associated with each reader's inability to reproduce her or his diagnosis of every case on repeated readings (16). In addition, we were not able to analyze the data for each radiologist separately because of data degeneracy as mentioned previously. The latter has diminished the statistical significance of our results obtained from the analysis of all data combined, because not all samples were completely independent.

Hence, for future ROC studies we plan to increase the number of cases to avoid degenerate data sets for the analysis and to increase the statistical power of the experiment.

Aside from statistical considerations and the cautious interpretation of the results of this study, we know that our prototype test bed software tool can be further optimized. To improve multiscale contrast enhancement the idea is to develop feature-specific enhancement protocols with different bases and associated nonlinear functions for each distinct mammographic feature, such as microcalcifications, masses, and spicular lesions. The enhancement protocol used for this experiment, dyadic spline wavelets with nonlinear sigmoidal function, was suggested to work best for microcalcifications according to our previous work with multiscale expansions (2,25). The results of this first ROC experiment seem to confirm our expectations.

Table 8 Binormal Parameters a, b, Area Under ROC Curve A_z with their Corresponding Standard Errors, 95% Confidence Intervals, and Correlation (a, b) for Condition 1 (with Enhancement) and Condition 2 (without Enhancement) Analyzed as Paired Data (Correlated Analysis)

Condition 1 (with enhancement)			Condition 2 (without enhancement)		
Binormal parameter a	Binormal parameter b	Area under ROC curve A_z	Binormal parameter a	Binormal parameter b	Area under ROC curve A_z
1.6084	0.6302	0.9132	1.0839	0.4172	0.8414
Standard error a	Standard error b	Standard error A_z	Standard error a	Standard error b	Standard error A_z
0.3137	0.2072	0.0327	0.233	0.1302	0.0474
95% confidence interval for a	95% confidence interval for b	95% confidence interval for A_z	95% confidence interval for a	95% confidence interval for b	95% confidence interval for A_z
(0.9936, 2.2232)	(0.2240, 1.0363)	(0.8304, 0.9613)	(0.6272, 1.5407)	(0.1620, 0.6724)	(0.7311, 0.9169)
	Correlation (a, b)			Correlation (a, b)	
	0.6506			0.4995	

Correlation of A_z for Condition 1 and A_z for Condition 2: -0.0922.

V. CONCLUSIONS AND FUTURE WORK

We have reported on the successful completion of the first ROC study to evaluate the benefits of contrast enhancement by means of overcomplete multiscale expansions of mammograms. The study was carried out in collaboration with radiologists at the Breast Imaging Center in Columbia-Presbyterian Medical Center and the Biomedical Imaging Laboratory of Columbia University.

In continuation of our previous work in digital mammography, an enhancement protocol using a dyadic spline wavelet as the basis for multiscale expansion and an associated nonlinear sigmoidal enhancement function was designed. Suspicious areas (ROIs) of digitized mammograms were decomposed onto a multiscale basis to obtain coefficients at distinct subbands. Coefficients were modified by applying a nonlinear sigmoidal function. Two parameters could be adjusted to change the nature of enhancement. Image reconstruction from modified coefficients occurred in nearly real time through an interactive interface running on a high-resolution digital mammography workstation. To visualize raw data of digitized mammograms at the highest possible contrast and spatial resolutions, 16-bit BARCO/Metheus framebuffers together with a dual-headed high-resolution MegaScan gray scale monitor were used in the hardware. We incorporated specialized software function calls to directly access the video framebuffer for fast/smooth image display and update.

To quantify the performance of our multiscale-based processing technique in terms of overall sensitivity and specificity, an ROC study was designed and conducted with three radiologists from Columbia-Presbyterian Medical Center specializing in mammography. Conventional ROC curves were generated and significant statistical parameters determined. The area under the ROC curve A_z was used as a summary index to quantify overall specificity and sensitivity of the two diagnostic systems (16). Unfortunately, it was not possible to analyze data sets for each of three mammographers separately because of data degeneracy. Nevertheless, analyzing all the data together yielded a slight increase (8.7%) in area A_z for diagnosis with enhancement compared with diagnosis without. Despite the limited statistical significance of this result, it encourages us to further investigate the application of multiscale methods for contrast enhancement of mammograms. More extensive ROC studies with a larger number of cases are planned to further evaluate the benefits of such processing techniques.

Ancillary to statistical results, we received very positive feedback from the participating radiologists, who expressed great interest in using the interactive display tool and acknowledged a marked improvement in image quality, when enhancement was applied.

The current enhancement protocol works best for the detection/enhancement of microcalcifications. Future directions of work include the expansion of the choice of enhancement protocols to a menu of feature-specific enhancement algorithms tailored for each mammographic feature, such as microcalcifications, masses, and spicular lesions (e.g., the application of brushlet functions) (47,48) to mammograms with spicular lesions. In addition, the investigation of a range of optimal enhancement parameters and the optimization of our interface software tool comprise further projects. Our "dream" is to present a clinical interface, in which specific enhancement protocols can be selected by a physician by only "pushing a button on the screen." We envision that through such a clinical interface the diagnostic performance of radiologists in screening digital mammograms could be substantially improved, both in terms of cost and quality.

ACKNOWLEDGEMENT

This work was supported by the Breast Cancer Research Program of the Department of Defense U.S. Army Medical Research and Material Command, Award Number DAMD17-93-J-3003 and the Whitaker Foundation.

REFERENCES

1. I Koren, A Laine. A discrete dyadic wavelet transform for multidimensional feature analysis. In: M Akay, ed. Time Frequency and Wavelets in Biomedical Signal Processing, IEEE Press Series in Biomedical Engineering. Piscataway, NJ: IEEE Press, 1998, pp 425–448.
2. AF Laine, S Schuler, J Fan, W Huda. Mammographic feature enhancement by multiscale analysis. IEEE Trans Med Imaging 13:725–740, 1994.
3. J Fan, AF Laine. Multiscale contrast enhancement and denoising in digital radiographs. In: A Aldroubi, M Unser, eds. Wavelets in Medicine and Biology. Boca Raton, FL CRC Press, 1996, pp 163–189.
4. D Brzakovic, XM Luo, P Brzakovic. An approach to automated detection of tumors in mammograms. IEEE Trans Med Imaging 9:233–241, 1991.
5. H Yoshida, K Doi, and RM Nishikawa, "Automated detection of clustered microcalcifications in digital mammograms using wavelet transform techniques," in *Proceedings of the SPIE,* vol. 2167, pp. 868–886, 1994.
6. H Yoshida, W Zhang, W Cai, K Doi, RM Nishikawa, and ML Giger, "Optimizing wavelet transform based on supervised learning for detection of microcalcifications in digital mammograms," in *Proceedings of the IEEE International Conference on Image Processing,* vol. 3, Washington, DC., pp. 152–155, 1995.
7. D Wei, H-P Chan, MA Helvie, B Sahiner, N. Classification of mass and normal breast tissue on digital mammograms: multiresolution texture analysis. Med Phys 22: 1501–1513, 1995.
8. L Li, W Qian, and LP Clark, "X-ray medical image processing using directional wavelet transform," in *Proceedings of the IEEE International Conference on Acoustics, Speech, and Signal Processing,* vol. 4, Atlanta, GA, pp. 2251–2254, 1996.
9. AF Laine, W Huda, D Chen, and J Harris, "Segmentation of masses using continuous scale representations," in *Proceedings of the Third International Workshop on Mammography,* Chicago, I.L., pp. 447–450, 1996.
10. RN Strickland, HI Hahn. Wavelet transforms for detecting microcalcifications in mammograms. IEEE Trans Med Imaging 15:218–229, 1996.
11. W Qian, LP Clarke, M Kallergi, and H-D Li, "Tree-structured nonlinear filter and wavelet transform for microcalcification segmentation in mammography," in *Proceedings of the SPIE: Biomedical Image Processing and Biomedical Visualization,* vol. 1905, San Jose, CA, pp. 520–590, 1995.
12. Y Xing, W Huda, AF Laine, and J Fan, "Simulated phantom images for optimizing wavelet-based image processing algorithms in mammography," in *Proceedings of*

the *SPIE: Mathematical Methods in Medical Imaging III,* vol. 2299, San Diego, CA, pp. 207–217, 1994.

13. Y Xing, W Huda, A Laine, J Fan, and B Steinbach, "Comparison of a dyadic wavelet image enhancement algorithm with unsharp masking and median filtering," in *Proceedings of the SPIE: Medical Imaging-Image Processing,* vol. 2434, San Diego, CA, pp. 718–729, 1995.

14. D Chen, C-M Chang, and A Laine, "Detection and enhancement of small masses via precision multiscale analysis," in *Proceedings of the Third Asian Conference on Computer Vision: Computer Vision-ACCV '98,* vol. 1, Hong Kong, PRC, pp. 192–199, 1998.

15. N Karssemeijer, GM teBrake. Detection of stellate distortions in mammograms. IEEE Trans Med Imaging 15:611–619, 1996.

16. CE Metz. ROC methodology in radiologic imaging. Invest Radiol 21:720–733, 1986.

17. BJ Betts, J Li, A Aiyer, SM Perlmutter, PC Cosman, RM Gray, RA Olshen, et al. Image Quality. Stanford University, Stanford, Final Report For U.S. Army Medical Research and Material Command, Fort Detrick, MD, November 18, 1998.

18. H Nab, N Karssemeijer, L Van Erning, J Hendriks. Comparison of digital and conventional mammography: a ROC study of 270 mammograms. Med Informatics 17:125–131, 1992.

19. W Qian, L Li, LP Clarke. Image feature extraction for mass detection in digital mammography: Influence of wavelet analysis. Med Physics 26:402–408, 1999.

20. H-P Chan, B Sahiner, R Wagner, and N Petrick, "Effects of sample size on classifier design for computer-aided diagnosis," in *Proceedings of the SPIE: Medical Imaging-Image Processing,* vol. 3338, pt. 1-2, San Diego, CA, USA, pp. 845–858, 1998.

21. M Unser, A Aldroubi. A review of wavelets in biomedical applications. Proc IEEE 84:626–638, 1996.

22. M Holschneider and R Kronland-Martinet, "A real-time algorithm for signal analysis with thehelp of the wavelet transform," in *Wavelets: Time-frequency Methods and Phase Space,* Berlin, Germany, pp. 286–304, 1990.

23. EP Simoncelli, WT Freeman, EH Adelson, DJ Heeger. Shiftable multiscale transforms. IEEE Trans Inform Theory 38:587–607, 1992.

24. SD Marco, J Weiss. M-band wavepacket-based transient signal detector using a translation-invariant wavelet. Opt Eng 33:2175–2182, 1994.

25. AF Laine, J Fan, W Yang. Wavelets for contrast enhancement of digital mammography. IEEE Eng Med Biol Soc Magazine 14:536–550, 1995.

26. AF Laine, J Fan, S Schuler. A framework for contrast enhancement by dyadic wavelet analysis. In: AG Gale, SM Astley, DR Dance, AY Cairns, eds. Digital Mammography. Amsterdam, The Netherlands: Elsevier, 1994, pp 91–100.

27. C-M Chang and AF Laine, "Enhancement of mammograms from oriented information," in *Proceedings of the IEEE International Conference on Image Processing,* vol. 3, Santa Barbara, CA, pp. 524–527, 1997.

28. S Mallat. A Wavelet Tour of Signal Processing. San Diego, CA: Academic Press, 1998.

29. PG Tahoces, J Correa, M Souto, CG. Enhancement of chest and breast radiographs by automatic spatial filtering. IEEE Trans Med Imaging 10:330–335, 1991.

30. I Daubechies. Ten Lectures on Wavelets. Philadelphia, PA: Siam, 1992.

31. S Mallat, S Zhong. Characterization of signals from multiscale edges. IEEE Trans Pattern Anal Machine Intell 14:710–732, 1992.
32. S Mallat, WL Hwang. Singularity detection and processing with wavelets. IEEE Trans Infor Theory 38:617–643, 1992.
33. I Koren, A Laine, F Taylor, and M Lewis, "Interactive wavelet processing and techniques applied to digital mammography," in *Proceedings of the IEEE International Conference on Acoustics, Speech, and Signal Processing,* vol. 3, Atlanta, GA, pp. 1415–1418, 1996.
34. WB Richardson Jr., "Nonlinear filtering and multiscale texture discrimination for mammograms," in *Proceedings of the SPIE: Mathematical Methods in Medical Imaging,* vol 1768, San Diego, CA, pp. 293–305, 1992.
35. DL Donoho and IM Johnstone, "Threshold selection for wavelet shrinkage of noisy data," in *Proc. 16th Annual Int. Conference of the IEEE Engineering in Medicine and Biology Society,* vol. 1, pp. A24–25, 1994.
36. DL Donoho, IM Johnstone. Ideal spatial adaptation via wavelet shrinkage. Biometrika 81:425–455, 1994.
37. DM Green, JA Swets. Signal Detection Theory and Psychophysics. New York: Wiley, 1966.
38. JA Swets. ROC analysis applied to the evaluation of medical imaging techniques. Invest Radiol 14:109–21, 1979.
39. BJ McNeil, JA Hanley. Statistical approaches to the analysis of receiver operating characteristic (ROC) curves. Med Decision Making 4:137–50, 1984.
40. JA Swets, RM Pickett. Evaluation of Diagnostic Systems: Methods from Signal Detection Theory. New York: Academic Press, 1982.
41. CE Metz. Some practical issues of experimental design and data analysis in radiological ROC studies. Invest Radiol 24:234–245, 1989.
42. CE Metz. ROCKIT 0.9B, Beta Version, Department of Radiology, University of Chicago, Chicago, IL, 1998.
43. CE Metz, BA Herman, CA Roe. Statistical comparison of two ROC curve estimates obtained from partially-paired datasets. Med Decision Making 18:110–121, 1998.
44. JA Swets. Form of empirical ROCs in discrimination and diagnostic tasks: implications for theory and measurement of performance. Psych Bull 99:181–198, 1986.
45. JA. Hanley. The robustness of the "binormal" assumptions used in fitting ROC curves. Med Decision Making 8:197–203, 1988.
46. KO Hajian-Tilaki, JA Hanley, L Joseph, J-P Collet. A comparison of parametric and nonparametric approaches to ROC analysis of quantitative diagnostic tests. Med Decision Making 17:94–107, 1997.
47. F Meyer, RR Coifman. Brushlets: A tool for directional image analysis and image compression. Appl Computational Harmonic Analysis 4:147–187, 1997.
48. E Angelini, A Laine, S Takuma, and S Homma, "Directional representations of 4D echocardiography for temporal quantification of LV volumes," in *Medical Imaging and Computer-Assisted Intervention-MICCAI'99,* Cambridge, England, pp. 430–440, 1999.

8
Detection of Masses in Mammograms

Nico Karssemeijer
University Medical Center, Nijmegen, Nijmegen, The Netherlands

I. INTRODUCTION

Nearly all breast cancers have an intraductal origin, and as long as a cancer remains inside the ductal system, mammography may only reveal it by the presence of microcalcifications. It is when an intraductal cancer becomes invasive that it will often appear as a mass in a mammogram. In this phase it should be detected as small as possible, because tumor size is a very important prognostic factor (1). Consequently, the success of breast cancer screening programs critically depends on the ability to detect nonpalpable invasive cancers, ideally when they are smaller than 1.5 cm, because only these are detected early enough to have a strong impact on overall mortality reduction. Masses smaller than 5 mm are rarely visible in mammograms, and detection of intraductal in situ cancers is less effective, because many of these do not get invasive during lifetime.

Detection of small masses in screening mammograms is difficult, because they may be hard to distinguish from normal fibroglandular tissue patterns. Moreover, in a screening population only three to six of a thousand women have breast cancer. It is this very large fraction of normal cases that makes screening into a complex visual task for radiologists. To avoid perception errors, radiologists need to be alert at a constant high level. That failures are not uncommon has been revealed by a number of retrospective studies. There is evidence that in current breast cancer screening programs radiologists do not detect around 25% of the cancers that are visible on retrospective review (2–7). An effective way to increase performance of radiologists in screening is double reading (8). Increases of sensitivity with 5% to 15% have been reported by having two independent readers.

However, implementation of double reading may be hard to organize because of time limitations. As an alternative, it has been suggested that computer programs that identify suspicious regions in mammograms can be used as a second reader. This approach turned out to be successful in a number of studies (9–12), but its success in practice will depend on the level of performance of detection algorithms in terms of both sensitivity and specificity.

In this chapter an overview of different approaches to computer-aided detection (CAD) of masses in mammograms will be presented. Masses in mammograms can be described as more or less compact areas that appear brighter than the tissue in which they are embedded because of a higher attenuation of x-rays. When the tissue surrounding a mass is fatty, the detection problem is relatively easy, and tumors as small as 5 mm can be detected. However, when a mass is projected in dense fibroglandular tissue, it may be very difficult to recognize. Even large masses may be completely obscured by dense tissue (13). This is one of the reasons for taking two different views of each breast, as is common practice in most screening programs. Usually, mediolateral oblique (MLO) and craniocaudal (CC) projections are recorded.

The appearance of masses can be circumscribed, fuzzy, or spiculated. In the latter case there is a radiating pattern of spicules surrounding the central mass area. Differentiation of masses from normal glandular tissue structures may be so difficult that one has to rely on distortion or asymmetry of the normal mammographic pattern. Stellate patterns of straight lines are especially suspect, as are straight retractions of the glandular tissue boundary. Bilateral asymmetry may form another important clue when a masslike area only appears in one breast. Furthermore, the location of a suspicious area sometimes plays a role. For instance, in a fatty area behind the glandular tissue, close to the chest wall, the presence of a mass is very suspect if it does not have a corresponding sign in the contralateral breast. Some examples of malign masses are shown in Fig. 1.

Detection of malignant masses in mammograms involves two tasks: search and interpretation. The problem of search is to locate mammographic regions suspected of containing a mass. The problem of interpretation is to classify mass lesions into predefined categories and to estimate how likely it is that a given mass is malignant. These categories include benign masses, like fibroadenomas and cysts, and projections of normal glandular tissue. In the literature on digital mammography, most of the research dealing with masses in mammograms has been focused on automated detection of suspicious areas. The classification stage involved in these methods is aimed at distinguishing real masses from normal breast tissue, and not on separating benign and malign abnormalities.

An adequate description of the detection problem requires analysis of the characteristics of normal parenchymal patterns and anatomical structures in the breast as imaged by mammography. In fact, it is the complex tissue pattern of nor-

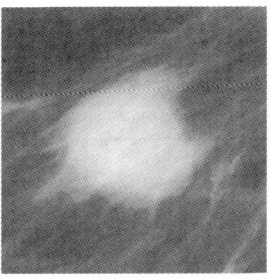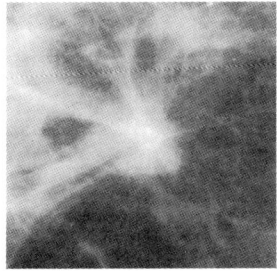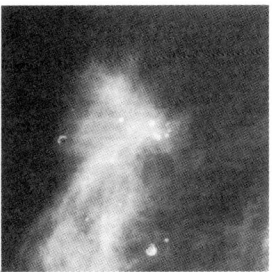

Fig. 1 Examples of malignant lesions: a circumscribed mass (left), a spiculated mass (middle), and an architectural distortion (right).

mal mammograms that makes detection difficult. Depending on breast composition and recording technique, normal breast tissue appears as a texture of many criss-crossing linear structures representing strands of connective tissue and the ductal pattern. Distinct areas in normal mammograms can be distinguished, and segmentation of these is an important problem. As a first step in classification of normal mammographic tissue, it has been suggested to segment fatty tissue from dense regions. Using such an approach, it should be realized that this is an ill-defined problem, because each pixel in a mammogram represents a column of tissue that may have more than one major component contributing to its value. Another distinct region in mammograms that can be segmented is the area in which the pectoral muscle is projected. When proper positioning techniques are used, the pectoral muscle should always be visible as a bright area in the upper corner of oblique views. Cancers may be located in the part of the pectoral muscle that partly overlaps the breast tissue. Often, the pectoral muscle is visible in CC views, as well at the chest wall boundary. Other anatomical structures that are visible in normal mammograms are blood vessels and the nipple.

In the next section common aspects of mass detection algorithms will be discussed, followed by a section on preprocessing methods used for segmentation and image normalization. An overview of methods for detection of masses in single views will be given in Sec. IV, and Sec. V discusses the use of multiple views. The chapter concludes with an example of the performance of different methods applied to the same database, aimed at giving an impression of current performance of mass detection schemes.

II. COMMON ASPECTS OF DETECTION ALGORITHMS

Detection of masses in mammograms has been investigated by many researchers, resulting in a great variety of different approaches. All these methods

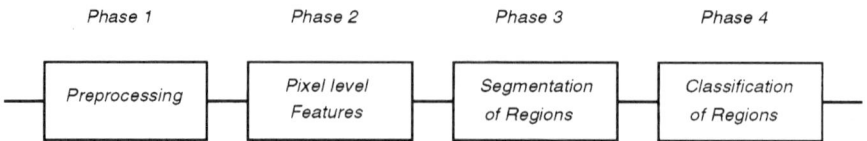

Fig. 2 A general framework for mass detection methods.

have some aspects in common, and it has been suggested that it is worthwhile to view them in a general framework that includes only a few different phases (14). Such a common scheme is depicted in Fig. 2. In the first phase, labeled as preprocessing, a digital mammogram is typically filtered and its gray scale normalized. Furthermore, areas that are to be processed differently (e.g., background, breast tissue, and the pectoral muscle) can be segmented. In the second phase, local image features are calculated at each pixel or at a set of regularly spaced points across the whole breast area. Using these features, pixels are grouped into regions by a segmentation scheme in phase three. In the last phase, features are calculated for each candidate region, and a classifier determines regions that are regarded as suspicious. Ideally, the output for each region is a measure of suspiciousness that can be thresholded at different levels to generate an FROC curve representing sensitivity as a function of the number of false positives per image.

Mass detection methods differ in the way they address and emphasize each of the different phases. Some apply very simple procedures to form many candidate regions and rely heavily on region classification to remove an abundance of false positives. Other approaches concentrate on designing features that can be computed directly from the pixel grid (e.g., without requiring a region boundary) and apply relatively simple segmentation and region classification techniques. Although it has been observed that the latter approach tends to result in better performance (14), it seems likely that optimal performance can only be achieved by paying careful attention to each of the four phases.

In both phase two and three a classifier is involved that respectively labels pixels as being part of a mass or background or labels regions as normal or abnormal. These classifiers can range from simple thresholding when only one measure is involved, to more complicated statistical classifiers, neural networks, or decision trees for classifying multidimensional samples. When many features are involved, genetic algorithms are sometimes used to find a best set of features. Details on construction of classifiers and their use are discussed elsewhere in this book. The focus of this chapter will be on definition and computation of features, preprocessing, and general design considerations.

III. PREPROCESSING

Digital mammograms can be obtained by digitization of conventionally recorded film screen mammograms or by using direct digital acquisition devices. It is good to realize that automated pattern recognition programs are often not very robust when images come from different sources. Each device has its own characteristics with respect to noise and contrast transfer, and the positioning of labels and markers on mammograms may differ. This may cause unexpected problems for computer programs that are often tuned to one particular image data set. To minimize such problems, it is important to develop methods that are invariant to resolution and gray scale conversions, and that use reliable methods for segmentation of breast tissue from the background. In this section various ways to normalize and convert mammograms with the aim of facilitating detection of mass lesions are discussed.

A. Image Segmentation

Segmentation of the breast tissue area is a step that is common to almost any breast image-processing technique. An obvious reason for initial labeling of the breast tissue area is the gain in computational speed, which can be achieved by avoiding time-consuming lesion detection operations to process the image background. Moreover, generation of false alarms outside the breast, for instance caused by film identification markers, should be avoided in practice to prevent the radiologist losing confidence in CAD. The necessity of knowing where the breast tissue boundary is located is also required by many mass detection algorithms to avoid inaccurate results caused by kernels overlapping the background or to warp corresponding images taken from different screenings of the same patient.

Mammography is a highly standardized technique. When mammograms are recorded or digitized with calibrated equipment, a fixed threshold can often be used to draw a boundary between tissue and background. Otherwise, a histogram of the image gray levels will provide a way to adaptively select a threshold for each image. This technique can be combined with edge detection to increase accuracy (15). Applying a threshold for segmentation will often generate more than one region because of markers or unexposed areas in the mammogram. In the resulting binary image, morphological operations like openings and closings are well suited to disconnect different areas that are only loosely connected, after which the largest region can be labeled as the breast. The whole process can be implemented in an efficient way by downsampling the image to a very low resolution. When an accurate determination of the skin line is needed in further processing steps, a local search near the detected breast boundary in the high-resolution image data may be implemented.

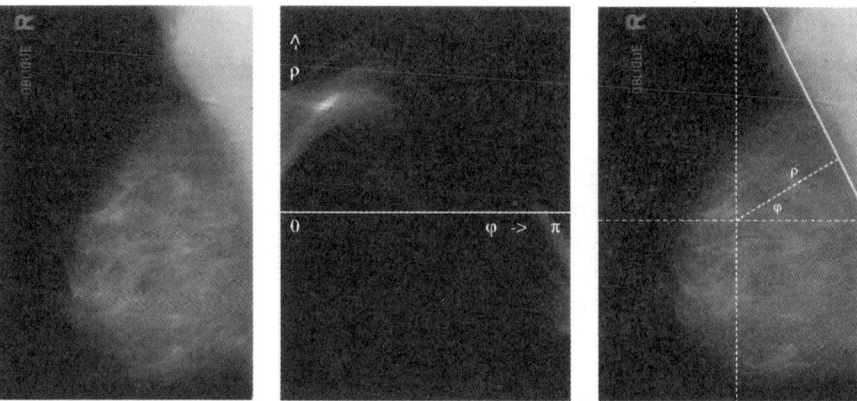

Fig. 3 The pectoral muscle in a mammogram is automatically recognized by detecting a peak in Hough space (middle) and transforming this back to the image (right).

In oblique or lateral views of the breast, the pectoral muscle will mostly be visible. Some methods for mass detection make use of the position of the pectoral muscle, for instance to guide a process of matching pairs of mammograms or to define different processing modes for the breast and the pectoral muscle. The boundary of the pectoral muscle as projected in a mammogram is normally imaged by strong gray level edges, which may induce problems for mass detection methods that are trained with more homogeneous background textures. Occasionally, a breast tumor may be projected in the lower areas of the pectoral muscle. Therefore, the pectoral area should not be excluded from processing by detection algorithms. An algorithm for determining the location of the pectoral boundary is described in Ref. 16. An example result of this Hough-transformed-based technique is shown in Fig. 3. A peak detected in Hough space represents a first approximation of the pectoral boundary as a straight line, which can be transformed back to the image space. When required, the shape and position of the boundary can be optimized, for instance by an active shape or contour model that uses the straight line boundary as an initial guess.

In some applications, it is required to determine the position of the nipple, for instance to guide a model-based search algorithm or to transform different views to a common coordinate frame. The nipple is the only well-defined landmark in the breast. In Ref. 17 a method is described that automatically determines the location of the nipple based on analysis of average gradient strength perpendicular to the skin-air interface.

B. Peripheral Enhancement

The standard procedure in mammography requires the breast to be compressed during exposure. This technique optimizes image quality for a number of reasons, including reduced scatter and motion blurring. Moreover, this procedure results in a more uniform exposure on the detector over the major part of the projected tissue area. This improves contrast visualization and allows more accurate image processing. Near the skin line, however, breast thickness rapidly decreases, causing a strong gradient of the image intensity perpendicular to the breast edge. Such a strong gradient may easily confuse a mass-detection algorithm in the area near the skin line. This is obvious when one realizes that operations used for detection of masses need to have a large supporting image area of at least the size of a mass, which will often overlap with the breast margin. To avoid this problem, image processing methods can be applied that correct for the decreasing image intensity near the breast edge. An example is shown in Fig. 4. In this case the mammogram has been smoothed with a large gaussian kernel and at all sites i, where the smoothed image had pixel values g_i lower than a threshold T, the original pixel values y_i were replaced by

$$y_i' = y_i - g_i + T \qquad (1)$$

The two parameters in this algorithm are the size of the gaussian smoothing kernel and the value of the threshold T. The latter was chosen here as the mean pixel value in the mammogram. This procedure has been applied as a preprocess-

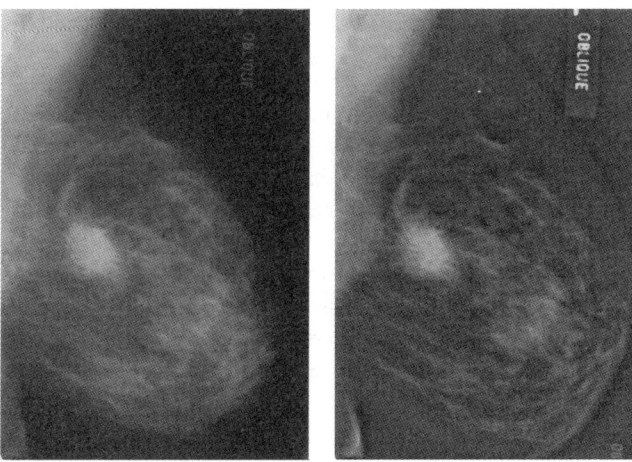

Fig. 4 Correction for breast thickness decrease in the peripheral zone of the breast.

ing step in an algorithm for detection of spiculated masses (18). Also Groshong and Kegelmeyer (19) correct for the brightness "roll-off" near the breast edge in a method for detecting circumscribed lesions.

A disadvantage of the simple approach described earlier is that ringing artifacts may be introduced near the boundary of bright areas in the image. If needed, these can be reduced by the use of nonlinear smoothing methods. Another approach for thickness equalizing in the periphery of the breast is described by Byng et al. (20), where the aim is reduction of the dynamic range to improved image display. Correction of the breast thickness differences also is an important part of a sophisticated image normalization procedure developed by Highnam et al. (21), which will be discussed in the next section.

C. Normalization of Gray Levels

Current methods for detection of masses in mammograms have been developed and tested using databases of digitized mammograms. Because of a lack of proper calibration data, most researchers do not attempt to normalize images in these databases with respect to variation in acquisition procedures. Unfortunately, it is true that reliable parameters that describe the physics of the recording process are hard to obtain for conventionally recorded series of mammograms. Ideally, there should be a known relation between pixel values and the underlying breast tissue attenuation. A major source of uncertainty is the breast thickness, which is usually not recorded by mammography technicians. Moreover, even in the same mammogram breast thickness may vary because of a tilt of the compression plate. A second source of variation is instability of the film development process. This variation is hard to deal with because of the strong nonlinear characteristics of the film/screen detector system. Direct digital mammography will solve part of these problems. Linearity of the transfer function and the availability of reliable calibration data will allow more quantitative assessment of parameters related to mammographic lesions.

Having available proper calibration data, it has been shown that mammograms can be normalized to a representation that reflects the amount of nonfatty tissue at each pixel (21–23). The basic idea behind this is the observation that in terms of linear attenuation for x-ray energy, two distinct types of breast tissues can be distinguished, namely fat and all other dense tissues, aside from calcifications. To obtain such a representation the scatter component of the mammographic image must be subtracted from the image data, and beam hardening should be taken into account. Estimation of the scatter component is only possible when the geometry of the imaging system and calibration data are known and when an accurate measurement or estimate of breast thickness is available (22). Other correction procedures that need to be carried out for image normalization should deal with divergence of the x-ray beam, the anode heel effect, and the inverse square law effect. It is expected that image analysis performed on normalized images can make detection and classification of breast masses more reliable and robust, but no studies have been performed yet that demonstrate this.

D. Reduction of Background Structure

Detection of masses is complicated by the rich structure of normal mammographic regions. A major component of this structure is composed of linear structures representing fibroglandular tissue, ducts, and blood vessels. Although these structures are very different in appearance from mammographic masses, they may easily reduce the performance of mass detection methods. A simple way to remove linear structures is smoothing. However, smoothing also reduces the edges of masses. To preserve the features related to a mass it has been suggested to remove curvilinear structure in a preprocessing step (24). A map of those pixels that are part of a linear structure is formed first, and by subtraction or interpolation the pixel values in this map are replaced by a local background estimates.

IV. DETECTION IN SINGLE VIEWS

A common phase in mass detection algorithms is generation of candidate regions that are suspicious enough to pass to the final classification stage (Fig. 2). Basically, there are two approaches in this phase. The first uses segmentation methods not specific to mammography but based on some general assumptions about the regions that are searched for. For instance, regions should be brighter than their surroundings, have a compact shape, and should be more or less homogeneous in intensity. The second approach uses more complex pixel-level features, often especially designed for mammography. These features are computed at each site, resulting in a multidimensional map that represents the local image characteristics relevant for mass detection in an explicit way. A classifier is usually applied to convert this map to an image representing the likelihood of abnormality at each site. Regions are subsequently segmented in this probability map instead of in the original image.

A disadvantage of more general segmentation schemes is that any bright region will be segmented, regardless of its shape. For true masses the regions that are formed may not correspond very well with the mass boundary because of parenchymal structures that overlap with the mass. Because of a lack of specificity in the initial detection stage, it may become very hard to classify regions in a second stage. Moreover, by using segmentation techniques that are merely based on local gray level statistics, speculated lesions that lack a clear central mass may not be found. More specific selection of suspicious areas in the initial detection stage requires computation of features that respond better to characteristic properties of mammographic masses. In this section, different methods for defining pixel level features will be discussed that were designed to find masses that are close to circular in shape or masses that have radiating line patterns surrounding them. Subsequently, approaches based on segmentation and features for classification of regions will be discussed. In the next section it will be described how features related to asymmetry can be computed. One of the consequences of using more complex features in the initial pixel-level stage is that the computations required will be more intensive. To increase speed, images can best be processed in a sampling mode, where features are computed at a sequence of regularly spaced test sites. These should be distributed densely enough to avoid missing small masses.

A. Features for Mass Detection

Features that signal masses in mammograms can be computed by band-pass filters that selectively enhance areas that are brighter than their surroundings. A technique that has been applied by a number of investigators, either in a single or multiresolution mode, is convolution of the image with a filter function that has a positive center and a negative surround (25–28). An example of such a filter function is the laplacian of the gaussian (LoG) function. To increase computational speed this function can be approximated by a difference of two gaussian (DoG) filters with a different scale. The latter approach, subtraction of two images that are somehow smoothed at a different spatial scale, is often referred to as a difference image technique. In Fig. 5 it is shown how a laplacian of the gaussian responds well to a mass when the size of the mass fits the dimension of the central part of the kernel and when the contrast of the mass is high enough. However, there is little reason to believe that application of this filter is a very good approach. In fact, the response to a mass with low contrast—also depicted in Fig. 5—is very poor. The shape of the convolution filter function influences the detection of lesions. It is hard, however, to tune this shape to mammographic masses because of their variability. In an application using a convolution neural network described in Ref. 27, a set of filter kernels is learned from example patterns during a training phase. However, optimization of a convolution filter for detection of mammographic mass lesions has not been studied in depth.

An important disadvantage of using convolution filters is that the filter output is proportional to the contrast of a given region. The contrast of true mass lesions may vary largely because of variation of size, tumor tissue properties, variability in exposure conditions, and nonlinearity of the contrast transfer of a film/screen imaging system. Small masses with low contrast may only give a modest signal compared with edges of the pectoral or glandular tissue boundary, as is shown in the bottom row of Fig. 5. To avoid direct dependence on contrast, template matching or area correlation can be used. This is a well-known technique in image processing in which the similarity between a model and the local image

Detection of Masses in Mammograms

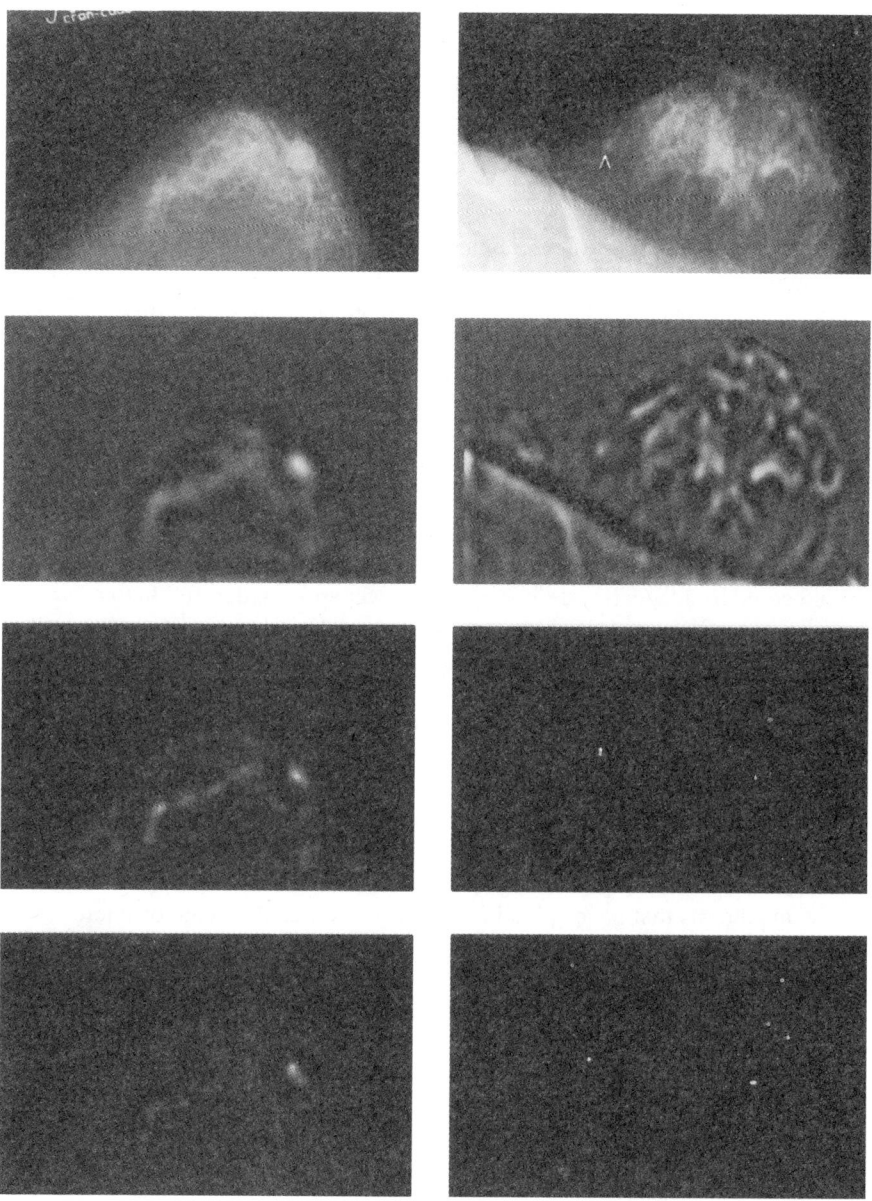

Fig. 5 Two mammograms with malignant mass lesions. From top to bottom feature maps computed by a DoG filter, area correlation, and a directional gradient filter are shown.

structure is determined by computing the cross-correlation (29). Let the shape model be described by a template $T(x,y)$ and the local image function by $f(x,y)$, then a similarity measure can be defined by the normalized cross-correlation $R(x,y)$ in a neighborhood S

$$R(x,y) = \frac{\Sigma_{(i,j) \in S}[T(i,j) - \overline{T}][f(x+i, y+j) - \overline{f}(x,y)]}{} \qquad (2)$$

with the variances of f and T computed within the support S of the filter. By using a number of templates of different sizes, this technique can been applied in a multiresolution scheme. The method was applied in some early articles on mass detection (30,31), where relatively simple mass templates with a uniform central region and a uniform surround were used. In Fig. 5 examples of area correlation are shown using a two-dimensional projection of a sphere as a template. The examples demonstrate that the correlation filter is superior to the DoG filter when a mass lesion has low contrast.

Template matching is a special case of the more general matched-filtering approach (e.g., Ref 29). This would be the optimal strategy for detecting a mass if the shape of the mass could be known exactly and if the mammographic background could be adequately described by a power spectral density. In that case the known shape of the mass should serve as the template, and a preprocessing filter should be implemented to prewhiten the background power spectrum. Unfortunately, in medical applications the shape of a lesion to be detected is unknown, and the background tissue patterns that are to be dealt with are not adequately described by simple statistical models. This makes the formal matched filtering approach less attractive.

Mass lesions occur over a wide range of sizes. For that reason investigators have suggested use of a multiscale approach for detection. Wavelets are especially popular tools for filtering out structures within a range of sizes of interest and to eliminate patterns that have spatial frequencies outside the range of interest. The use of wavelets for contrast enhancement and detection of masses in mammography has been explored by several authors (32,33). As pointed out by Miller and Ramsey (34), however, the motivation for using wavelets is not very strong. They propose the use of a nonlinear method of multiscale analysis. It is argued that assigning an optimal set of low-frequency modes to a mammogram can best be treated as an inverse problem, when it is desired that these low-frequency modes correlate well with imaged physical objects like masses. Maximum entropy is used in combination with a positivity constraint to decompose a mammogram into subimages representing structure at different spatial scales. A simple adaptive thresholding approach is used to detect masses at a selected set of resolution levels. A disadvantage of inverse filtering is the high computational load, especially when judged in comparison with the wavelet transform, which can be implemented with great computational efficiency.

Detection of Masses in Mammograms

An alternative approach to mass detection is based on analysis of gradient patterns. The idea behind this is that in a neighborhood surrounding the center of a mass, most of the brightness gradient vectors will be oriented toward the center, especially when a mass is approximately circular. This property was used by Groshong and Kegelmeyer (19) in a method based on the generalized Hough transform for circles. By using an edge detector, the strongest edges in the image are transformed to a Hough accumulator, in which each element represents a circle with given radius and location. By normalizing the peak heights and by measuring an additional image contrast component for circular areas corresponding to the peaks, masses are detected. Another approach using gradient orientation was described by Te Brake and Karssemeijer (35). Instead of using the generalized Hough transform, a statistical analysis of local gradient orientation patterns is performed. Given that computations are carried out at site i, of all pixels j that are located within a distance r_{ij} from i, with $r_{ij} \in [r_{min}, r_{max}]$, the orientation is evaluated (Fig. 6). Denoting the number of pixels oriented to the center by n_i and the total number of pixels in the neighborhood by N_i, a feature g_i representing gradient ori-

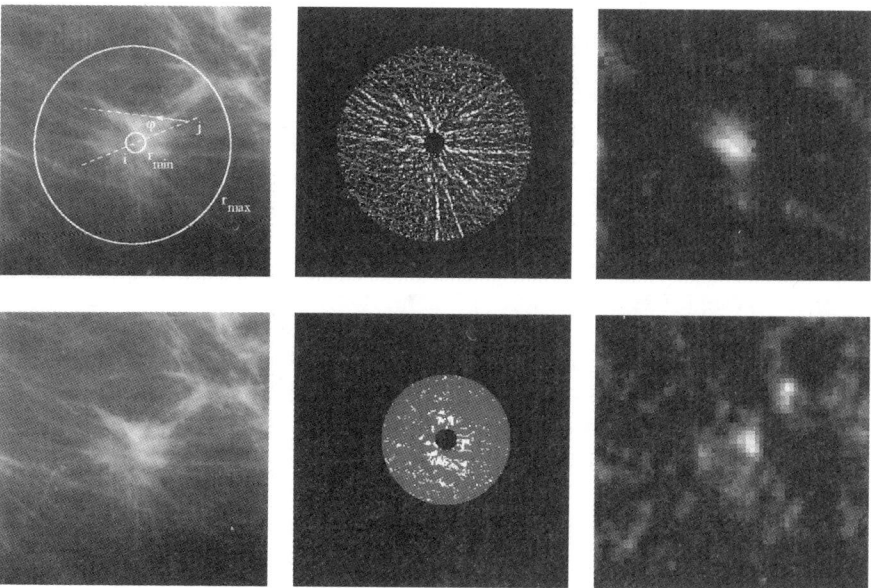

Fig. 6 Detection of a spiculated mass using line (top) and gradient orientation (bottom) maps. The figures in the central column show the labels allocated to pixels based on their orientations, when the window is centered at the tumor. Pixels are marked white when they are oriented toward the center or gray when they are not. The right-most column represents the output of the feature detector.

entation convergence is computed as

$$g_i = \frac{n_i - pN_i}{\sqrt{N_i p(1-p)}} \qquad (3)$$

with p the mean probability that a pixel is oriented toward the center in a random background. By this definition, the feature is normalized by an expected value and variance estimated for random noise patterns. In this way problems at the breast edge are avoided, and parameters can be changed adaptively. Application to the images in Fig. 5 demonstrate good performance for both bright and faint masses.

The use of texture features to distinguish masses from normal mammographic tissue has been proposed in a number of articles, either for supporting detection of potentially suspect sites in an early processing stage (36) or as part of a region description in a later stage aimed at removing false alarms. The use of multiresolution texture analysis was investigated by Wei et al. (37). In this study large numbers of texture features were computed in fixed size rectangular windows, using either the original image or wavelet coefficients as input. Texture features were based on the co-occurrence matrix, and the performance of different feature combinations was measured. Results were presented for small regions of interest only.

B. Features for Detection of Spicules

Malignant masses are often surrounded by a radiating pattern of linear spicules. Several methods have been proposed to construct features that respond to such patterns. Kegelmeyer (12,36) describes a method for detection of such stellate lesions that is based on analysis of local histograms of gradient orientations. These histograms are computed in a square moving window 3 cm wide. Stellate patterns will give rise to histograms that are more or less flat, whereas normal breast tissue is assumed to generate less uniform histograms, because of a ductal pattern that is oriented from the chest wall to the nipple. In addition to this feature, the more general Law's texture measures are used. The features are combined using a binary decision tree to label pixels as normal or abnormal. Impressive results were reported by the author, but other researchers were not able to reproduce these (14,38). It seems that the method is not specific enough because of a feature definition that does not incorporate the idea of a center with respect to which convergence of orientations is measured. Also the use of first-order derivative orientation seems suboptimal. When one is interested in orientation of linear spiculation, the use of a second-order line orientation measure is more appropriate.

Methods that do analyze local orientation patterns with respect to a center have been proposed by Ng et al. (31). Several methods are described, all based on a variation of the Hough transform. The idea is that extrapolating straight lines through selected edge points in the direction normal to the local gradient vector will yield a peak of line density at centers of radiating structures. Because of edges at the mass boundary, however, the response of this filter is rather poor. To improve performance the authors attempt to detect spicules first on the basic of their characteristic microstructure. It seems, however, that the resolution of their images was too low to justify such an approach. Detection of spicules and subsequent accumulation of evidence for the presence of spiculated masses is also the goal of a method described by Parr et al. (39,40). Their approach is based on a statistical representation of line patterns and principal component analysis. A method for detecting stellate lesions by texture analysis in Hough space is described in Ref. 41.

Detection of stellate patterns by a statistical analysis of linear orientation patterns is described by Karssemeijer (18,25). A feature that measures the degree of convergence of pixel orientations is defined in a way similar to the gradient orientation method for mass detection described earlier, with a live-based orientation measure in place of gradient orientations. This feature represents the normalized number of pixels with directions pointing to a test area (Fig. 6). A second feature measures the homogeneity of the orientation pattern surrounding the test site. This allows a classifier to distinguish radiating patterns from crossing lines or vessel structures. Both features are statistically normalized by a variance, and the expected value is computed for random noise patterns. In this way, problems at the chest or skin line boundary are avoided. Furthermore, it allows the features to be computed in a multiresolution mode, in which window size changes adaptively to increase sensitivity for lesions of varying diameters. Fig. 7 gives an example of the response of the orientation convergence filter to a stellate lesion without a clear central mass. The method critically depends on creation of a map of local

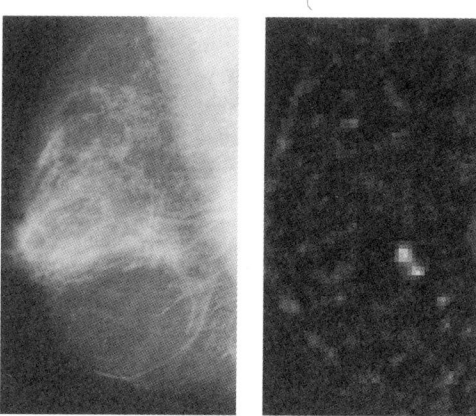

Fig. 7 A stellate lesion and a feature designed for detecting radiating line patterns.

line orientations, using second-order directional gaussian derivatives (18). This method of orientation estimation is an example of a more general approach known as steerable filters (42), which allows the output of a directional filter at any orientation to be computed from the filter output at a limited set of orientations, only three in the preceding application.

C. Detection and Segmentation of Regions

By using image segmentation, it is possible to generate candidate regions directly, without time-consuming computation of pixel level features by operators with large support. The term "segmentation" is used here for techniques that subdivide images into regions that are homogeneous with respect to some property, usually the pixel value or brightness itself. The assumption that is made is that masses in mammograms are brighter than their surroundings and have a relatively uniform intensity level inside. Brzakovic et al. (43,44) use a multiresolution segmentation scheme called fuzzy pyramid linking to identify regions. Woods and Bowyer (45) use region growing, in which local maxima in the image intensity distribution are used as seeds. A method based on adaptive thresholding, followed by a refinement stage using a Markov Random Field model, is described by (46) Li et al. By use of spatial interactions defined by the Markov model, this segmentation method can iteratively guide the segmentation process to a solution that is composed of larger connected structures only. Constraints on the shape of these regions, however, cannot be imposed. Region growing is also used by Chang et al. (47) in a method in which results of a number of different segmentation processes are combined by use of the overlap of detected regions. Yin and Giger (48) use local gray-level thresholding based on histograms in subimages. A segmentation method based on edge detection, after a contrast enhancement step, is used by Petrick et al. (49).

When more complex features, as described in the previous section, are used that respond directly to circular shapes and spiculation patterns, a segmentation step is required to identify suspicious regions. The common approach is that features are computed at a sample of sites across the image and are susequently used to classify each individual site independently as normal or abnormal. In general, these more complex features are computed with a support that is large enough to cover a typical circumscribed lesion or stellate mass. Therefore, evidence about the presence of a mass is accumulated at each site, which allows features to be combined into a map that represents the likelihood that a mass is present. For feature combination schemes there are many possible choices, such as neural networks, binary decision trees, or bayesian classifiers (18,50). A discussion of these falls outside the scope of this chapter. Having the likelihood representation available, a simple peak detection procedure is sufficient to generate potentially suspicious sites. Starting from these sites, regions can be segmented in the original image or in feature space, using techniques such as region growing, active contours, or random field models.

D. Classification of Regions

Once reliable boundaries of a potential mass area have been obtained, region-based measures representing size, shape, texture, and contrast can be computed to classify structures as normal, benign, or malign. Measures that have been used include morphological features like compactness, irregularity of the boundary, and gray-level statistics computed inside the segmented region of interest. Most of these techniques are not specific to mammography and can be found in textbooks on image processing. Exceptions are formed by measures that are defined to signal spiculation or a halo. Giger et al. (51) define two spiculation measures using a blurred lesion contour determined by the margin fluctuation and the difference in area of the processed and unprocessed contour. More recently, it was suggested by the same group to use a method termed "radial edge gradient analysis," that is derived from histograms of edge orientations taken relative to the center of the mass (52). The method was applied to distinguish malignant masses from benign ones. Analysis of tumor boundary characteristics to measure spiculation was also investigated by Pohlman et al. (53). They show that the results of their method depend strongly on spatial resolution of the mammograms. A feature aimed at measuring a dark halo that is often visible around masses is described in Ref. 54.

An interesting question is: Do some region-based features have a clear benefit over others in terms of statistical power for discrimination of malign masses from normal tissue or benign lesions. Unfortunately, this question is hard to answer by reviewing the literature on this subject. The problem is that optimizing a region-based feature space cannot be studied without taking the segmentation method being used into account and that different segmentation methods yield regions with very different boundary characteristics. Another problem is that most authors use a large number of region-based features in combination, for instance more than 200 in Ref. 37, and in many articles only overall measures of the performance of feature combinations are presented as results. Individual features that have been shown to have good discriminating power for malign structures are mostly related measures of spiculation or roughness of the extracted region boundary. In general, features related to contrast measures seem to perform less well, perhaps because of improper calibration of the gray levels. In Ref. 37, it is remarked that texture analysis of detail images generated by a wavelet transform is not effective using measures based on the co-occurrence matrix.

V. DETECTION USING MULTIPLE VIEWS

Masses may be easily obscured by the fibroglandular tissue, especially when a lesion is still small. For this reason radiologists are trained to compare left and right images and to compare a mammogram with previous screening images of the same breast. Changes of the parenchymal pattern may reveal tumor growth. However, comparing densities in two different images is difficult for the human eye. Moreover, corresponding mammograms often differ significantly because of variation of positioning, compression, and x-ray exposure during recording, whereas other changes are due to natural changes in the breast over time. For left/right comparison, there is an additional difference caused by anatomical variability. Therefore, correspondence between positions in two views can only be determined by approximation. Once correspondence has been established, asymmetry features can be computed by comparing local texture or brightness measures in the two views, for instance by subtraction. To avoid generating false asymmetries because of inadequate registration, an alternative approach to asymmetry detection was suggested by Miller and Astley (55). They found that many of the radiologists' comparisons have a regional basis, considering four breast quadrants and the glandular region. Because most cancers are located in the glandular region, radiologists pay special attention to the shape of the glandular disc. Based on this, they suggest a method that determines more global features related to shape, brightness, and topology of the glandular tissue area. In their method, the glandular tissue area is automatically segmented from the fatty regions of the breast. It seems that the reliability of this segmentation step is a critical issue. A disadvantage of this approach might be that these global asymmetry measures do not give a direct clue as to where to find the origin of the asymmetry itself, which hampers combination of the asymmetry measure with other features computed for regions.

Various approaches to establish correspondence between different views have been proposed. Yin and Giger (48,56,57) apply a relatively simple rigid body transformation to align the skin line of two breast images. More elaborate methods generate a set of corresponding landmarks or control points in each breast and apply some form of nonlinear interpolation. Lau and Bisschof (58) use a set of three control points defined on the skin line, including the estimated location of the nipple, in a method for asymmetry detection. Sallam and Bowyer (59) apply a more general warping technique in a method for detecting changes with respect to previous screenings of the same breast. In their approach, landmarks are generated over the whole breast area by an algorithm that determines maximum curvature points at the outline of dense tissue regions. In a second stage, landmarks inside the dense tissue area are used as well. Correspondence between the points is established by minimizing a cost function. They also introduce the use of thin-plate splines (60) as a model for deforming the tissue area between the control points in the mapping stage. Vujovic et al. (61,62) also use automatically generated control

Detection of Masses in Mammograms

points in the breast in a method for detection of cancerous changes. In their method, control points are selected from a set of cross-sections of prominent ducts and vessels. An example of registration using landmarks defined on the breast outline and thin-plate spline interpolation is shown in Fig. 8.

Once correspondence has been established, features can be computed that respond to bilateral asymmetry or abnormal changes with respect to previous screenings. Asymmetrical regions can be found by bilateral subtraction and

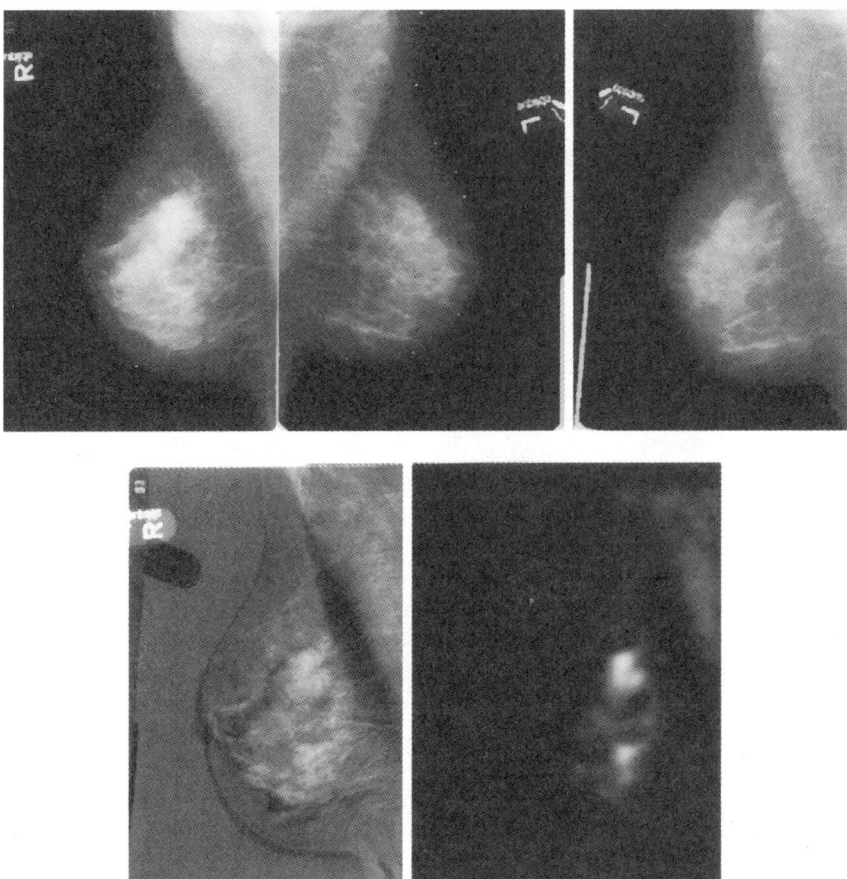

Fig. 8 Registration of a pair of mammograms using landmarks defined on the breast outline and thin plate spline mapping. The image of the left breast is mapped to the right. The bottom row shows the subtraction image, and a feature map representing bilateral asymmetry, obtained by smoothing the subtraction image.

smoothing (58). Some form of normalization of the gray levels is appropriate before applying this technique, because exposure conditions may vary. In Ref. 58, mammograms are normalized to the same levels of mean intensity and variance. To deal with variation of compression, a thickness correction in the peripheral zone of the breast should be implemented. Ideally, gray levels should be calibrated by a rigorous approach, taking all aspects of image acquisition into account (21–23). Fig. 8 shows an example of bilateral subtraction. The example demonstrates that in oblique views misalignment of the pectoral muscle may be a source of false asymmetries. To avoid this, more accurate registration is needed with the use of additional landmarks on the pectoral boundary.

The subtraction itself can also be performed in a nonlinear way, for instance as described in Refs. 48 and 56, in which multiple thresholds are used before subtraction, setting pixels below the threshold to a constant value. From the set of subtraction images thus obtained, suspicious regions are extracted by a linking scheme. In addition to subtraction of intensity levels, images representing texture differences in corresponding regions of an image pair can be computed as well (58). It has been suggested that slight textural changes can be used to predict early stages of cancer. Using advanced statistical methods, this is investigated by Priebe (63).

VI. EXPERIMENTAL RESULTS AND DISCUSSION

Because of the complexity of normal fibroglandular patterns in the breast and the variability in appearance of mass lesions, a straightforward and simple approach to detect mass lesions in mammograms does not exist. A great variety of approaches have been proposed in the literature, but it seems that for a successful approach a number of techniques need to be combined. This is demonstrated by an experiment, in which current versions of mass detection methods developed at our institute were combined. Fig. 9 and 10 show FROC curves representing detection performance measured on a series of 71 cancers detected in the breast cancer screening program in Nijmegen, The Netherlands, from 1993 to 1996. In total this set consisted of 132 mammograms with a cancer and 132 bilateral normal mammograms. In 10 cases only oblique views had been taken at screening. All cases detected by screening in the selected period were included, with the exception of those that only showed microcalcifications. Thus, the set can be regarded as representative for cancers detected by screening mammography. The results show the performance of a method that is almost entirely based on pixel-level features. The only region-based feature that was used is the size of the detected suspicious area. Regions were simply obtained by thresholding the output of a neural network classifier used to combine features for masses, spiculation, and asymmetry. Gradient and line orientation filters were used for detecting masses and spiculation (18, 35).

Detection of Masses in Mammograms

Bilateral subtraction was used for asymmetry detection, using thin-plate spline interpolation with landmarks on the breast boundary. The results show that the methods designed to detect each of the individual features have only a modest performance compared with the classifier in which the different approaches are combined. It is also shown that the value of using asymmetry computed by bilateral subtraction is limited compared with mass detection by gradient orientation analysis in single views.

Having more views per breast available, there are in fact two valid approaches to compute detection sensitivity. In the curves shown in Figs. 9 and 10, true positives were counted independently in each mammogram, except for the case-based curve in Fig. 10. The latter was computed by counting a true positive whenever a cancer was detected in view of the two or in both views. One might argue that this is more realistic, because in some of the cases a cancer is hardly visible in one of the views. Had that view been the only one available at screening, the cancer would probably not have been detected. It could only be annotated, because a clear sign in the other view at a corresponding location was visible. Therefore, a case-based analysis is more appropriate when a comparison with human detection performance is made. When doing this, it is clear that, at present, methods only achieve a high sensitivity at the cost of a false-positive rate that is an order of magnitude higher than that of radiologists in breast cancer screening. A simple calculation makes this clear. Assuming a radiologist has a positive predictive value of 20% in a population-based screening with an incidence of 0.3%, it can be calcu-

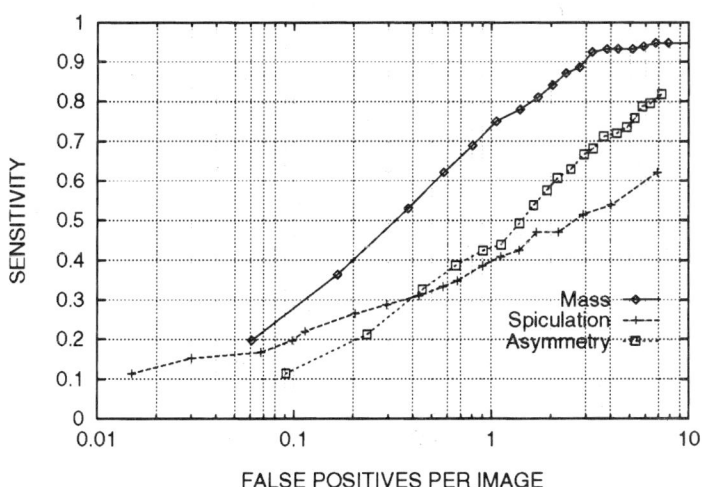

Fig. 9 Froc curves computed on database of 71 cases using single image mass and spiculation features, and asymmetry.

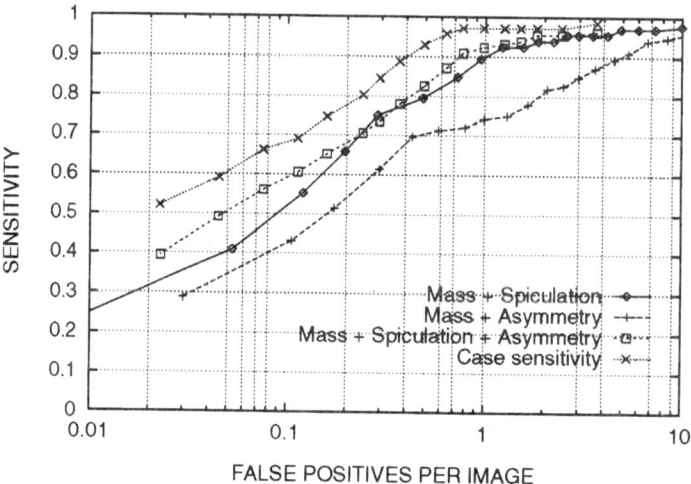

Fig. 10 Froc curves obtained by combination of features using a neural network. Also a case-based measure of sensitivity was used for the combined feature set, counting a true positive whenever a lesion is hit in at least one view. This leads to a higher FROC curve.

lated that this radiologist reports only about 12 false positives per 1000 cases. This corresponds to only 0.003 FP/image when there are four mammograms recorded per case, which is well below the range of performance measured in Fig. 10. Still, application of mass detection method at this stage is likely to be very useful when they are used to alert radiologists to potentially suspicious mammographic regions. It should be kept in mind that the estimated sensitivity of radiologists in breast cancer screening is around 75%. Furthermore, radiologists not only detect lesions but also distinguish benign from malign types. The latter is not reflected in the FROC curves of the computer performance. Retrospective studies have shown that a significant number of cancers missed in screening are due to oversight. Such errors may well be prevented by using a computer as second reader.

REFERENCES

1. L Tabar, G Fagerberg, NE Day. Breast cancer treatment and natural history: new insights from results of screening. Lancet, 339:412–414, 1992.
2. CJ Baines, DV McFarlane, and AB Miller. The role of the reference radiologist: estimates of inter-observer agreement and potential delay in cancer detection in the national breast screening study. Invest Radiol 25:971–976, 1990.

3. RE Bird, TW Wallace, BC Yankaskas. Analysis of cancers missed at screening mammography. Radiology 184:613–617, 1992.
4. JAM van Dijck, LM Verbeek, JHCL Hendriks, R Holland. The current detectability of breast cancer in a mammographic screening program. Cancer 72:1933–1938, 1993.
5. JE Harvey, LL Fajardo, CA Inis. Previous mammograms in patients with impalpable breast carcinoma: retrospective vs blinded interpretation. AJR 161:1167–1172, 1993.
6. A Gale, ARM Wilson, EJ Roebuck. Mammographic screening: radiologic performance as a precursor to image processing. SPIE 1905:458–464, 1993.
7. CJ Savage, AG Gale, EF Pawley, ARM Wilson. To err is human; to compute divine? In AG Gale, SM Astley, DR Dance, AY Cairns, eds. Digital Mammography. Amsterdam: Elsevier, 1994, pp 405–414.
8. EL Thurfjell, KA Lernevall, AAS Taube. Benefit of independent double reading in a population-based mammography screening program. Radiology 191:241–244, 1994.
9. IW Hutt, SM Astley, CRM Boggis. Prompting as an aid to diagnosis in mammography. In AG Gale, SM Astley, DR Dance, AY Cairns, ed. Digital Mammography. Amsterdam: Elsevier, 1994, pp 389–398.
10. HP Chan, K Doi, CJ Vyborny, RA Schmidt, CE Metz, KL Lam, T Ogura, Y Wu, H Macmahon. Improvement in radiologist's detection of clustered microcalcifications on mammograms. Invest Radiol 25:1102–1110, 1990.
11. S Astley, I Hutt, S Adamson, P Rose, P Miller, C Boggis, C Taylor, T Valentine, J Davies. Automation in mammography: computer vision and human perception. SPIE 1905:716–730, 1993.
12. WP Kegelmeyer, JM Pruneda, PD Bourland, A Hillis, MW Riggs, ML Nipper. Computer-aided mammographic screening for spiculated lesions. Radiology 191:331–337, 1994.
13. PB Dean. Overview of breast cancer screening. In: K Doi, ML Giger, RM Nishikawa, RA Schmidt, eds. Digital Mammography. Amsterdam: Elsevier, 1996, pp 19–26.
14. K Woods, K Bowyer. general view of detection algorithms. In: K Doi, ML Giger, RM Nishikawa, RA Schmidt, eds, Digital Mammography. Amsterdam: Elsevier, 1996, pp 385–390.
15. M Abdel-Mottaleb, CS Carman, CR Hill, S Vafai. Locating the boundary between the breast skin edge and the background in digitized mammograms. In: K Doi, ML Giger, RM Nishikawa, RA Schmidt, ed. Digital Mammography. Amsterdam: Elsevier, 1996, pp 467–470.
16. N Karssemeijer. Automated classification of parenchymal patterns in mammograms. Phys Med Biol, 43:365–378, 1998.
17. R Chandrasekhar, Y Attikiouzel. A simple method for automatically locating the nipple in mammograms. IEEE Trans Med Imag 16:483–494, 1997.
18. N Karssemeijer, GM te Brake. Detection of stellate distortions in mammograms. IEEE Trans Med Imag 15:611–619, 10 1996
19. BR Groshong, WP Kegelmeyer. Evaluation of a Hough transform method for circumscribed lesion detection. In: K Doi, ML Giger, RM Nishikawa, RA Schmidt, eds. Digital Mammography Amsterdam: Elsevier, 1996, pp 361–366.
20. JW Byng, JP Critten, MJ Yaffe. Thickness-equalization processing for mammographic images. Radiology 203:564–568, 1997.

21. RP Highnam, JM Brady, BJ Shepstone. A representation for mammographic image processing. Med Imag Analysis 1:1–18, 3 1996.
22. RP Highnam, JM Brady, BJ Shepstone. Computing the scatter component of mammographic images. IEEE Trans Med Imag 13:301–313, 1994.
23. JH Smith, SM Astley, J Graham, AP Hufton. The calibration of grey levels in mammograms. In: K Doi, ML Giger, RM Nishikawa, and RA Schmidt, eds. Digital Mammography. Amsterdam: Elsevier, 1996, pp 195–200.
24. N Cerneaz, JM Brady. Enriching digital mammogram image analysis with a description of the curvi-linear structures. In: AG Gale, SM Astley, DR Dance, AY Cairns, eds. Digital Mammography. Amsterdam: Elsevier, 1994, pp 297–306.
25. N Karssemeijer. Recognition of stellate lesions in digital mammograms. In: AG Gale, SM Astley, DR Dance, AY Cairns, eds. Digital Mammography. Amsterdam: Elsevier, 1994, pp 211–220.
26. SL Kok, JM Brady, L Tarrasenko. The detection od abnormalities in mammograms. In: AG Gale, SM Astley, DR Dance, AY Cairns, eds. Digital Mammography. Amsterdam: Elsevier, 1994, pp 261–270.
27. B Sahiner, HP Chan, N Petrick, D Wei, MA Helvie, DD Adler, MM Goodsitt. Classification of mass and normal breast tissue: a convolution neural network classifier with spatial domain and texture images. IEEE Trans Med Imag 15:598–610, 10 1996.
28. B Zheng, YH Chang, D Gur. Computerized detection of masses in digitized mammograms using single image segmentation and a multi-layer topographic feature analysis. Acad Radiol 2:959–966, 1995.
29. AK Jain. Fundamentals of Digital Image Processing. Englewood Cliffs, NJ: Prentice-Hall 1989.
30. SM Lai, X Li, WF Bischof. On techniques for detecting circumscribed masses in mammograms. IEEE Trans on Med Imag 8:377–386, 1989.
31. SL Ng, WF Bischof. Automated detection and classification of breast tumors. Comput Biomed Res 25:218–237, 1992.
32. AF Laine, S Schuler, J Fan, W Huda. Mammographic feature enhancement by multiscale enhancement. IEEE Trans on Med Imag 13:725–740, 1994.
33. A Laine, W Huda, DW Chen, J Harris. Segmentation of masses using continuous scale representations. In: K Doi, ML Giger, RM Nishikawa, RA Schmidt, eds. Digital Mammography. Amsterdam: Elsevier, 1996, pp 447–450.
34. L Miller, N Ramsey. The detection of malignant masses by non-linear multiscale analysis. In: K Doi, ML Giger, RM Nishikawa, RA Schmidt, eds. Digital Mammography. Amsterdam: Elsevier, 1996, pp 335–340.
35. GM te Brake, N Karssemeijer. Detection of stellate breast abnormalities. In: K Doi, ML Giger, RM Nishikawa, RA Schmidt, eds. Digital Mammography. Amsterdam: Elsevier, 1996, pp 341–346.
36. WP Kegelmeyer. Computer detection of stellate lesions in mammograms. SPIE 1660:446–454, 1992.
37. D Wei, HP Chan, MA Helvie, B Sahiner, N Petrick, DD Adler, MM Goodsitt. Classification of mass and normal breast tissue on digital mammograms: multiresolution texture analysis. Med Phys 22:1501–1513, 9 1995.
38. GM te Brake, N Karssemeijer. Automated detection of breast carcinomas that were not detected in a screening program. Radiology (in press), 1998.

39. TC Parr, SM Astley, CJ Taylor, CRM Boggis. Model based classification of linear structures in digital mammograms—(automatic detection and model based classification of anatomically different linear structures in digital mammograms). In: K Doi, ML Giger, RM Nishikawa, RA Schmidt, eds. Digital Mammography. Amsterdam: Elsevier 1996, pp 351–356.
40. TC Parr, CJ Taylor, SM Astley, CRM Boggis. Statistical representation of pattern structure for digital mammography. In: K Doi, ML Giger, RM Nishikawa, RA Schmidt, eds. Digital Mammography. Amsterdam: Elsevier 1996, pp 357–360.
41. M Zhang, ML Giger. Automated detection of spiculated lesions and architectural distortions in digitized mammograms. SPIE 2434:846–855, 1995.
42. WT Freeman, EH Adelson. The design and use of steerable filters. IEEE PAMI. 13(9):891–906, 1991.
43. D Brzakovic, XM Luo, P Brzakovic. An approach to automated detection of tumors in mammograms. IEEE Trans on Med Imag 9:233–241, 1990.
44. D Brzakovic, M Nescovic. Mammogram screening using multiresolution based image segmentation. Int J Pattern Recognition AI 7(6):1437–1460, 1992.
45. KS Woods, KW Bowyer. Computer detection of stellate lesions. In: AG Gale, SM Astley, DR Dance, AY Cairns, eds. Digital Mammography. Amsterdam: Elsevier, 1994, pp 221–230.
46. HD Li, M Kallergi, LP Clarke, VK Jain, RA Clark. Markov random field for tumor detection in digital mammography. IEEE Trans on Med Imag 14:565–576, 1995.
47. YH Chang, B Zheng, D Gur. Computerized identification of suspicious regions for masses in digitized mammograms. Invest Radiol 31:146–153, 1996.
48. FF Yin, ML Giger, CJ Vyborny, K Doi, RA Schmidt. Comparison of bilateral-substraction and single-image processing techniques in the computerized detection of mammographic masses. Invest Radiol 6:473–481, 1993.
49. N Petrick, HP Chan, B Sahiner, D Wei. An adaptive density-weighted contrast enhancement filter for mammographic breast mass detection. IEEE Trans Med Imag 15:59–67, 1996.
50. WP Kegelmeyer, MC Allmen. Dense feature maps for detection of calcifications. In: AG Gale, SM Astley, DR Dance, AY Cairns, eds. Digital Mammography. Amsterdam: Elsevier 1994, pp 3–12.
51. ML Giger, CJ Vyborny, RA Schmidt. Computerized characterization of mammographic masses: analysis of spiculation. Cancer Lett 77:201–211, 1994.
52. Z Huo, ML Giger, CJ Vyborny, U Bick, P Lu, DE Wolverton, RA Schmidt. Analysis of spiculation in the computerized classification of mammographic masses. Med Phys 22:1569–1579, 10 1995.
53. S Pohlman, KA Powell, NA Obuchowski, WA Chilcote, S Grundfest-Broniatowski. Quantitative classification of breast tumors in digitized mammograms. Med Phys 23:1337–1345, 1996.
54. RP Highnam, JM Brady, BJ Shepstone. A quantitative feature to aid diagnosis in mammography. In: K Doi, ML Giger, RM Nishikawa, RA Schmidt, eds. Digital Mammography. Amsterdam: Elsevier, 1996, pp 201–206.
55. P Miller, SM Astley. Automated detection of mammographic asymmetry using anatomical features. Int. J Pattern Recognition AI 7(6):1461–1476, 1992.
56. FF Yin, ML Giger, K Doi, CE Metz, CJ Vyborny, RA Schmidt. Computerized de-

tection of masses in digital mammograms: Analysis of bilateral substraction images. Med Phys 18:955–963, 1991.
57. ML Giger, P Lu, Z Huo, U Bick, CJ Vyborny, RA Schmidt, W Zhang, CE Metz, D Wolverton, RM Nishikawa, W Zouras, K Doi. Cad in digital mammography: computerized detection and classification of masses. In: AG Gale, SM Astley, DR Dance, AY Cairns, eds. Digital Mammography. Amsterdam: Elsevier, 1994, pp 281–288.
58. TK Lau, WF Bischof. Automated detection of breast tumors using the asymmetry approach. Comp Biomed Res 24:273–295, 1991.
59. M Sallam, KW Bowyer. Registering time-sequences of mammograms using a two-dimensional unwarping technique. In: AG Gale, SM Astley, DR Dance, AY Cairns, eds. Digital Mammography. Amsterdam: Elsevier, 1994, pp 121–131.
60. FL Bookstein. Principal warps: thin-plate splines and the decomposition of deformations. IEEE PAMI 11(6):567–585, 1989.
61. N Vujovic, D Brzakovic, K Fogarty. Detection of cancerous changes in mammograms using intensity and texture measures. Proc SPIE 2434:37–47, 1995.
62. N Vujovic, D Brzakovic. Establishing the correspondence between control points in pairs of mammographic images. IEEE Trans Image Proc 6(10):1388–1399, 1997.
63. CE Priebe, RA Lorey, DJ Marchette, JL Solka. Nonparametric spatio-temporal change point analysis for early detection in mammography. In: AG Gale, SM Astley, DR Dance, AY Cairns, eds. Digital Mammography. Amsterdam: Elsevier, 1994, pp 111–120.

9
Region-Based Adaptive Contrast Enhancement

Rangaraj M. Rangayyan, Liang Shen, and Yiping Shen, M. Sarah Rose
University of Calgary, Calgary, Alberta, Canada

J. E. Leo Desautels, Heather E. Bryant, Timothy J. Terry, and Natalka Horeczko[†]
Alberta Program for the Early Detection of Breast Cancer, Calgary, Alberta, Canada

The fundamental enhancement needed in mammography is an increase in contrast, especially for dense breasts. Contrast between malignant tissue and normal dense tissue may be present on a mammogram, albeit below the threshold of human perception. As well, microcalcifications in a sufficiently dense mass may not be readily visible because of low contrast. Although many enhancement techniques reported are able to enhance specific details, they typically produce disturbing artifacts. An adaptive enhancement method* is proposed in this chapter to enhance the contrast of features of mammograms and improve the visibility of diagnostic details without creating significant artifacts (1–4).

---

* Based on "Improvement of sensitivity of breast cancer diagnosis with adaptive neighborhood contrast enhancement of mammograms," by R.M. Rangayyan, L. Shen, Y. Shen, J.E.L. Desautels, H. Bryant, T.J. Terry, N. Horeczko, and M.S. Rose, which appeared in IEEE Transactions on Information Technology in Biomedicine, 1(3):161–170, September 1997. ©1997 IEEE.
† Deceased

I. ENHANCEMENT OF MAMMOGRAMS

Accurate diagnosis depends on the quality of mammograms; in particular, on the visibility of small, low-contrast objects within the breast image. Unfortunately, contrast between malignant tissue and normal tissue is often so low that detection of malignant tissue becomes difficult. Hence, the fundamental enhancement needed in mammography is an increase in contrast, especially for dense breasts.

Dronkers and Zwaag (5) suggested the use of reversal film rather than negative film for the implementation of a form of photographic contrast enhancement for mammograms. They found that the image quality produced was equal to that of conventional techniques without the need for special mammographic equipment. A photographic unsharp masking technique for mammographic images was proposed by McSweeney et al. (6). This procedure includes two steps: first, a blurred image is produced by copying the original mammogram through a sheet of glass or clear plastic that diffuses the light; then, by using subtraction print film, the final image is formed by subtracting the blurred image from the original mammogram. Although these photographic techniques improve the visualization of mammograms, they have not been widely adopted, possibly because of the variability in the image reproduction procedure.

Askins et al. (7) investigated autoradiographic enhancement of mammograms by use of thiourea labeled with ^{35}S. In this instance, mammograms underexposed as much as 10-fold could be autoradiographically intensified so that the enhanced impage was comparable to a normally exposed film. The limitations to routine use of autoradiographic techniques include cost, processing time, and disposal of radioactive solutions.

Digital image enhancement techniques have been used in radiography for more than two decades. [See Bankman (8) for a section including discussions on several enhancement techniques.] Ram (9) stated that images considered unsatisfactory for medical analysis may be rendered usable through various enhancement techniques and further indicated that application of these techniques in a clinical situation may reduce the radiation dose by about 50%. Rogowska et al. (10) applied digital unsharp masking and local contrast stretching to chest radiographs and reported that the quality of images was improved. Chan et al. (11) investigated unsharp-mask filtering for digital mammography: according to their receiver operating characteristics (ROC) studies, the simple unsharp masking procedure could improve the detectability of calcifications on digital mammograms. However, this method also increased image noise and enhancement of artifacts.

Algorithms based on adaptive neighborhood image processing to enhance mammographic contrast were first reported by Gordon and Rangayyan (12). Rangayyan and Nguyen (13) defined a tolerance-based method for growing foreground regions, which could have arbitary shapes rather than squares. Morrow et al. (1,14) further developed this approach with a new definition for background regions. Dhawan et al. (15) investigated the benefits of various contrast transfer functions, including $\sqrt{C}$, $\ln(1 + 3C)$, $1 - e^{-3C}$, and $\tanh(3C)$, where C is the original contrast, but used square adaptive neighborhoods. They found that although a suitable contrast function was important to bring out features of interest in mammograms, it was difficult to select such a function. Later, Dhawan and Le Royer (16) proposed a tunable contrast enhancement function to better enhance mammographic features. Although the adaptive neighborhood enhancement techniques have been successful in enhancing the diagnostic information on mammograms, accompanying enhancement of noise continues to be a problem; thus further modification to this procedure may be necessary.

Emphasis has recently been directed toward image enhancement based on the characteristics of the human visual system (17), leading to innovative methods using nonlinear filters, scale-space filters, multiresolution filters, and wavelet transforms. Attention has been paid to designing algorithms to enhance the contrast and visibility of diagnostic features while maintaining control on noise enhancement. Laine et al. (18) presented a method for nonlinear contrast enhancement based on multiresolution representation and the use of dyadic wavelets. A software package named MUSICA (19) (MUlti-Scale Image Contrast Amplification) has been produced by Agfa-Gevaert. Belikova et al. (20) discussed various optimal filters for enhancement of mammograms. Qu et al. (21) used wavelet techniques for enhancement and evaluated the results using breast phantom images. Tahoces et al. (22) presented a multistage spatial filtering procedure for nonlinear contrast enhancement of chest and breast images. Qian et al. (23) reported on tree-structured nonlinear filters based on median filters and an edge detector. Chen et al. (24) proposed a regional contrast enhancement technique based on unsharp masking and adaptive density shifting.

The various mammogram enhancement algorithms that have been reported in the literature may be sorted into three categories: algorithms based on conventional image processing methods (10,11,20,22,25,26), adaptive algorithms based on principles of human visual perception (1,12,15–17,24,27), and multiresolution enhancement algorithms (18,21,23,28–31). To evaluate the diagnostic usefulness of an enhancement algorithm, an ROC study has to be conducted. However, few of the aforementioned methods (3,11,25,27,28) have been tested with ROC procedures.

In their ROC study to evaluate the effects of digitization and unsharp-mask filtering on the detection of calcifications, Chan et al. (11) used 12 images with calcifications and 20 normal images. The digitization was performed at a spatial resolution of 0.1 mm/pixel, and the enhanced images were printed on film. Nine radiologists interpreted the images. They found that detectability of calcifications in the digitized mammograms was improved by unsharp-mask filtering, although both the unprocessed digitized and the processed mammograms provided lower accuracy than the conventional mammograms. Kimme-Smith et al. (25) compared contact, magnified, and television-enhanced mammographic images of 31 breasts for diagnosis of calcifications. The interpretation was performed by three experienced radiologists and three radiology residents. The television enhancement procedure used the Wallis filter, which is similar to unsharp masking. They concluded that television enhancement could not replace microfocal spot magnification and could lead to misdiagnosis by inexperienced radiologists. Experienced radiologists showed no significant improvement in performance with the enhanced images. Nab et al. (32) performed ROC analysis comparing 270 mammographic films with $2K \times 2K$ 12-bit digitized versions (at 0.1 mm/pixel) displayed on monitors. The task for the two radiologists in the study was to indicate the presence or absence of tumors or calcifications. No significant difference in performance was observed between the use of films and their digitized versions.

Kallergi et al. (28) conducted an ROC study with 100 mammograms and four radiologists, including the original films, digitized images (105-μm pixel size) displayed on monitors, and wavelet-enhanced images displayed on monitors (limited to 8-bit gray scale). The diagnostic task was limited to detection and classification of calcifications. Although they observed a statistically significant reduction in the area under the ROC curve with the digitized images, the difference between reading the original films and the wavelet-enhanced images displayed on monitors was not significant. They also noted that interobserver variation was reduced with the use of the wavelet-enhanced images. They concluded that filmless mammography with their wavelet-based enhancement method is comparable to screen–film mammography for detecting and classifying calcifications.

It is important to distinguish between the evaluation of the detection of the presence of features such as microcalcifications in an image and the evaluation of the diagnostic conclusion about a subject. Although some enhancement techniques may enhance the visibility of features such as calcifications, they may also distort their appearance and shape characteristics, which may lead to misdiagnosis (please refer to our article (1) on contrast enhancement using adaptive neighborhoods for a discussion on this topic). A similar observation was made by Kimme-Smith et al. (25), who stated that "Studies of digitally enhanced mammograms should examine the actual ability to form diagnostic conclusions from the enhanced images, rather than the ability merely to report the increased numbers of clusters of simulated microcalcifications that it is possible to detect. Radiologic evaluation obviously begins with the detection of an abnormality, but if the image of the abnormality is distorted, an incorrect diagnosis may result."

II. REGION GROWING METHODS

A. Additive Tolerance Region Growing

A commonly used region growing scheme is pixel aggregation (1,33). It compares the properties of neighboring pixels (i.e., pixels that are spatially connected to the

Region-Based Adaptive Contrast Enhancement

pixels belonging to the region) with those of the starting or "seed" pixel; the properties used are determined by homogeneity criteria. For intensity-based image segmentation, the simplest property is the pixel gray value. The term "additive tolerance level" stands for the permitted absolute gray level difference between the neighboring pixels and the seed pixel: a neighboring pixel, $p(i, j)$, is appended to the region if its absolute gray level difference with respect to the seed pixel μ is within the additive tolerance level T:

$$|p(i,j) - \mu| \leq T \tag{1}$$

Fig. 1 shows a simple example of additive tolerance region growing using different seed pixels in a 5 × 5 image. The additive tolerance level T used in the example is 3. It is seen that two different regions are obtained by starting with two seeds at different locations as shown in Fig. 1b and Fig. 1c. To overcome this dependence of the region shape on seed pixel selection, we define the following

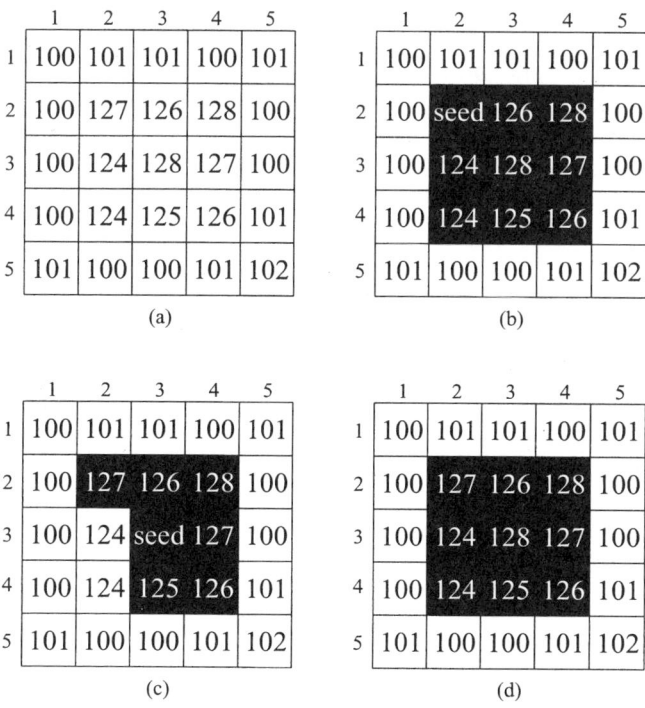

Fig. 1 A simple example of additive tolerance region growing using different seed pixels ($T = 3$). (a) Original image. (b) The result of region growing with the seed pixel at (2, 2). (c) The result of region growing with the seed pixel at (3, 3). (d) The result of region growing with the modified algorithm with any seed pixel within the highlighted region.

modified criterion to determine whether a neighboring pixel should be included in a region or not. Instead of comparing the incoming pixel with the gray level of the seed, the gray level of a neighboring pixel is now compared with the mean gray level (called the *running mean*) or average gray level (called the *running average*) of the region being grown at its current stage, R_c. This method can also be represented by Eq. (1), with the parameter μ replaced by

$$\mu = \frac{1}{N_c} \sum_{(x,y) \in Rc} p(x, y) \qquad (2)$$

where N_c is the number of pixels in R_c. Fig. 1d shows the result obtained with this modified scheme by using the same additive tolerance level as before ($T = 3$). With the new criterion, no matter which pixel is selected as the seed, the same final region will be obtained by this method as long as the seed pixel is within the region that is the central highlighted area in this illustration (Fig. 1d).

In the simplest scheme described earlier [Eq. (1)], the seed pixel is always used to check the incoming neighboring pixels, even though most of them are not spatially close to the seed. Such a region growing procedure may fail when a seed pixel is inappropriately located at a noisy pixel.

In addition to the running-mean/average-based method that may prove to be a solution, another alternative modification is to use the current center pixel as the reference instead of the seed pixel. For example, the shaded area shown in Fig. 2 represents a region being grown. When the pixel $N0$ is appended to the region, its 4-connected neighbors (labeled as Ni, $i = 1, 2, 3, 4$) or 8-connected neighbors (marked as Ni, $i = 1, 2, \ldots, 8$) should be checked for inclusion in the region, using

$$|Ni - N0| \leq T \qquad (3)$$

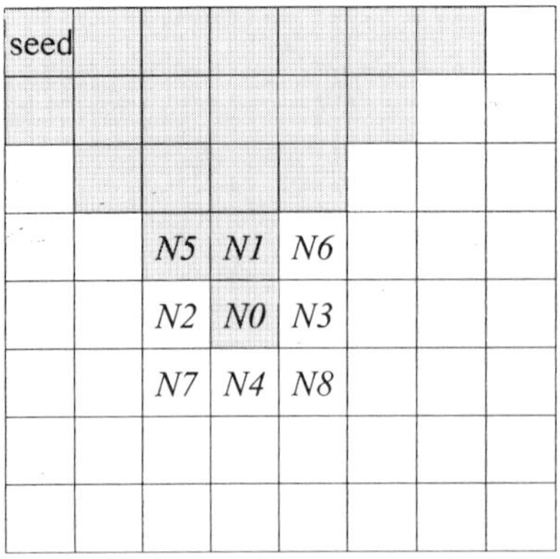

Fig. 2 Illustration of the concept of the "current" center pixel.

Region-Based Adaptive Contrast Enhancement

However, because some of the neighbor pixels are already included in the region, only $N2$, $N3$, and $N4$ in the case of 4-connectivity or $N2$, $N3$, $N4$, $N6$, $N7$, and $N8$ in the case of 8-connectivity are compared with their current center pixel $N0$ for region growing, rather than with the seed pixel. This procedure generates the same result as shown in Fig. 1d without the dependence on the location of the seed pixel when using the same additive tolerance level ($T = 3$).

B. Multiplicative Tolerance Region Growing

In addition to the sensitivity of the region to seed pixel selection with the additive tolerance region growing method, the additive tolerance level (or absolute difference in gray level) is not a good criterion for region growing; an additive tolerance level of 3, although appropriate for a seed pixel value (or running mean/average) of 127, may not be suitable when the seed pixel gray level (or running mean/average) is at a different level (e.g., 230).

To address this concern, a relative difference (called *the Multiplicative Tolerance Level*) τ could be used. Then, the criterion for region growing could be defined as

$$\frac{|p(i,j) - \mu|}{\mu} \leq \tau \tag{4}$$

or

$$2\frac{|p(i,j) - \mu|}{p(i,j) + \mu} \leq \tau \tag{5}$$

Both additive and multiplicative tolerance levels determine the maximum gray level deviation allowed within a region, and any deviation less than this level is considered to be an intrinsic property of the region or to be noise. Multiplicative tolerance is meaningful when related to the signal/noise ratio (SNR) of a region (or image), whereas additive tolerance has a direct connection with the standard deviation (SD) of the pixels within the region or a given image.

C. Analysis of Region Growing

A mathematical analysis of the additive and multiplicative tolerance-based algorithms may provide some insight and establish their need and theoretical basis. Assume that any image I can be modeled as an ideal image R plus a pure noise image N, where R consists of a series of strictly uniform disjoint or nonoverlapping regions R_i, $i = 1, 2, \ldots, k$, and N includes their corresponding noise parts N_i, $i = 1, 2, \ldots, k$. Mathematically, the image can be expressed as

$$I = R + N \tag{6}$$

where
$$R = \bigcup_i R_i; \quad i = 1, 2, \ldots, k \tag{7}$$
and
$$N = \bigcup_i N_i; \quad i = 1, 2, \ldots, k \tag{8}$$
A strictly uniform region R_i is composed of a set of connected pixels $p(x, y)$ at positions (x, y) whose values equal a constant P_i, i.e.
$$R_i = \{(x, y) \mid p(x, y) = P_i\} \tag{9}$$
The set of regions R_i, $i = 1, 2, \ldots, k$, is what we expect to obtain as the result of region growing or segmentation. Suppose the noise parts N_i, $i = 1, 2, \ldots, k$, are composed of white noise with zero mean and standard deviation σ_i; then, we have
$$I = \bigcup_i (R_i + N_i); \quad i = 1, 2, \ldots, k \tag{10}$$
and
$$R = \bigcup_i R_i = I - \bigcup_i N_i; \quad i = 1, 2, \ldots, k \tag{11}$$
Because I is the given image, some knowledge of the white-noise components N_i has to be available to obtain the segmentation result R. As a special case when all the noise components have the same standard deviation σ, i.e.,
$$\sigma_1 = \sigma_2 = \cdots = \sigma_k = \sigma \tag{12}$$
and
$$N_1 \simeq N_2 \simeq \cdots \simeq N_k \simeq N \tag{13}$$
(where the symbol $\simeq$ represents statistical similarity), the image I can be described as
$$I \simeq \bigcup_i R_i + N; \quad i = 1, 2, \ldots, k \tag{14}$$
and
$$R = \bigcup_i R_i \simeq I - N; \quad i = 1, 2, \ldots, k \tag{15}$$
The additive tolerance region growing method is well suited for segmentation of this special type of image, and an additive tolerance level solely determined by σ can be used globally over the image. However, such special cases are rare in real images. A given image generally has to be modeled as Eq. (10), in which case multiplicative tolerance region growing may be more suitable, with the expectation that a global multiplicative tolerance level can be derived for all the regions in a given image. Because the multiplicative tolerance level could be made a function of σ_i/P_i (related to SNR, which can be defined as $10 \log_{10} P_i^2/\sigma_i^2$ in dB) for each individual region i, such a global tolerance level can be found if and only if
$$\frac{\sigma_1}{P_1} = \frac{\sigma_2}{P_2} = \cdots = \frac{\sigma_k}{P_k} \tag{16}$$

D. Region Growing Criteria

A region growing procedure is used in our contrast-enhancement algorithm for the purpose of identifying nearly homogeneous regions in the image. The procedure relies on one of the multiplicative tolerance region-growing algorithms introduced in Sec IIB. The region-growing procedure starts with the pixel to be processed, called the seed. The eight neighbors of the seed are checked to see whether their gray level values are within a specified deviation from the seed [τ set to be 0.05 and μ set equal to the seed pixel as in Eq. (4)]. Pixels that meet the criterion for inclusion in the region are labeled. The neighbors of the labeled pixels are then checked for inclusion, and so on. A region thus grown is labeled as the foreground layer. The foreground stops growing when it is surrounded by a layer of pixels that do not meet the criterion for inclusion in the foreground. This layer of pixels is labeled as the background, which may be increased to a specified size (e.g., 3-pixel width) by further region growing, molded to the foreground region in shape. Fig. 3 illustrates the concepts of the foreground and the background. Note that the criterion for background growing is as simple as checking whether the pixel is already labeled as a foreground pixel.

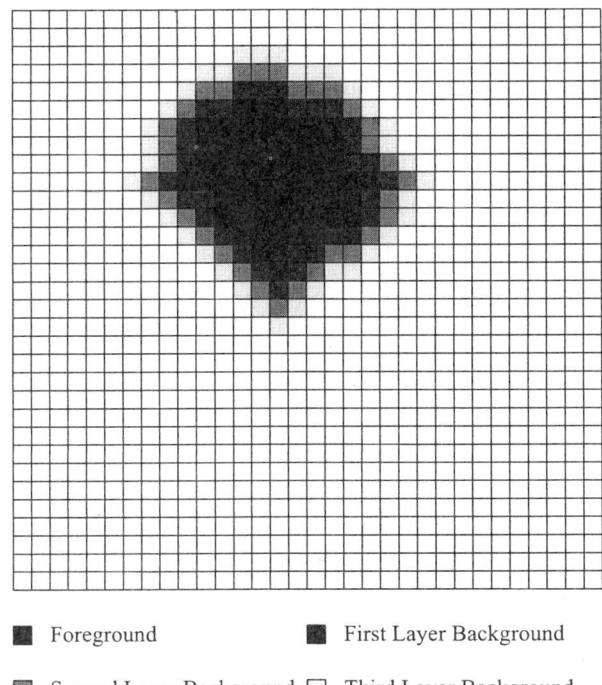

■ Foreground　　　■ First Layer Background

▨ Second Layer Background　☐ Third Layer Background

Fig. 3 Illustration of the concepts of the foreground and the background.

III. ADAPTIVE CONTRAST ENHANCEMENT

The adaptive neighborhood contrast enhancement (ANCE) method (1) is an image-enhancement technique designed to improve the perceptibility of objects or features in an image. The technique may be summarized as follows. First, nearly homogeneous regions in the image are identified by the region growing procedure. The visual contrast of each region is then computed by comparing the intensity of the region with the intensity of its surroundings. The region's contrast is selectively increased by modifying its intensity if the following conditions are met:

- The region's contrast is low [C as defined in Eq. (17) being in the range 0.02 to 0.4].
- The pixels in the region's background have a standard deviation normalized with respect to their mean of less than 0.1.

The first condition is imposed so as to not enhance low-level noise or regions already with high contrast; the second is used to rule out enhancement of regions surrounded by a variable or "busy" background. This approach is applied sequentially at each pixel in the image to enhance the contrast of all objects and features in the image.

In the ANCE procedure, the contrast C is calculated from groupings of pixels using the optical contrast definition (34)

$$C = \frac{f - b}{f + b} \tag{17}$$

where f and b are the foreground and background densities. Letting N_f and N_b be the numbers of pixels in the foreground and background, respectively, and $p(i, j)$ be the pixel value at the location (i, j), f and b can be obtained as

$$f = \frac{1}{N_f} \sum_{(i,j) \in \text{foreground}} p(i, j) \tag{18}$$

and

$$b = \frac{1}{N_b} \sum_{(i,j) \in \text{background}} p(i, j) \tag{19}$$

The groupings of pixels are referred to as neighborhoods, and a neighborhood is determined for each pixel in the image. Thus, ANCE is based on the contextual details in the image around each pixel. Note that each pixel in the image is treated in turn as the seed for region growing and processing for enhancement.

The basic objective of ANCE is to increase the contrast of specific regions that may be of radiological interest and need enhancement, without changing the rest of the image significantly. This is realized by selectively assigning a new con-

Region-Based Adaptive Contrast Enhancement

trast C' to those regions that are of interest, and then determining from C' the desired value of the foreground (seed pixel) as

$$f' = b \frac{1 + C'}{1 - C'} \qquad (20)$$

A specific relationship between C' and C, as shown in Fig. 4, was designed to obtain clinically useful enhancement.

Because the ANCE algorithm works on the basis of adaptive neighborhoods, it can enhance the visibility of features of varying shape and size. The general comments of the radiologist who interpreted the original and enhanced images of eight biopsy-proven cases with different types of mammographic features and presentation (1) indicated that the enhanced images "... suggested carcinoma as the origin of both lesions much more strongly than the unenhanced mammogram"; "... dense nodule appeared to be connected to the spiculated mass, suggesting a much further advanced carcinoma than that suspected from the unenhanced mammogram"; "... the details in the internal architecture of the breast appeared clearer, adding further weight to the diagnosis of benign lesions"; "... provided stronger evidence of carcinoma with poor margins of the lesion, a greater number of calcifications, and inhomogeneity in the density of the calcium"; "... showed the same detail as the unenhanced mammogram with the additional finding of some microcalcifications."

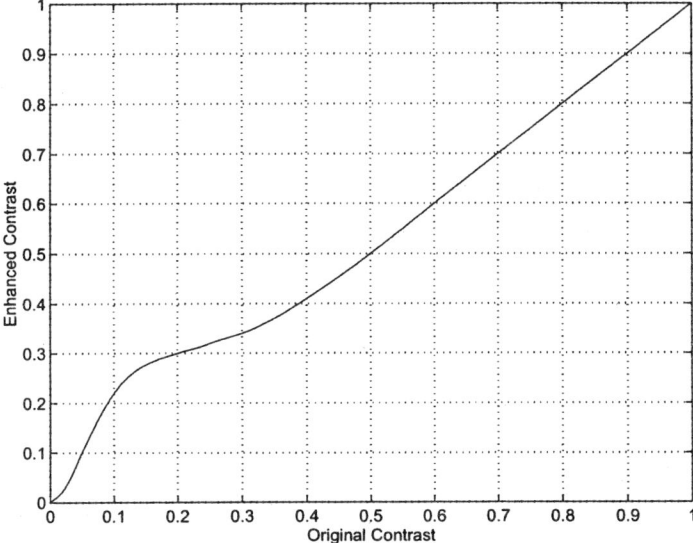

Fig. 4 Relationship between original contrast C and enhanced contrast C'.

IV. CASE SELECTION, DIGITIZATION, AND PRESENTATION

To evaluate the diagnostic usefulness of the ANCE technique, two ROC studies were conducted using two different databases: *Difficult Cases* and *Interval Cancer Cases*. The Difficult Cases data set is a collection of cases for which the radiologist had been unsure enough to call for a biopsy. The cases were difficult in terms of both detection of the abnormality present and the diagnosis as normal, benign, or malignant. The investigation to be described here was conducted to test whether ANCE could be used to distinguish benign cases from their malignant counterparts (2). Interval Cancer Cases are cases in a screening program where cancer is detected before a scheduled return screening visit; they may be indicative of the inability to detect an already present cancer or an unusually rapid-growing cancer. In these cases, the radiologist had declared that there was no evidence of cancer on the previous mammograms. The purpose of the study to be described next was to test whether interval cancers could be detected earlier with appropriate digital enhancement and analysis (3).

It should be noted that the goal of interpretation in this study was screening, and not detection of signs such as calcifications or masses; as such, no record was maintained of the number or sizes of signs [as done by Kallergi et al. (28) and Nishikawa et al. (35)].

A. Difficult Cases

An experienced radiologist selected 21 difficult cases (related to 14 subjects with benign breast disease and seven subjects with malignant disease) for this study from files covering the period 1987 to 1992 at the Foothills Hospital, Calgary, Canada. Four films (two views: MLO—Mediolateral oblique and CC—Craniocaudal, of each breast) were available for each of 18 cases, whereas only two films (of one breast) were available for each of three cases, leading to a total of 78 screen–film mammograms. Biopsy results were also available for each subject, on which our ROC evaluation was based.

Each film was digitized using an Eikonix 1412 scanner (Eikonix Inc., Bedford, MA) to 4096 by about 2048 pixels (the second index value depends on the size of the image in the mammogram; the sizes of the digitized images were thus different from case to case) with 12-bit gray-scale resolution. This sampling represents a spot size on the film of about 0.062 mm $\times$ 0.062 mm. Films were illuminated by a Plannar 1417 lightbox (Gordon Instruments, Orchard Park, NY). Although the lightbox is designed to have a uniform light intensity distribution, it was necessary to correct for nonuniformities in illumination. After correction, pixel gray levels were determined to be accurate to 10 bits, with a dynamic range of approximately 0.02 to 2.52 optical density units (36).

The digital images were down-sampled by a factor of two for processing and display for interpretation on a MegaScan 2111 monitor (Advanced Video Products Inc., Littleton, MA.). Although the memory buffer of the Megascan system is $4096 \times 4096 \times 12$ bits, the display buffer is limited to $2560 \times 2048 \times 8$ bits, with panning and zooming facilities. The original screen—film mammograms used in the study were presented to the radiologists using a standard mammogram film viewer.

Six radiologists from the Foothills Hospital interpreted the original, the unprocessed digitized, and the enhanced mammograms separately. Only one of the radiologists had prior experience with digitized and enhanced mammographic images. The images were presented in random order and the radiologists were given no additional information about the patients. The radiologists ranked each case as (1) definitely or almost definitely benign, (2) probably benign, (3) possibly malignant, (4) probably malignant, (5) definitely or almost definitely malignant.

B. Interval Cancer Cases

Two hundred twenty-two screen–film mammograms of 28 interval cancer patients and six control patients with benign disease were selected for this study from files over the period 1991 to 1995 at the Screen Test Centres of the Alberta Program for the Early Detection of Breast Cancer. Some of the cases of cancer were diagnosed by physical examination or mammography performed after the initial (or previous) visit to the screening program but before the next scheduled visit. Note that the radiologists reading the mammograms taken before diagnosis of the cancer had declared that there was no evidence of cancer on the films. The small number of benign cases were included to prevent "overdiagnosis"; the radiologists were not informed of the proportion of benign to malignant cases in the set. Most of the files include multiple sets of films taken at different times; all sets except one have at least four films each (two views: MLO and CC, of each breast) in the database. (More specifically, the database includes 52 four-film sets, one 3-film set, one 5-film set, and one 6-film set). Previous films of all the interval cancer cases had initially been reported as being normal. Biopsy results were available for each subject.

The aim of this study was to investigate the possibility of earlier detection of interval breast cancer with the aid of appropriate image-processing techniques. Because a few sets of films taken at different times were available for each subject, we labeled the sets of mammograms of each subject as separate cases. All films of the subjects with malignant disease within the selected period were labeled as being malignant, even though the cases had not been previously interpreted as such. By this process, 55 cases were obtained, of which 47 were malignant and eight were benign (the numbers of subjects being 28 with malignant disease and six with benign disease).

The films were digitized as described in the previous section and processed using the ANCE technique with the full digitized resolution available. The digitized version and the ANCE-processed version were printed on film using a KODAK XL 7700 Digital Continuous Tone Printer (Eastman Kodak Company, Rochester, NY) with pixel arrays up to 2048 × 1536 (8-bit pixels). Gray-level remapping (10 bits/pixel to 8 bits/pixel) and downsampling by a factor of two were applied before a digitized/enhanced mammogram image was sent for printing with two different look-up tables (LUTs).

Three reference radiologists from the Screen Test Program separately interpreted the original films of the involved side, their digitized versions, and their ANCE-processed versions on a standard mammogram film viewer. Only one of the radiologists had prior experience with digitized and enhanced mammographic images. Interpretation of the digitized images (without ANCE processing) was included in the test to evaluate the effect on diagnostic accuracy of digitization and printing with the resolution and equipment used. The images were presented in random order, and the radiologists were given no additional information about the patients. The radiologists ranked each case as (1) definitely or almost definitely benign, (2) probably benign, (3) indeterminate, (4) probably malignant, (5) definitely or almost definitely malignant. Note that the diagnostic statement for rank (3) is different in this study from that described in the previous section. This was done based on comments from the radiologists involved in the Difficult Cases study.

In both studies the objective was screening and not localization of disease. The radiologists had to find lesions, if any, and assess them for the likelihood of malignancy, but did not have to mark their locations on the films.

Images were interpreted in random order by the radiologists. Images were presented in the same random order to each radiologist individually. Each radiologist interpreted all of the images in a single sitting. Multiple sets of films of a given subject (taken at different times) were treated as different cases and interpreted separately to avoid the development of familiarity and bias. The original, digitized, and enhanced versions of any given case were mixed for random ordering, treated as separate cases, and interpreted separately to prevent the development of familiarity and bias. All available views of a case were read together as one set. Note that the initial (original) diagnosis of the cases was performed by different teams of radiologists experienced in the interpretation of screening mammograms, which further limits the scope of bias in this study.

V. ROC AND STATISTICAL ANALYSIS

In this study, ROC analysis (37,38) is used to compare the radiologists' performance in detecting abnormalities in the various images. The maximum likelihood estimation method (39) was used to fit a binormal ROC curve to each radiologist's confidence rating data for each set of mammograms. The slope and intercept parameters of the binormal ROC curve (when plotted on normal probability scales) were calculated for each fitted curve. To estimate the average performance of the group of radiologists on each set of images, composite ROC curves (37) were calculated by averaging the slope and the intercept parameters of the individual ROC curves. Finally, the area under the binormal ROC curve (as plotted in the unit square) was computed, which represents the overall abnormality detection accuracy for each type of image.

In addition to ROC analysis of the interval cancer cases, McNemar's test of symmetry (40,41) was performed on a series of 3 × 3 contingency tables obtained by cross-tabulating (a) diagnostic confidence using the original mammograms (categories 1 or 2, 3, and 4 or 5) against the diagnostic confidence using the digitized mammograms, and (b) diagnostic confidence using the digitized mammograms against the diagnostic confidence using the enhanced mammograms. Separate 3 × 3 tables, as illustrated in Fig. 5, were formed for the malignant cases and the benign cases. Cases in which there is no change in the diagnostic confidence will fall on the diagonal (upper left to lower right, labeled as D in Fig. 5) of the table. For the malignant cases, improvement in the diagnostic accuracy is illustrated by a 3 × 3 table with most cases in the three upper right-hand cells (labeled as U in Fig. 5). Conversely, for the benign cases, improvement in the diagnostic accuracy will be illustrated by a 3 × 3 table with most cases in the three lower left-hand cells (labeled as L in Fig. 5). The hypothesis of significant improvement can be tested statistically using McNemar's test of symmetry (40,41), namely that the probability of an observation being classified into a cell $[i, j]$ is the same as the probability of being classified into the cell $[j, i]$.

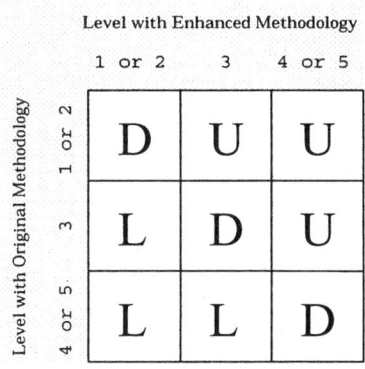

Fig. 5 Illustration of the table for McNemar's test.

The validity of McNemar's test depends on the assumption that the cell counts are at least moderately large. To avoid limitations caused by this factor and also to avoid the problem of excessive multiple comparisons, the data across the individual radiologists were combined in two different ways before applying McNemar's test. The first method (referred to as "averaged") averaged the radiologists' diagnostic ratings before forming the 3 × 3 tables. In the second method (referred to as "combined"), the 3 × 3 tables for each of the radiologists were formed first and then combined by summing the corresponding cells.

Because this analysis involves multiple p values, the Bonferroni correction was used to adjust the p values (42). When multiple p values are produced, the probability of making a type I error increases. (Rejection of the null hypothesis when it is true is called a type I error.) The Bonferroni method for adjusting multiple p values requires that when k hypothesis tests are performed, each p value is multiplied by k, so that the adjusted p value is $p^* = kp$.

To reduce the number of p values, it was decided to test symmetry for each situation (malignant/benign and averaged/combined) for the two tables original-to-digitized and digitized-to-enhanced, but not the original-to-enhanced (which follows from the other two).

VI. RESULTS

Fig. 6 shows a part of a mammogram with malignant calcifications (left) and the corresponding image after processing by the ANCE procedure (right). It is seen that increased contrast in the enhanced image has improved the visibility of the calcifications.

A. ROC Analysis of Difficult Cases

Because the population involved in this study was such that the original mammograms were sufficiently abnormal to cause the initial attending radiologist to call for biopsy, the aim of this study was to test whether specificity could be improved with the ANCE method.

The composite ROC curves representing breast cancer diagnosis by the six radiologists in this study are compared in Fig. 7. Several points are clearly illustrated by Fig. 7. First, the process of digitization (and downsampling to an effective pixel size of 0.124 mm × 0.124 mm) degrades the quality of images and therefore makes the radiologists' performance worse, especially in the low false-positive fraction (FPF) range. However, better performance of the radiologists is seen with the digitized images at high FPFs (better sensitivity with worse specificity). Second, it should be noticed that the ANCE method improves the radiologists' performance at all ranges of FPF (more significantly in the low FPF range)

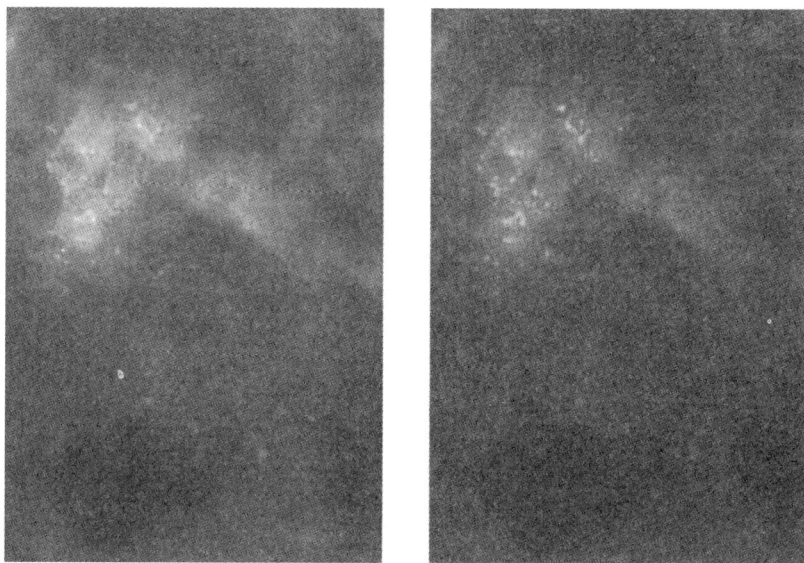

Fig. 6 A part of a mammogram with malignant calcifications (left) and its ANCE-processed version (right).

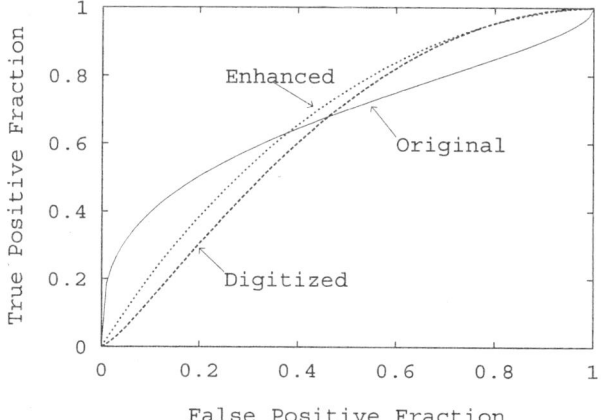

Fig. 7 Comparison of composite ROC curves for detection of abnormalities by interpreting the original, unprocessed digitized, and enhanced images of 21 difficult cases. Reproduced with permission from Rangayyan et al. (4). ©IEEE 1997.

compared with the unprocessed digitized images, although it is still lower than that with the original films in the low range of FPF. The values of the area parameter (A_z) for the original, digitized, and enhanced mammograms were computed to be 0.6735, 0.6259, and 0.6745, respectively. (Note that Kallergi et al. (28) also observed a drop in the area under the ROC curve when digitized images were interpreted from monitor display compared with the original films; their wavelet-based enhancement method provided an improvement over the digitized version, although the enhanced images did not provide any statistically significant benefit over the original films.) The area values are lower than those normally encountered in the literature (in the range 0.9–0.98), because the cases selected were difficult enough to call for biopsy. Larger area values could have been obtained by adding a large number of obvious or easy cases, but this approach was not taken in this work. Regardless, the numerical results confirm our observations and indicate that the ANCE technique improves the radiologists' overall performance, especially over unprocessed digitized mammograms, and allows the radiologists to discriminate between the two populations slightly better while interpreting the enhanced mammograms compared with the original films.

B. McNemar's Tests on Difficult Cases

Tables 1 and 2 contain details of the radiologists' diagnostic performance variations for malignant cases and benign cases with this database. (NOTE: in the tables, B refers to Benign, U to Undecided or Indeterminate, and M to Malignant ratings.) For almost every table for individual readers, the numbers were too small to perform the McNemar chi-square test (including the average). In other cases, the numbers would be too small to detect a statistically significant difference. Therefore, the data were combined for the six readers by simply summing the 3×3 matrices.

For the benign cases (combined), p values of 0.004, 0.5319, and 0.0225 were obtained for original-to-digitized, digitized-to-enhanced, and original-to-enhanced, respectively. For the malignant cases (combined), the p values were 0.1577, 0.3618, and 0.6858 for original-to-digitized, digitized-to-enhanced, and original-to-enhanced, respectively. The p values represent no evidence of improvement in the diagnostic accuracy for any of the three tables (original-to-digitized, digitized-to-enhanced, and original-to-enhanced) for the malignant cases in the Difficult Cases data set. However, for the benign cases, there is a statistically significant improvement in the diagnostic accuracy ($p = 0.004$, Bonferroni adjusted value $p^* = 0.024$). There is no evidence of a significant improvement from digitized to enhanced, and although there is a significant improvement from the original to the digitized category (but not significant after Bonferroni adjustment, $p^* = 0.135$), this is entirely caused by the improvement in moving from the original to the digitized category.

Region-Based Adaptive Contrast Enhancement

Table 1 Details of Radiologists' Diagnostic Performance Variations with Original Mammograms (Orig), Unprocessed Digitized Mammograms (Digt), and ANCE-processed Digitized Mammograms (Enhn) for the Seven Malignant Cases in the Difficult Cases Database. (NOTE: To Obtain the Average Values, the Individual Diagnostic Confidence Levels were Averaged First.)

Radiologist	Image types	Change of diagnostic confidence level					
		B: level 1 or 2;		U: level 3;		M: level 4 or 5	
		B → U (U → B)	U → M (M → U)	B → M (M → B)	B → B	U → U	M → M
#1	Orig → Digt	1 (1)	0 (2)	0 (0)	1	0	2
	Digt → Enhn	1 (0)	1 (0)	0 (0)	1	2	2
	Orig → Enhn	0 (0)	0 (2)	1 (0)	1	1	2
#2	Orig → Digt	0 (0)	0 (1)	0 (0)	1	1	4
	Digt → Enhn	0 (0)	0 (0)	0 (0)	1	2	4
	Orig → Enhn	0 (0)	0 (1)	0 (0)	1	1	4
#3	Orig → Digt	1 (0)	1 (2)	0 (0)	0	2	1
	Digt → Enhn	0 (1)	0 (0)	0 (0)	0	4	2
	Orig → Enhn	1 (1)	1 (2)	0 (0)	0	1	1
#4	Orig → Digt	0 (1)	0 (1)	0 (1)	1	0	3
	Digt → Enhn	1 (0)	1 (0)	0 (0)	2	0	3
	Orig → Enhn	0 (0)	0 (0)	0 (1)	1	1	4
#5	Orig → Digt	0 (0)	1 (0)	0 (0)	1	2	3
	Digt → Enhn	1 (0)	1 (1)	0 (0)	0	1	3
	Orig → Enhn	1 (0)	2 (1)	0 (0)	0	1	2
#6	Orig → Digt	0 (1)	0 (0)	0 (2)	1	0	3
	Digt → Enhn	0 (0)	0 (1)	2 (0)	2	0	2
	Orig → Enhn	0 (0)	1 (1)	0 (1)	1	0	3
Average	Orig → Digt	0 (0)	0 (2)	0 (0)	1	1	3
	Digt → Enhn	0 (0)	1 (0)	0 (0)	1	2	3
	Orig → Enhn	0 (0)	1 (2)	0 (0)	1	0	3

C. ROC Analysis of Interval Cancer Cases

Fig. 8 shows the variation of the ROC curves among the three radiologists who interpreted the same set of unprocessed digitized mammograms of interval cancers. Similar variation was observed with the sets of the original film mammograms and the enhanced mammograms. Details of the radiologists' diagnostic performance variations with the original mammograms, unprocessed digitized mammograms, and ANCE-processed mammograms are listed in Table 3 and 4 for the 47 malignant and eight nonmalignant cases, respectively.

It is seen from Table 3 that, on the average (average of individual diagnostic confidence levels), almost half (21) of the 47 malignant cases, which were originally diagnosed as benign (average diagnostic confidence level of less than 2.5) by the three radiologists with the original films, were relabeled as malignant (average diagnostic confidence level of greater than 3.5) with the ANCE-processed

Table 2 Details of Radiologists' Diagnostic Performance Variations with Original Mammograms (Orig), Unprocessed Digitized Mammograms (Digt), and ANCE-processed Digitized Mammograms (Enhn) for the 14 Benign Cases in the Difficult Cases Database. (NOTE: To Obtain the Average Values, the Individual Diagnostic Confidence Levels were Averaged First.)

Radiologist	Image types	B: level 1 or 2;		U: level 3;		M: level 4 or 5	
		U → B (B → U)	M → U (U → M)	M → B (B → M)	B → B	U → U	M → M
#1	Orig → Digt	3 (1)	2 (0)	0 (0)	2	3	3
	Digt → Enhn	1 (2)	0 (1)	0 (1)	2	4	3
	Orig → Enhn	2 (1)	2 (1)	0 (1)	1	3	3
#2	Orig → Digt	1 (0)	0 (1)	0 (0)	5	4	3
	Digt → Enhn	0 (0)	0 (0)	0 (0)	6	4	4
	Orig → Enhn	1 (0)	0 (1)	0 (0)	5	4	3
#3	Orig → Digt	3 (1)	1 (2)	0 (1)	4	1	1
	Digt → Enhn	1 (1)	1 (0)	0 (0)	6	2	3
	Orig → Enhn	2 (1)	1 (2)	0 (0)	5	2	1
#4	Orig → Digt	4 (0)	0 (1)	2 (0)	5	1	1
	Digt → Enhn	0 (2)	0 (0)	0 (0)	9	1	2
	Orig → Enhn	3 (1)	0 (1)	2 (0)	4	2	1
#5	Orig → Digt	3 (1)	1 (1)	1 (1)	2	2	2
	Digt → Enhn	2 (0)	1 (1)	1 (1)	5	1	2
	Orig → Enhn	3 (0)	1 (2)	1 (0)	4	1	2
#6	Orig → Digt	5 (0)	0 (1)	2 (0)	5	0	1
	Digt → Enhn	0 (1)	0 (0)	0 (2)	9	0	2
	Orig → Enhn	4 (1)	0 (2)	2 (1)	3	0	1
Average	Orig → Digt	5 (1)	1 (1)	1 (0)	3	1	1
	Digt → Enhn	1 (1)	0 (1)	0 (0)	8	1	2
	Orig → Enhn	4 (0)	1 (2)	1 (0)	4	1	1

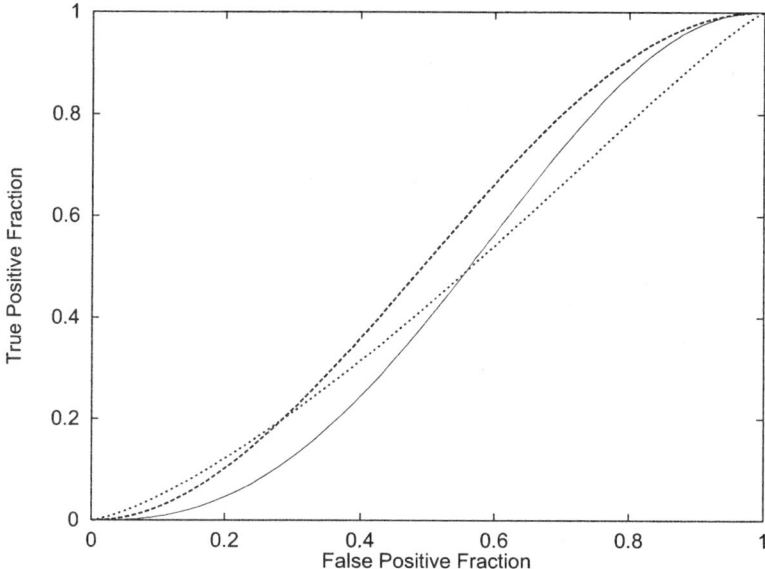

Fig. 8 Variation of conventional ROC curves among three radiologists interpreting the same set of unprocessed digitized mammograms from the Interval Cancer Cases dataset. Reproduced with permission from Rangayyan et al. (4). ©IEEE 1997.

versions. Only three malignant cases whose original average diagnostic confidence levels were greater than 3.5 had their average confidence levels reduced to the range of 2.5 to 3.5 while interpreting the enhanced mammograms. However, in general, no significant changes are observed for the benign cases (Table 4) with the ANCE procedure.

Composite ROC curves for breast cancer diagnosis with the original, unprocessed digitized, and enhanced images are plotted in Fig. 9. The following facts, similar to those described earlier, may be observed in Fig. 9. First, the radiologists' performance with the enhanced versions is the best among the three, especially when FPF is more than 0.3. This is reasonable, because most of the cancer cases in this database were difficult and were initially diagnosed as normal while interpreting the original films. Therefore, the FPF level has to be increased to achieve good sensitivity (high true-positive fraction or TPF). Second, the digitized versions seem to provide better diagnostic results when compared with the original films. This is likely because two printouts for each digitized image with two different print tables (unchanged and lighten2) were provided to the radiologists; the lighten2 table (Fig. 10) provided by Kodak performs some enhancement. Two print tables were used, because the radiologists did not favor the use of the hyperbolic tangent (sigmoid) function, which is an approximate model of an x-ray film system, during initial setup tests. Finally, the values of the area parameter A_z for the original, digitized, and enhanced mammograms were computed to be 0.3906, 0.4682, and 0.5407, respectively. These numbers are much lower than the commonly encountered area values, because the cases selected are difficult cases, and—more importantly—because signs of earlier stages of the interval cancers were either not present on the previous films or were not visible. (The radiologists interpreting the mammograms taken before diagnosis of the cancer had declared that the there was no evidence of cancer on the films; hence the improvement indicated by the ROC curve is significant in terms of diagnostic outcome. This also explains why the area parameter is less than 0.5 for the original and digitized mammograms.) The area parameter could be increased by expanding the set of cases by adding easy-to-diagnose normal cases; this was not done in this study to maintain focus on interval cancer. Regardless, the numerical results confirm our observations and indicate that the ANCE technique can improve sensitivity, thereby allowing the radiologists to diagnose cancer at earlier stages.

Table 3 Details of Radiologists' Diagnostic Performance Variations with Original Mammograms (Orig), Unprocessed Digitized Mammograms (Digt), and ANCE-processed Digitized Mammograms (Enhn) for the 47 Malignant Cases in the Interval Cancer Cases Database. (NOTE: To Obtain the Average Values, the Individual Diagnostic Confidence Levels were Averaged First.)

		Change of diagnostic confidence level					
		B: level 1 or 2;		U: level 3;		M: level 4 or 5	
Radiologist	Image types	B → U (U → B)	U → M (M → U)	B → M (M → B)	B → B	U → U	M → M
#1	Orig → Digt	8 (0)	4 (0)	15 (1)	2	1	16
	Digt → Enhn	0 (0)	9 (0)	2 (0)	0	1	35
	Orig → Enhn	1 (0)	5 (1)	24 (0)	0	0	16
#2	Orig → Digt	8 (0)	7 (0)	5 (0)	4	7	16
	Digt → Enhn	1 (1)	12 (2)	3 (0)	0	3	25
	Orig → Enhn	4 (1)	13 (1)	13 (0)	0	0	15
#3	Orig → Digt	7 (1)	0 (1)	4 (3)	9	6	16
	Digt → Enhn	5 (2)	8 (3)	2 (1)	6	4	16
	Orig → Enhn	6 (0)	4 (3)	8 (3)	6	3	14
Average	Orig → Digt	9 (0)	2 (4)	10 (0)	4	4	14
	Digt → Enhn	1 (0)	14 (2)	3 (0)	0	3	24
	Orig → Enhn	2 (0)	5 (3)	21 (0)	0	1	15

Table 4 Details of Radiologists' Diagnostic Performance Variations with Original Mammograms (Orig), Unprocessed Digitized Mammograms (Digt), and ANCE-processed Digitized Mammograms (Enhn) for the Eight Benign Cases in the Interval Cancer Cases Database. (NOTE: To Obtain the Average Values, the Individual Diagnostic Confidence Levels were Averaged First.)

		Change of diagnostic confidence level					
		B: level 1 or 2;		U: level 3;		M: level 4 or 5	
Radiologist	Image types	U → B (B → U)	M → U (U → M)	M → B (B → M)	B → U	U → M	M → M
#1	Orig → Digt	0 (0)	1 (4)	0 (0)	1	0	2
	Digt → Enhn	0 (1)	1 (0)	0 (0)	0	1	5
	Orig → Enhn	0 (1)	1 (3)	0 (0)	0	1	2
#2	Orig → Digt	0 (0)	1 (0)	0 (0)	1	2	4
	Digt → Enhn	0 (1)	0 (1)	0 (0)	0	2	4
	Orig → Enhn	0 (1)	1 (1)	0 (0)	0	1	4
#3	Orig → Digt	0 (0)	1 (0)	0 (1)	2	1	1
	Digt → Enhn	0 (0)	0 (1)	0 (1)	1	1	1
	Orig → Enhn	0 (0)	0 (0)	0 (2)	1	1	2
Average	Orig → Digt	0 (0)	1 (2)	0 (0)	1	1	3
	Digt → Enhn	0 (1)	1 (1)	0 (0)	0	1	4
	Orig → Enhn	0 (1)	1 (2)	0 (0)	0	1	3

D. McNemar's Tests on Interval Cancer Cases

For the benign cases (averaged) and for the original-to-enhanced, the numbers were too small to provide a valid chi-square statistic for McNemar's test. Therefore, for the benign cases, two tables (digitized-to-enhanced and original-to-enhanced) combined over the three radiologists were tested. No significant difference in diagnostic accuracy was found for the benign cases for either the digitized-to-enhanced table with $p = 0.097$ (Bonferroni adjusted p value $p^* = 0.582$) or for the original-to-enhanced table with $p = 0.0833$ ($p^* = 0.50$).

For each of the four tables for the malignant cases, a significant improvement was observed in the diagnostic accuracy. The various p values are original-to-digitized (combined) $p < 0.001$, $p^* < 0.001$; digitized-to-enhanced (combined) $p = 0.0001$, $p^* = 0.0006$; original-to-digitized (averaged) $p = 0.002$, $p^* = 0.012$; digitized-to-enhanced (averaged) $p = 0.0046$, $p^* = 0.0276$.

In summary, no significant changes were seen in the diagnostic accuracy for the benign control cases. For the malignant cases, a significant improvement was

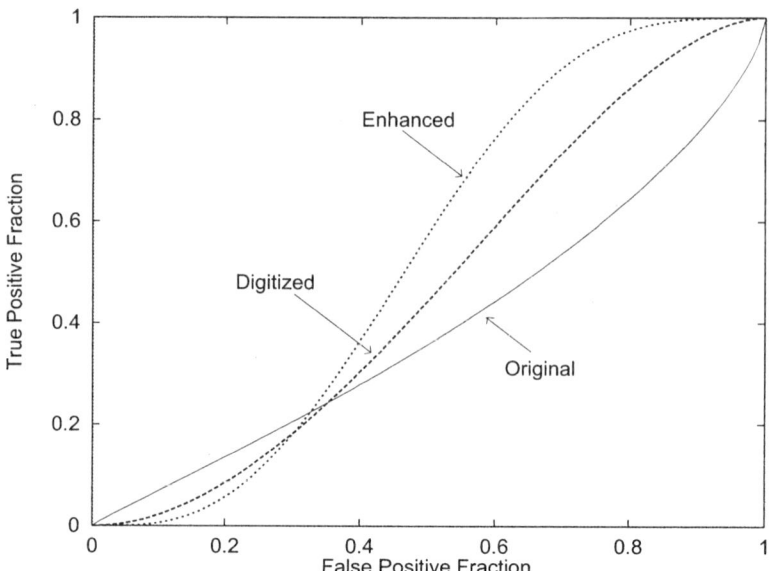

Fig. 9 Comparison of composite ROC curves for the detection of abnormalities by interpreting the original, unprocessed digitized, and enhanced images from the Interval Cancer Cases dataset. Reproduced with permission from Rangayyan et al. (4). ©IEEE 1997.

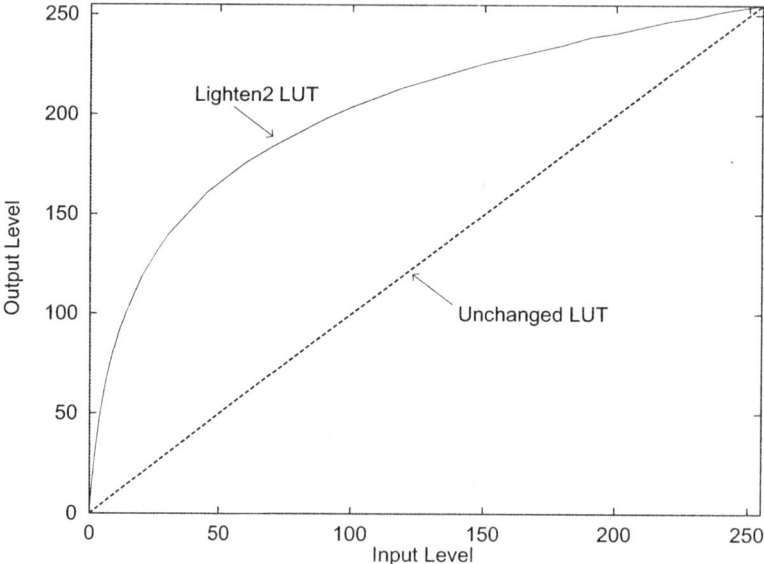

Fig. 10 The two Look-Up-Tables (LUT) used for printing. Reproduced with permission from Rangayyan et al. (4). ©IEEE 1997.

VII. DISCUSSION

The results of the Interval Cancer Cases study indicate that the ANCE method has a positive impact on the interpretation of mammograms in terms of early detection of breast cancer (improved sensitivity). The ANCE-processed mammograms increased the detectability of malignant signs at earlier stages (of the interval cancer cases) compared with the original and unprocessed digitized mammograms. In terms of the average diagnostic confidence levels of three experts, 19 of 28 interval cancer patients were not diagnosed during their earlier mammography tests with the original films only. However, had the ANCE procedure been used, all of these cases would have been diagnosed as malignant at the corresponding earlier times. Only one of six patients initially labeled as having benign disease with the original mammogram films was interpreted as malignant after enhancement. Although the resultant high sensitivity (TPF) comes with increased FPF of more than 0.3, such an improvement in the detection of breast cancer at early stages is important. With the specific Interval Cancer Cases database used, the ANCE technique leads to 38% improvement in overall diagnostic efficiency compared with original films.

Results with the set of Difficult Cases were not as conclusive as the results with the Interval Cancer Cases. Three reasons for this could be (a) lack of familiarity of five of the six radiologists with digitized and enhanced mammographic images; (b) reading the images on a monitor; and (c) use of downsampled images at a lower resolution of 124 µm. Better results may be achieved if the mammograms are digitized and processed with the desired spatial resolution of 50 µm and dynamic range of 0 to 3.0 optical density units and printed at full resolution on film. (No monitor is as yet available to display images of the order of 4096 × 4096 pixels at 12 bits/pixel.)

Results of statistical analysis using McNemar's tests have shown (more conclusively than ROC analysis) that the ANCE procedure has resulted in a statistically significant improvement in the diagnosis of interval cancer cases, with no significant effect on the benign control cases. Statistical tests such as McNemar's test complement ROC analysis in certain circumstances, such as those in this study, involving small numbers of difficult cases. Both methods are useful, because they analyze the results from different perspectives: ROC analysis provides a measure of the accuracy of the procedure in terms of sensitivity and specificity, whereas McNemar's test analyzes the statistical significance and consistency of the change (improvement) in performance. ROC analysis could include a chi-square test of statistical significance, but this was not possible in this study because of the small numbers of cases.

In the study with the Difficult Cases dataset, both the ROC study and statistical analysis using McNemar's tests have shown that the digital versions have led to some improvements in distinguishing benign cases from malignant cases (specificity). However, the improvement in the unprocessed digitized mammograms may have come from the availability of a zooming utility.

The ANCE method was recently used in a preference study comparing the performance of mammographic enhancement algorithms (43). The other methods used in the study were adaptive unsharp masking, contrast-limited adaptive histogram equalization, and wavelet-based enhancement. In most cases with microcalcifications, the ANCE algorithm provided the most preferred results. In the set of images with masses, the unenhanced images were preferred in most of the cases.

Further investigation needs to be conducted by using the hyperbolic tangent (sigmoid) function for printing images, because some visual problems were noticed with the use of two print LUTs in this study. New versions of laser printers (such as the Kodak 8600) can print images of the order of 4096×4096 pixels; this could lead to improved quality in the reproduction of the enhanced images and consequent improved interpretation by radiologists.

Although the ANCE algorithm includes procedures to control noise enhancement, increased noise has been observed in the processed images. Improvements in this direction should lead to better specificity while increasing the sensitivity of breast cancer detection.

The results could also be improved by interpreting a combination of the original or digitized mammograms with their enhanced versions; increased familiarity with the enhanced mammograms may assist the radiologists in the detection of abnormalities. (This was the first experience with digitized mammograms for two of the three reference radiologists involved in the Interval Cancer Cases study and for five of the six experienced radiologists with the Difficult Cases study; no training was provided with the digitized images before the study.)

Digital image enhancement has the potential to dramatically improve the accuracy of breast cancer diagnosis and lead to earlier detection of breast cancer. Investigations are in progress to develop parallel computing strategies to make the ANCE technique applicable in a screening program (44–47).

VIII. SUMMARY

Breast cancer is a leading cause of death among women. Mammography is the best established procedure for breast cancer screening and early diagnosis. However, mammograms are difficult to interpret, especially in cancers at their early stages. The effectiveness of the ANCE technique in increasing breast cancer diagnosis sensitivity was demonstrated in this chapter. The results of ROC analysis show that the radiologists' performance with the ANCE-processed images is the best among the three sets of images (original, digitized, and enhanced) in terms of the area under the ROC curve and that diagnostic sensitivity is improved by the ANCE algorithm. All of the 19 interval cancer cases not detected with the original films of earlier mammographic examinations were diagnosed as malignant with the corresponding ANCE-processed versions, whereas only one of six benign patients initially labeled correctly with the original mammograms was interpreted as malignant after enhancement. McNemar's tests of symmetry indicate that the diagnostic confidence for the Interval Cancer Cases was improved by the ANCE procedure with a high level of statistical significance (p values of 0.0001–0.005) with no significant effect on the diagnosis of the benign control cases (p values of 0.08–0.1). This study demonstrates the potential of diagnostic performance improvement for early detection of breast cancer with appropriate digital image enhancement.

ACKNOWLEDGMENT

This work was supported by the Alberta Breast Cancer Foundation, the Alberta Heritage Foundation for Medical Research, and the Natural Sciences and Engineering Research Council of Canada.

REFERENCES

1. WM Morrow, RB Paranjape, RM Rangayyan, JEL Desautels. Region-based contrast enhancement of mammograms. IEEE Trans Med Imag 11(3):392–406, 1992.
2. RM Rangayyan, L Shen, RB Paranjape, JEL Desautels, JH MacGregor, HF Morrish, P Burrowes, S Share, FR MacDonald. An ROC evaluation of adaptive neighborhood contrast enhancement for digitized mammography. Proceedings of 2nd International Workshop on Digital Mammography, York, UK, July 1994, pp 307–313.
3. L Shen, Y Shen, RM Rangayyan, JEL Desautels, H Bryant, TJ Terry, N Horeczko. Earlier detection of interval breast cancers with adaptive neighborhood contrast enhancement of mammograms. Proceedings of SPIE on Medical Imaging 1996: Image Processing, volume SPIE-2710, Newport Beach, CA, February 1996, pp 940–949.
4. RM Rangayyan, L Shen, Y Shen, JEL Desautels, H Bryant, TJ Terry, N Horeczko, MS Rose. Improvement of sensitivity of breast cancer diagnosis with adaptive neighborhood contrast enhancement of mammograms. IEEE Trans Inform Tech Biomed 1(3):161–170, 1997.
5. DJ Dronkers, HV Zwaag. Photographic contrast enhancement in mammography. Radiol Clin Biol 43:521–528, 1974.
6. MB McSweeney, P Sprawls, RL Egan. Enhanced-image mammography. In: Recent Results in Cancer Research, Vol. 90. Berlin Heidelberg; Springer-Verlag, 1984, pp 79–89.

7. BS Askins, AB Brill, GUV Rao, GR Novak. Autoradiographic enhancement of mammograms. Diagn Radiol 130:103–107, 1979.
8. IN Bankman, ed. Handbook of Medical Imaging: Processing and Analysis. San Diego, CA: Academic Press, 2000.
9. G Ram. Optimization of ionizing radiation usage in medical imaging by means of image enhancement techniques. Med Phys 9(5):733–737, 1982.
10. J Rogowska, K Preston, D Sashin. Evaluation of digital unsharp masking and local contrast stretching as applied to chest radiographs. IEEE Trans Biomed Eng 35(10):817–827, 1988.
11. HP Chan, CJ Vyborny, H MacMahon, CE Metz, K Doi, EA Sickles. ROC studies of the effects of pixel size and unsharp-mask filtering on the detection of subtle microcalcifications. Invest Radiol 22:581–589, 1987.
12. R Gordon, RM Rangayyan. Feature enhancement of film mammograms using fixed and adaptive neighborhoods. Appl Opt 23(4):560–564, 1984.
13. RM Rangayyan, HN Nguyen. Pixel-independent image processing techniques for enhancement of features in mammograms. IEEE/Eighth Annual Conference of the Engineering in Medicine and Biology Society, 1986, pp 1113–1117.
14. WM Morrow. Region-based image processing with application to mammography. Master's thesis, Department of Electrical Engineering, The University of Calgary, Calgary, Alberta, Canada, December 1990.
15. AP Dhawan, G Buelloni, R Gordon. Enhancement of mammographic features by optimal adaptive neighborhood image processing. IEEE Trans Med Imag MI-5(1):8–15, 1986.
16. AP Dhawan, E Le Royer. Mammographic feature enhancement by computerized image processing. Comput Methods Programs Biomed 27:23–35, 1988.
17. TL Ji, MK Sundareshan, H Roehrig. Adaptive image contrast enhancement based on human visual properties. IEEE Trans Med Imag 13(4):573–586, 1994.
18. AF Laine, S Schuler, J Fan, W Huda. Mammographic feature enhancement by multiscale analysis. IEEE Trans Med Imag 13(4):725–740, December 1994.
19. P Vuylsteke, E Schoeters. Multiscale image contrast amplification (MUSICA). Proceedings of SPIE on Medical Imaging 1994: Image Processing, volume SPIE-2167, 1994, pp 551–560.
20. T Belikova, V Lashin, I Zaltsman. Computer assistance in the digitized mammogram processing to improve diagnosis of breast lesions. Proceedings of the 2nd International Workshop on Digital Mammography. York, England, 10–12 July 1994, pp 69–78.
21. G Qu, W Huda, A Laine, B Steinbach, J Honeyman. Use of accreditation phantoms and clinical images to evaluate mammography image processing algorithms. Proceedings of the 2nd International Workshop on Digital Mammography. York, England, 10–12 July 1994, pp 345–354.
22. PG Tahoces, J Correa, M Souto, C Gonzalez, L Gomez, JJ Vidal. Enhancement of chest and breast radiographs by automatic spatial filtering. IEEE Trans Med Imag 10(3):330–335, September 1991.
23. W Qian, LP Clarke, M Kallergi, RA Clark. Tree-structured nonlinear filters in digital mammography. IEEE Trans Med Imag 13(4):25–36, March 1994.

24. J Chen, MJ Flynn, M Rebner. Regional contrast enhancement and data compression for digital mammographic images. Proceedings of SPIE on Biomedical Image Processing and Biomedical Visualization, volume SPIE-1905. San Jose, CA, February 1993, pp 752–758.
25. C Kimme-Smith, RH Gold, LW Bassett, L Gormley, C Morioka. Diagnosis of breast calcifications: Comparison of contact, magnified, and television-enhanced images. Am J Roentgenol 153:963–967, 1989.
26. K Simpson, KW Bowyer. A comparison of spatial noise filtering techniques for digital mammography. Proceedings of the 2nd International Workshop on Digital Mammography. York, England, 10–12 July 1994, pp 325–334.
27. RM Rangayyan, L Shen, RB Paranjape, JEL Desautels, JH MacGregor, HF Morrish, P Burrowes, S Share, FR MacDonald. An ROC evaluation of adaptive neighborhood contrast enhancement for digitized mammography. Proceedings of the 2nd International Workshop on Digital Mammography. York, England, 10–12 July 1994, pp 307–314.
28. M Kallergi, LP Clarke, W Qian, M Gavrielides, P Venugopal, CG Berman, SD Holman-Ferris, MS Miller, RA Clark. Interpretation of calcifications in screen/film, digitized, and wavelet-enhanced monitor-displayed mammograms: A receiver operating characteristic study. Acad Radiol 3:285–293, 1996.
29. A Laine, J Fan, S Schuler. A framework for contrast enhancement by dyadic wavelet analysis. Proceedings of the 2nd International Workshop on Digital Mammography. York, England, 10–12 July 1994, pp 91–100.
30. A Laine, J Fan, WH Yan. Wavelets for contrast enhancement of digital mammography. IEEE Eng Med Biol Magazine 14(5):536–550, September/October 1995.
31. W Qian, LP Clarke, BY Zheng. Computer assisted diagnosis for digital mammography. IEEE Eng Med Biol Magazine 14(5):561–569, September/October 1995.
32. HW Nab, N Karssemeijer, LJTHO van Erning, JHCL Hendriks. Comparison of digital and conventional mammography: A ROC study of 270 mammograms. Med Informat 17:125–131, 1992.
33. RC Gonzalez, RE Woods. Digital Image Processing. Reading, MA: Addison-Wesley Publishing Company, Inc., 1992.
34. EL Hall. Computer Image Processing and Recognition. New York: Academic Press, 1979.
35. RM Nishikawa, ML Giger, K Doi, CE Metz, FF Yin, CJ Vyborny, RA Schmidt. Effect of case selection on the performance of computer-aided detection schemes. Med Phys 21:265–269, 1994.
36. GR Kuduvalli, RM Rangayyan. Performance analysis of reversible image compression techniques for high-resolution digital teleradiology. IEEE Trans Med Imag 11(3):430–445, 1992.
37. JA Swets, RM Pickett. Evaluation of Diagnostic Systems: Methods from Signal Detection Theory. New York: Academic Press, 1982.
38. CE Metz. ROC methodology in radiologic imaging. Invest Radiol 21:720–733, 1986.
39. DD Dorfman, E Alf. Maximum likelihood estimation of parameters of signal detection theory and determination of confidence intervals—rating method data. J Math Psychol 6:487–496, 1969.

40. JL Fleiss. Statistical Methods for Rates and Proportions. 2nd ed. New York: Wiley, 1981.
41. JH Zar. Biostatistical Analysis. 2nd ed. Englewood Cliffs, NJ: Prentice-Hall, 1984.
42. DG Altman. Practical Statistics for Medical Research. London: Chapman & Hall, 1991.
43. R Sivaramakrishna, NA Obuchowski, WA Chilcote, G Cardenosa, KA Powell. Comparing the performance of mammographic enhancement algorithms: A preference study. Am J Roentgenol 175:45–51, 2000.
44. WM Morrow, RM Rangayyan. Implementation of adaptive neighborhood image processing algorithm on a parallel supercomputer. In: Pelletier M, ed. Proceedings of the Fourth Canadian Supercomputing Symposium. Montreal, PQ, Canada, 1990, pp 329–334.
45. RB Paranjape, WA Rolston, RM Rangayyan. An examination of three high performance computing systems for image processing operations. Proceedings of the Supercomputing Symposium. Montreal, PQ, Canada, 1992, pp 208–218.
46. H Alto, D Gavrilov, RM Rangayyan. Parallel implementation of the adaptive neighborhood contrast enhancement algorithm. Proceedings of SPIE on Parallel and Distributed Methods for Image Processing Vol. 3817. 1999, pp 88–97.
47. RM Rangayyan, H Alto, D Gavrilov. Parallel implementation of the adaptive neighborhood contrast enhancement technique using histogram-based image partitioning. J Elect Imag pp 10(3): 804–813, 2001.

10
Computerized Detection of Lung Nodules

Maryellen L. Giger, Samuel G. Armato III, Heber MacMahon, and Kunio Doi
The University of Chicago, Chicago, Illinois

I. INTRODUCTION

Lung cancer is the leading cause of cancer death among both American women and men. The disease is expected to claim the lives of 157,400 Americans in 2001, a figure that represents 25% of cancer deaths among women and 31% of cancer deaths among men (1). Moreover, an anticipated 169,500 new lung cancer cases (13% of all new cancer cases) will be diagnosed in the United States in 2001 (1). Unfortunately, clinical symptoms of lung cancer, such as shortness of breath, chronic cough, and hemoptysis, usually do not occur until the disease has reached a more advanced stage, when patient prognosis is especially poor. The 5-year survival rate for lung cancer patients is only 13% (2).

The primary noninvasive modes for lung cancer detection include sputum cytology, chest radiography, and thoracic computed tomography (CT). Although CT is considered the most sensitive imaging modality for the detection of lung nodules (3), radiation dose and economic considerations maintain chest radiography as the dominant modality for the initial diagnosis of lung cancer, although the use of low-dose helical CT as a lung cancer screening modality is gaining acceptance. Because resection of certain lung cancers at an early stage has been shown to significantly improve survival rate (4), timely radiographic detection of pulmonary nodules is important to the proper management of patients with lung cancer.

The chest radiograph is one of the most challenging radiographs to produce technically and to interpret diagnostically (5,6). The thorax contains anatomical structures that greatly vary in their attenuation of diagnostic-energy x-ray photons. These structures range from air-filled alveoli on one end of the attenuation spectrum to bones and dense soft-tissue structures on the other end. Once this range of normal anatomy is captured by an imaging system with appropriate brightness and contrast, the complex background presented by normal anatomy creates "structured noise" that hinders the detection and interpretation of pulmonary nodules. Nodules may be missed because of obscuration by overlying ribs, bronchi, blood vessels, the cardiac silhouette, or other normal anatomical structures (7–10).

In a study of missed bronchogenic carcinoma at chest radiography, anatomical structures (predominantly bones) obscured the missed cancer in all 27 patients (10). When the radiographs were shown to six independent radiologists who were told that the cases represented missed cancers, 73% of the lesions were missed by at least one of these radiologists. The average miss rate for the radiographic detection of early lung nodules is estimated to be about 30% (11). In a lung cancer screening study, 90% of identified peripheral lung carcinomas were visible in retrospect even though three physicians had interpreted previous radiographs acquired at 4-month intervals as normal (7). Of these retrospectively identifiable lesions, 40% had been visible for more than one year prior to the time of initial diagnosis. Clearly, radiographic diagnosis poses a difficult challenge for radiologists.

Nodule detection errors have been attributed to faulty processing of image information in the perception and cognition domains of the observer (12). Reasons for failure to detect nodules have been categorized as scanning errors, recognition errors, and decision-making errors (12). A scanning error occurs when the observer fails to fixate a nodule within the visual field of view. Even when the nodule is scanned by the visual field, however, the observer may not recognize the abnormal features contained within the field. The result is an error in recognition. A decision-making error will occur when the abnormal features of the fixated region are recognized by the observer but then rejected as insignificant. It is within this psychological paradigm of fixation, recognition, and decision making that human observers must operate to successfully perform a detection task.

It has been shown that visual dwell times can predict the location of nodules in chest radiographs (13–15). Gaze durations for missed nodules were significantly longer than for regions with no lesion present. This perception-based method to facilitate the recognition of pulmonary nodules was then investigated as an aid to nodule detection (16). The computer-assisted method indicated regions on chest images that had received prolonged visual attention during the initial viewing of each image. Results from the observer study demonstrated a 16% improvement in nodule-detection performance when, during a second viewing of the images, observers were provided with dwell-time feedback.

Image analysis may also be performed by computers for the purpose of detecting signals (i.e., lung nodules) on complex backgrounds (i.e., normal anatomy). Indeed, the very nature of the radiological process, from the technical, image acquisition aspect to the clinical, diagnostic evaluation aspect, makes it uniquely amenable to the logic used by computers. The quantitative processing of a computer is inherently distinct from the qualitative nature of the human eye–brain system so that a computerized scheme may be designed to exploit characteristics of a structure in an image even though these characteristics may not be normally recognized by human observers. Consequently, computers have the potential to complement human observers. Thus, the interpretation of radiographical chest images may benefit from image processing and computer-aided diagnostic methods that direct radiologists' attention to suspect regions in an attempt to overcome scanning and recognition errors.

Computer-aided diagnosis (CAD) can be defined broadly as a diagnosis made by an individual who incorporates output from a computer into his or her medical decision-making process. Such computer output could take the form of a processed (i.e., enhanced) version of an original image, a superimposed symbol such as an arrow that indicates the location of a suspected lesion in the image, a numerical value that indicates, for example, the likelihood of malignancy of a suspected lesion, text that describes characteristics of the lesion as "seen" by the computer, a visual presentation of other lesions from a standardized database that have similar characteristics to the lesion in question, or a suggested diagnosis based on clinical and image data.

Potchen and Austin have stated that "despite attempts to improve on the imaging system, the ability to systematically detect pulmonary nodules in large screening series has not changed much" (17). They suggest a focus on the human factors that play a role in radiographic interpretation. Computerized approaches to image analysis address this issue by directing radiologists' attention to computer-identified regions of suspicion. Use of image processing techniques and CAD systems have been shown to improve radiologists' detection accuracy for lung nodules in chest radiographs (18,19), as well as for breast masses and clustered microcalcifications in mammograms (20,21). Today, the availability of high-speed computers and high-quality, high-resolution digital image acquisition systems (i.e., film digitizers, computed radiography [CR], and digital "flat panel" detectors) make possible near-real-time processing of chest images to facilitate their interpretation.

In this chapter, we present an overview of current research for the improvement of lung nodule detection through enhanced (processed) images for human vision and through automated image analysis for computer vision.

II. IMAGE PROCESSING TECHNIQUES FOR LUNG NODULE ENHANCEMENT

Image processing refers to manipulation of the gray level information contained within the pixels of a digital image. The result is image output intended for either human interpretation or further computer analysis. The latter option effectively results in the automation of the detection task and is termed "computer vision." One goal of medical image processing is to increase the conspicuity of a lesion or region of interest within the image, where lesion conspicuity may be defined as the ratio of the lesion contrast to the complexity of the surround (22). Accordingly, a computerized method may be developed that either preferentially increases the relative contrast of nodule like structures in an image or reduces the apparent complexity of the surrounding background anatomy. Once processed, the enhanced image may be viewed by a radiologist either as soft copy on a computer monitor or as hard copy on film. This section presents examples of some common image processing techniques that have been investigated for use in chest radiography for subsequent image display and human interpretation.

A. Exposure Correction

Computerized methods for the correction of underexposed and overexposed chest radiographs have been developed to decrease the number of repeat exposures that may be required (23–25), thereby reducing dose to patients and costs to radiology departments. Such techniques are especially useful for hospital intensive care units in which correct exposure levels are more difficult to obtain with portable radiography equipment, and daily chest films for a patient are required. By normalizing the optical densities of each film, variation between sequential images is reduced. The resulting consistency among the radiographs also facilitates the day-to-day comparison of sequential films for the evaluation of temporal change.

Thoracic anatomy poses technical challenges for plain film chest radiography. In particular, the presence of tissues with a wide range of attenuation properties requires a screen-film system with a wide exposure latitude. For a given range of film optical densities, however, wide latitude is achieved at the expense of contrast. Moreover, an improperly exposed radiograph could force a lung nodule to appear in the nonlinear "toe" or "shoulder" regions of the screen-film system's characteristic curve. A nodule in one of these regions would demonstrate severely reduced contrast that may render the nodule imperceptible. Automated compensation for such exposure errors could serve to bring pulmonary structures (including nodules) within the linear portion of the characteristic curve and improve detectability.

One exposure correction technique involves initial digitization of a conventional radiograph. Next, a nonlinear density-correction technique, based on the characteristic curves of both the original radiographic film and the digitizer, is used to compensate for improperly exposed radiographs. Fig. 1 illustrates the comparison of gray-level histograms of the same "phantom" radiograph acquired at three different exposure levels. It should be noted that the three histograms will have the same shape in terms of "logarithm of relative exposure," but they will differ in terms of pixel values because of the nonlinear relationship between exposure and pixel value as expressed by the characteristic curve. A "lookup table" can be created to represent this nonlinear relationship (25). Fig. 2 illustrates (a) an original portable chest radiograph that was overexposed 400% relative to the proper level and (b) the digitized chest image after correction (23). Similarly, Fig. 3 illustrates (a) an original portable chest radiograph with an underexposure equivalent to 50% of the proper exposure level and (b) the digitized chest image after correction (23).

The problem of limited exposure latitude in screen/film combinations is solved with CR systems based on storage phosphor technology (26). The physical phenomenon of storage phosphor systems is referred to as photostimulable luminescence, and the intensity of the stimulated luminescence is proportional to the number of x-ray photons absorbed by the storage phosphor. Storage phosphor systems have an exposure latitude that spans a factor of approximately 10,000 (27) compared with approximately 50 to 200 for screen/film systems. Therefore, CR systems are used widely for portable chest radiography to compensate for the

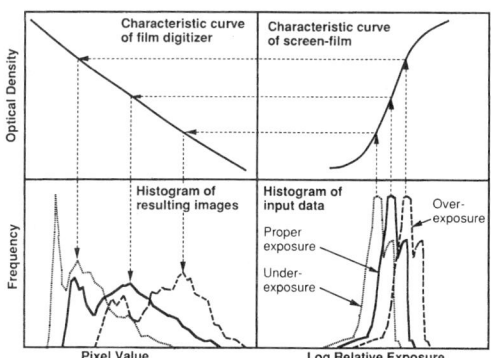

Fig. 1 Schematic diagram illustrating the comparison of pixel value histograms for the same patient radiographs from acquired at three different exposures. Reprinted with permission from Ref. 25 (Fig. 1).

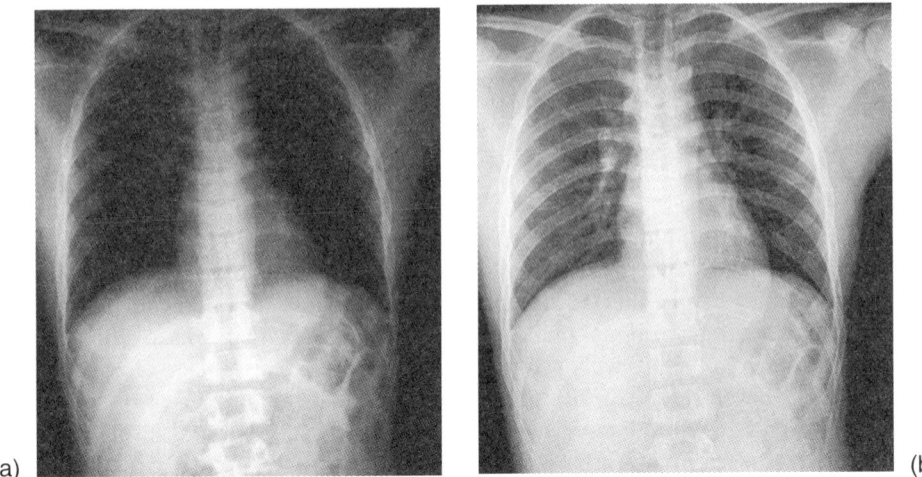

Fig. 2 (a) Original portable chest radiograph with an overexposure level of 400% of the proper level. (b) Digitized processed chest radiograph that provides markedly improved diagnostic quality. Reprinted with permission from Ref. 23 (Fig. 2).

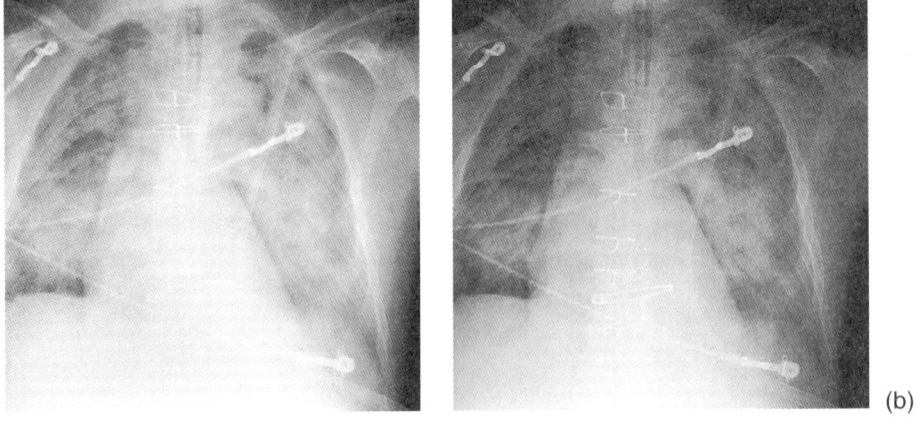

Fig. 3 (a) Original portable chest radiograph with an underexposure level of 50% of the proper exposure level. (b) Digitized processed chest radiograph that is diagnostically superior, especially for mediastinal and upper abdominal detail. Reprinted with permission from Ref. 23 (Fig. 3).

overexposure and underexposure errors that commonly occur. Similar benefits are offered by solid-state image capture devices that have become commercially available. These technologies include systems based on amorphous selenium and amorphous silicon (28–30).

B. Unsharp Mask Filtering

Digital unsharp mask filtering is a technique that is routinely used in computed radiography systems to increase local contrast and enhance the visibility of fine-detail structures (31,32). It is most extensively used in digital chest radiography.

The linear form of unsharp mask filtering can be expressed as:

$$D_p(x,y) = D_o(x,y) + K [D_o(x,y) - D_{us}(x,y)]$$

where $D_o(x,y)$ corresponds to the original two-dimensional digital image, and $D_p(x,y)$ corresponds to the final processed image. $D_{us}(x,y)$ refers to a blurred version (an "unsharp mask") of $D_o(x,y)$ and includes mainly the low spatial frequency components of the original image. The size of the kernel used to produce the unsharp image determines the spatial frequency range that is enhanced, and the weighting factor, K, determines the magnitude of enhancement. Fig. 4 shows (a) an original digitized chest radiograph and (b) the same image highly enhanced with linear unsharp masking. Note that the highly enhanced image (b) amplifies the interstitial lung texture to such a degree that incorrect image interpretation may result.

To compensate for overenhancement of certain anatomical regions, some investigators have found it advantageous to perform nonlinear unsharp mask filtering in which the degree of enhancement depends on the original local optical density of the film. Accordingly, enhancement is dependent on the underlying anatomy, so that maximum processing would be applied to low optical density regions such as the mediastinum, and minimum processing would be applied to high optical density regions such as the peripheral lung region. Fig. 4c illustrates such processing on the chest image from Fig. 4a. More recently, multiscale unsharp masking techniques have been developed to selectively enhance detail across the image at different resolutions (33), and dynamic range control techniques have been implemented to restore visible detail in high- or low-density regions (34).

C. Temporal Subtraction

In conventional clinical practice, radiologists commonly refer to a patient's previous chest films while interpreting the current radiographs to identify changes over time (35). This approach aids in the identification of new disease. Such sequential radiographs also provide a means for assessing the progression or the re-

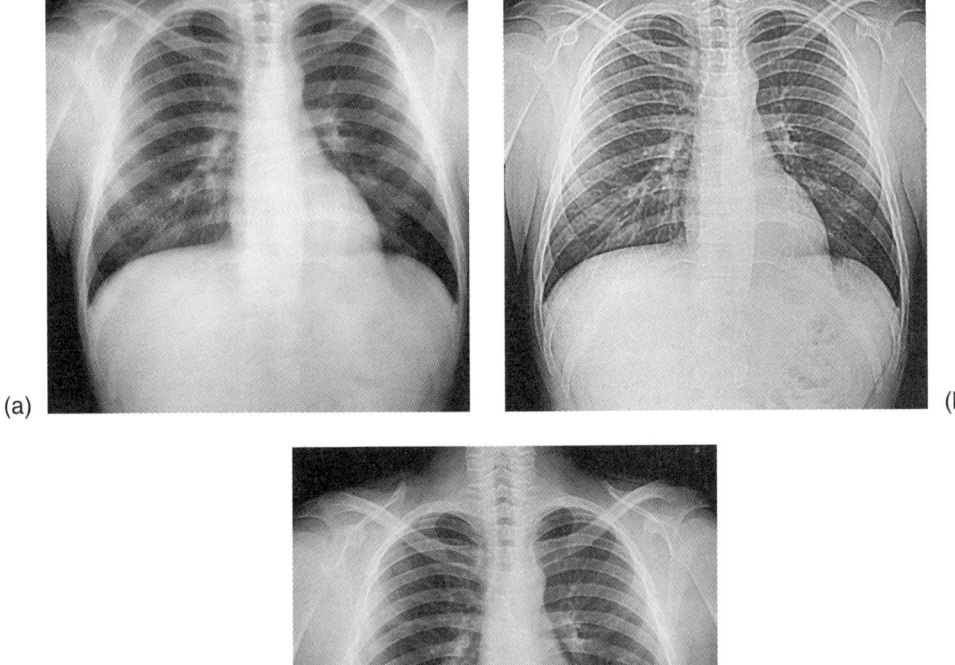

Fig. 4 Example of (a) an original digitized chest radiograph, (b) the same image processed with linear unsharp masking, and (c) the same image processed with moderate nonlinear unsharp masking.

sponse to treatment of a known abnormality. Comparison among sequential radiographs may be facilitated through introduction of a "difference image" into the decision-making process. Once previous and current chest images are obtained in digital format (either directly through, for example, a CR system or indirectly through the digitization of analog films), the previous chest radiograph can be registered with and subtracted from the current chest radiograph. The resulting difference image tends to enhance areas of temporal change by suppressing the background on which abnormalities are superimposed.

Various investigators have reported on such difference imaging techniques (36–38). Kano et al. (37) developed a subtraction method for sequential chest radiographs that consists of an automatic registration technique based on nonlinear geometric warping followed by digital subtraction. Initially, the chest images are processed by the density-correction method described earlier. Next, regions of interest (ROIs) are located in each of the two subsampled chest images (500 × 500-pixel matrix, 0.7-mm effective pixel dimension). A local cross-correlation technique is used to locally match the ROIs. The associated shifts between the (x,y) coordinates of the two chest images are subjected to a two-dimensional curve-fitting algorithm with 10th-order polynomials. The fitted shift values are used to create a warped version of the previous chest image, which is then subtracted from the current chest image. Fig. 5 shows original digital images of (a) a current chest film and (b) a previous chest film of the same patient (37). Fig. 5c contains the subtraction image after use of the nonlinear warping technique. A subtle nodule is more easily perceived in the subtraction image. The usefulness of this technique is its potential to enhance the appearance of subtle lesions that may develop during the time between acquisition of the previous and current radiographs.

In a receiver operating characteristic (ROC) study (39), Difazio et al. (40) evaluated the effects of temporal subtraction images on the detection of interval change. Observers' performances when viewing paired digitized chest radiographs (the current and previous radiographs) were compared with their performances when the paired digitized chest radiographs were viewed together with a temporal subtraction image. Statistically significant improvement was reported in the detection of abnormalities greater than 1 cm in size when the observers were given the paired chest radiographs (current and previous) together with the temporal subtraction image (Fig. 6). In addition, the mean interpretation time decreased by 19% when the temporal subtraction images were used (40).

D. Dual-Energy Imaging

A recurrent theme in radiography is that visual perception of lesions in radiographic images may be limited because of overlying normal anatomical structures. Another means of suppressing "structured noise" caused by the normal anatomical background is dual-energy imaging. In dual-energy imaging, two images of the patient are obtained simultaneously (or nearly so), each produced by x-ray beams with effectively different mean energies. These individual images are then combined to form tissue-selective images such as a soft-tissue image or a bone image (41–44). In a soft-tissue-selective image, for example, calcium-containing

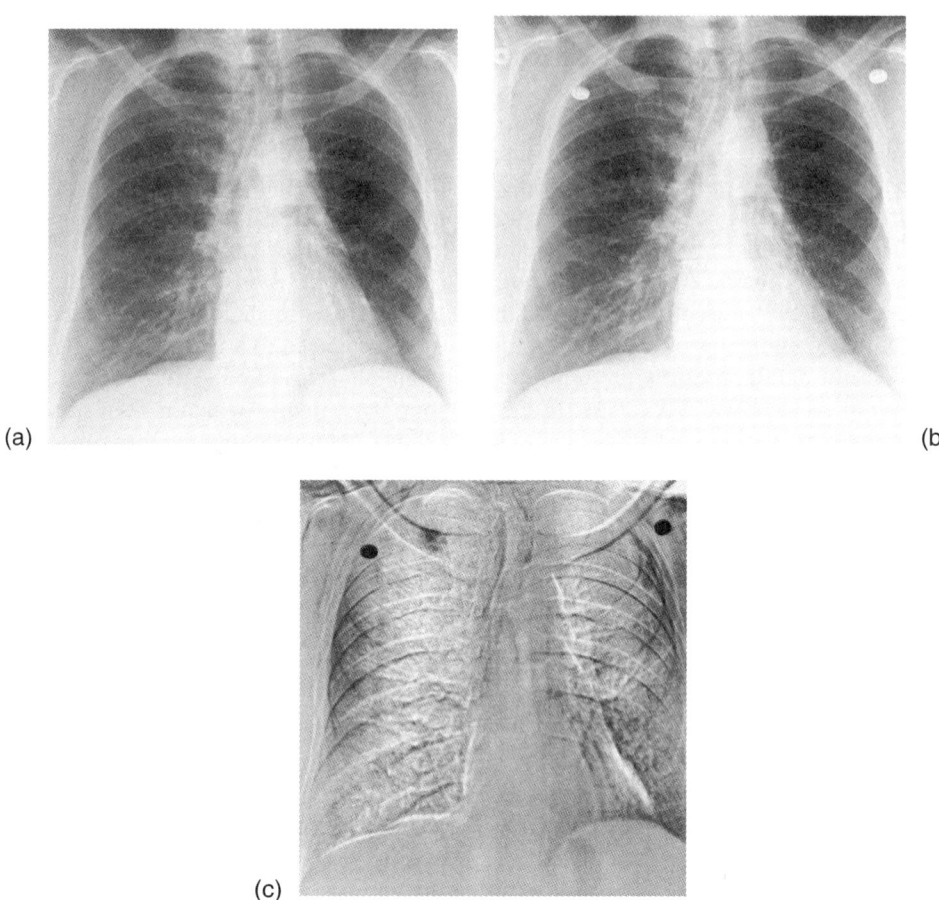

Fig. 5 A chest radiograph (a) shows a faint right upper lobe nodule. A previous radiograph (b) was used as a subtraction mask to produce a difference image (c). The nodule is substantially more conspicuous in the subtraction image (c) than in the current image. Reprinted with permission from Ref. 40 (Fig. 2).

structures such as the ribs and vertebral bodies are suppressed to yield improved visualization of the lungs. This technique has the potential to greatly improve the detectability of nodules. Furthermore, dual-energy imaging is uniquely able to assist in the identification of calcified lesions, which may aid radiologists in diagnosing detected lung nodules as either benign or malignant.

The energy separation needed for dual-energy imaging can be obtained through either (a) a double-exposure technique in which the peak x-ray energy is changed or (b) a single-exposure technique that uses paired detectors (such as photostimulable phosphor plates) separated by a beam-attenuating filter (41). The front detector records the low-energy component of the beam, and, after the filter serves to harden the x-ray beam, the rear detector records the high-energy component of the beam. Methods for combining the low- and high-energy images include scatter correction techniques, improved basis material decomposition algorithms, and noise suppression techniques (45).

Various researchers have applied dual-energy imaging to chest radiography to improve the detection of pulmonary nodules and to distinguish between malignant and benign lesions (41,43). Fig. 7 illustrates a set of dual-energy CR images for a patient with a left-upper-lobe pulmonary nodule: (a) the conventional chest radiograph, (b) the soft-tissue image, and (c) the bone image. These images were acquired from a CR system with photostimulable phosphor plates.

In an ROC study, investigators compared conventional chest radiography with dual-energy CR (43). In this study involving five observers and images from 60 patients, significant improvements were found in the observers' ability to diagnose pulmonary nodules and to characterize calcified nodules with dual-energy CR. In another observer study in which a chest phantom was used, investigators compared conventional chest radiography with the two types of dual-energy chest radiography (i.e., the single-exposure technique and the double-exposure tech-

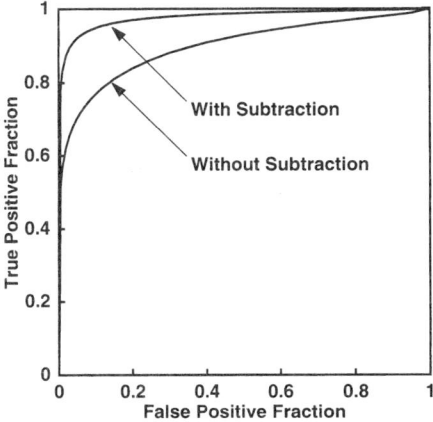

Fig. 6 ROC curves illustrating the statistically significant improvement in radiologists' performance when the radiologists used the temporally subtracted chest image during their interpretation. Reprinted with permission from Ref. 40 (Fig. 7).

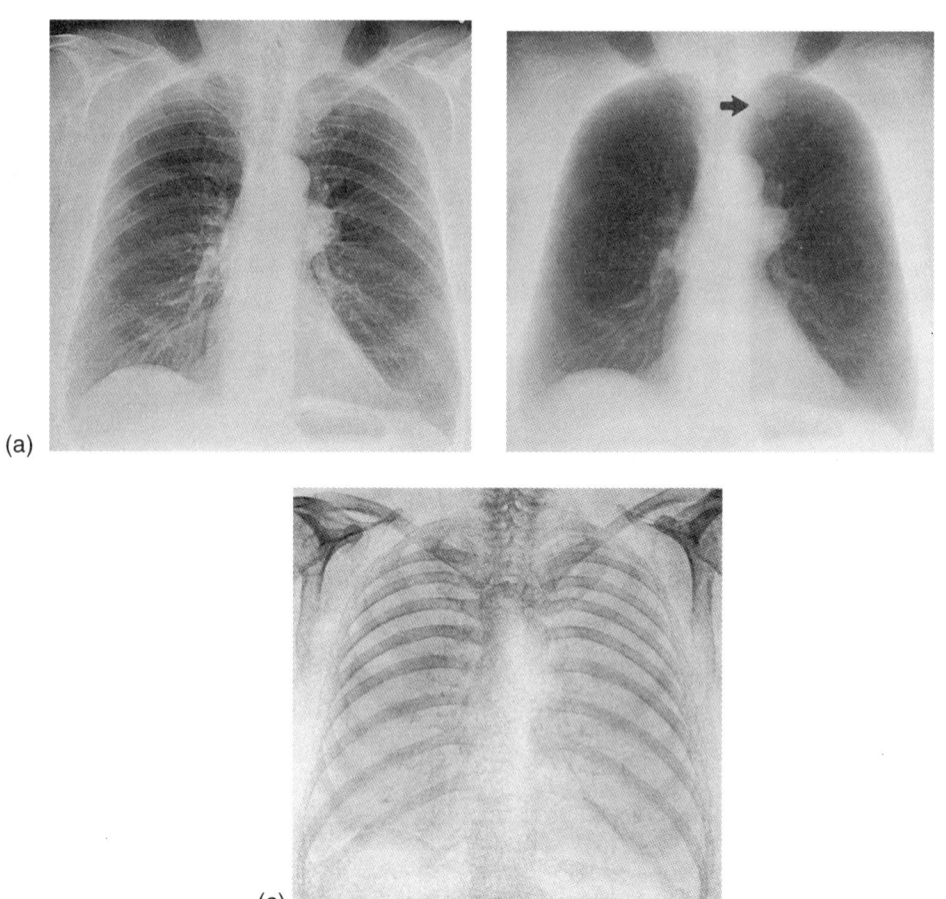

Fig. 7 A set of dual-energy computed radiography images obtained from a single-exposure system for a patient with a left upper lobe pulmonary nodule. (a) The image captured by the photostimulable phosphor plate closest to the patient is virtually equivalent to a standard chest radiograph, (b) tissue-selective image showing the nodule without obscuration from overlying ribs, and (c) bone-selective image in which the noncalcified nodule cannot be visualized.

nique) (46). They found that both dual-energy techniques yielded observer performances superior to conventional chest radiography. Although differences between the single- and double-exposure dual-energy techniques did not achieve statistical significance, these investigators preferred the single-exposure technique for reasons such as ease of implementation, reduced patient exposure, and reduced motion artifacts.

III. COMPUTERIZED DETECTION OF LUNG NODULES

Computer vision seeks to automate a particular detection task. Through the integration of image processing, image segmentation, feature extraction, and decision analysis techniques (47), computerized medical image analysis systems attempt to identify normal and abnormal structures based on their radiographic characteristics in a digital image. The development of computer vision methods requires information about the physical properties of the radiographic image acquisition system and the range of expected radiographic appearances of both the abnormality under investigation and the associated anatomical background on which the abnormality is expected to be superimposed. Thus, a database composed of a large number of cases is needed to cover the broad range of abnormal and normal patterns.

The development of CAD methods is timely in the sense that digital chest radiography is routinely used in some medical centers and is on the threshold of widespread clinical use. Thus, CAD techniques that have been developed for images derived from digitized film may be calibrated instead for images that have been acquired digitally. These computerized schemes then may be automatically and routinely applied to the images between the time of acquisition and interpretation. The potential significance of CAD lies in the fact that if the detectability of cancer and other diseases can be increased through computerized methods designed to assist radiologists, then the treatment of patients can be initiated earlier with an anticipated concomitant improvement in prognosis.

Many investigators are involved in the development and evaluation of CAD methods for chest radiography. In the following sections, a few examples are used to illustrate the potential use of CAD for the detection of lung nodules in chest radiographs and in thoracic CT images.

A. Lung Segmentation

Segmentation of the lung fields in chest radiographs initiates most computerized schemes developed for the detection of pulmonary disease, including lung nodules (Fig. 8). Because nodule-detection methods are effectively trained to recognize specific deviations from the normal radiographic appearance of pulmonary anatomy, application of these schemes to regions outside the lungs would provide meaningless information and would greatly increase computation time. Investigators have developed a variety of lung segmentation schemes for posteroanterior (PA) (48–59) and lateral chest radiographs (60,61). In one such method, an itera-

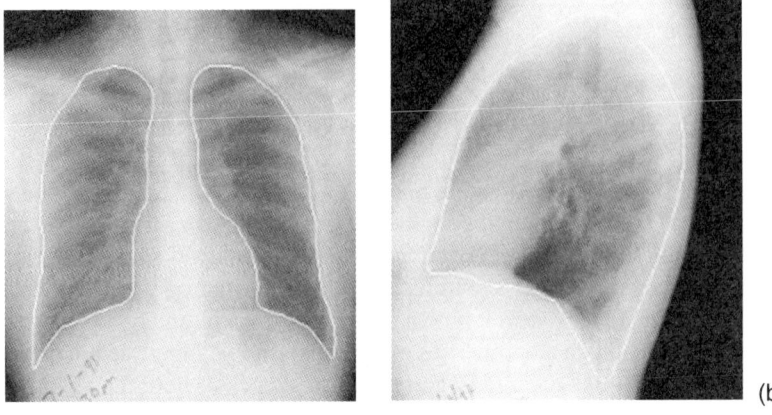

Fig. 8 Example of accurately segmented lung regions in (a) a PA chest image and (b) a lateral chest image. (a) reprinted with permission from Ref. 58 (Fig. 12).

tive global gray-level thresholding scheme was used to identify an initial set of lung segmentation contours (58). To more completely capture the aerated lung regions, local gray-level thresholding was then applied within regions of interest placed along these initial contours. Another method analyzed the first and second derivatives of gray-level profiles to delineate the rib cage edge (55). Polynomial functions were then fit to these initially detected edges.

B. Plain Chest Radiographs

Among the first computerized analyses of chest radiographs for the detection of lung tumors were techniques based on edge detection and contrast enhancement (62,63) and methods based on a hierarchical process that incorporated a ladderlike decision tree (64,65). Since then, many investigators have developed and evaluated computerized lung nodule detection methods for single-projection chest radiographs based on mathematical morphology (66,67), fractal analysis (68), artificial neural networks (69–73), rule-based methods (74), multiscale approaches (75,76), and wavelet-based deformable contour methods (77). Toriwaki et al. (63) and Hashimoto et al. (78) used edge detection approaches in conjunction with gray-level thresholding to locate suspect lesions in chest images. Giger et al. (79,80) initially reported on a background suppression approach for the computerized detection of lung nodules in digitized chest radiographs. This technique, which involved creation of a signal-enhanced version and a signal-suppressed version of the original image, attempted to remove the structured anatomical background before application of feature analysis. Fig. 9 illustrates (a) an original digitized chest radiograph, (b) the corresponding difference image, and (c) the difference image after a

Computerized Detection of Lung Nodules

specific gray-level threshold has been applied (80). The arrow indicates the location of an actual nodule. The number of false-positive detections from the computerized scheme was substantially reduced through the combination of rule-based classifiers and an artificial neural network (ANN) that merged various geometric- and edge-gradient-orientation–based features (66,73,81).

A radiographic feature that has been successfully used to differentiate nodules from false-positive detections is the edge-gradient orientation (Fig. 10) (81).

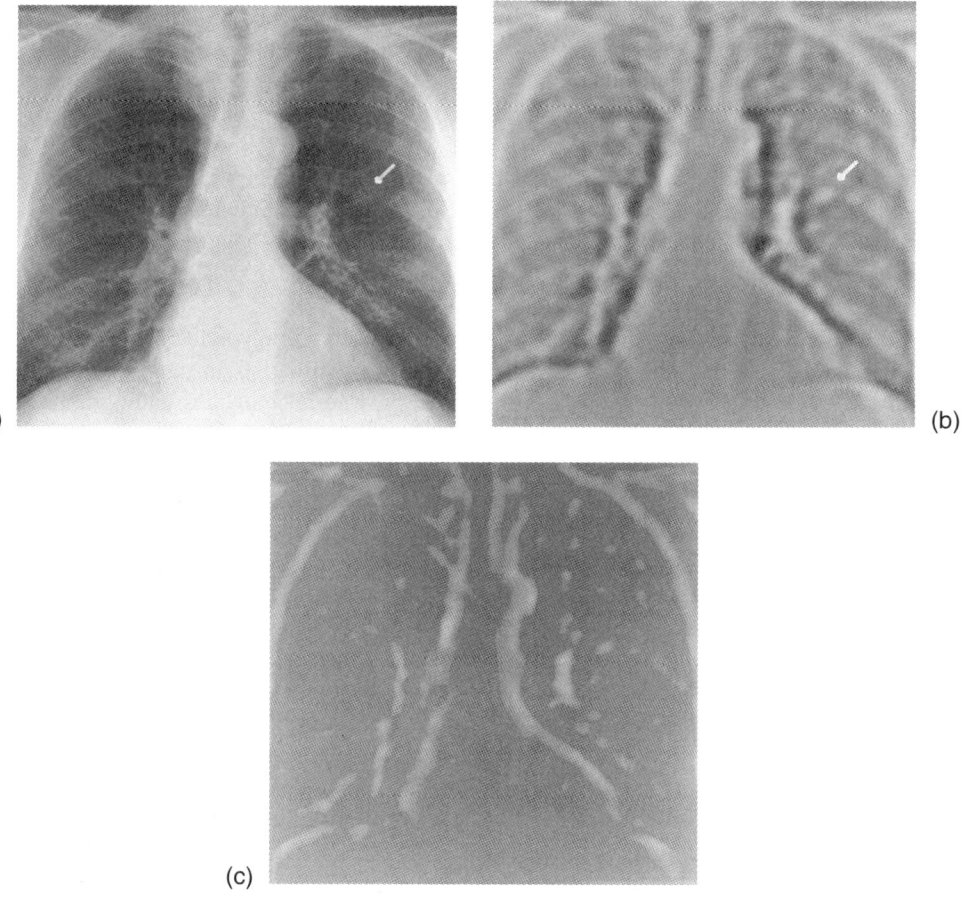

Fig. 9 Example of (a) an original digitized chest radiograph with a 1-cm nodule in the left lung (arrow), (b) the difference image obtained using a 9-mm-diameter nodule-matched filter and an 18-mm ring-shaped averaging filter for enhancement and suppression, respectively, and (c) the difference image after gray-level thresholding. Reprinted with permission from Ref. 80 (Figs. 3a, d, and 5b).

The center of a suspected nodule is automatically identified, and the magnitude and direction of the maximum edge gradient is computed for each pixel within a 50 × 50-pixel ROI. A histogram of accumulated edge gradients as a function of the angle (with respect to the x-axis) associated with this gradient direction is then constructed. Trends in the shape of such a cumulative edge-gradient–orientation histogram are used to determine whether the suspected region is actually a nodule. Fig. 10 shows the cumulative edge-gradient–orientation histograms (c and d) for (a) a lung nodule and (b) the intersection of a rib and the clavicle (81). The peaks in the edge-gradient–orientation histogram for the rib crossing correspond to the strong gradients along the rib edges. More recently, a similar technique based on radial edge-gradient analysis (82) has been used to improve the specificity of lung nodule detection methods (83).

The ultimate test of any computerized analysis scheme will be its ability to actually improve radiologists' performance when used as a clinical aid. CAD uses the computer as a "second opinion," not as a stand-alone reader; therefore, a computerized method need not be perfect to be useful. A CAD scheme may be beneficial even with an overall accuracy less than that of a radiologist, because the lesions detected by the computer will typically not coincide completely with those detected by the human observer.

Observer performance studies have been carried out in which output from a computer detection scheme was incorporated by radiologists in their decision-making process. In the task of detecting pulmonary nodules in chest radiographs, a statistically significant improvement was obtained when the locations of computer-suspected nodules were provided to radiologists during their interpretation (19). In that study, the computer performed at a sensitivity of 75% with approximately one false-positive detection per image. Fig. 11 shows a comparison of the areas under the ROC curve (denoted A_z) for all observers in the study. Gray shading represents A_z values when only the conventional chest radiographs were interpreted, and diagonal stripes correspond to the increase in A_z values attained in conjunction with the CAD method. The gain in performance achieved through the use of CAD was larger for residents than it was for thoracic and general radiologists. Fig. 12 shows a comparison of average reading time for the observers. Overall, reading time decreased slightly when the computer aid was used (Fig. 12). The observation of decreased reading time is notable, because it counters the perceived notion that CAD will increase interpretation time caused by the additional information that radiologists must assimilate.

To facilitate introduction of CAD results into the routine clinical interpretive process, investigators are developing intelligent workstations that incorporate CAD results derived from chest radiographs (84,85). Images and their corresponding CAD results are displayed in a format that can be reviewed rapidly in conjunction with conventional interpretation. Radiographs are either digitized or digital radiographs are transferred from sources such as CR systems or image archives. CAD analyses are then run automatically using distributed computing

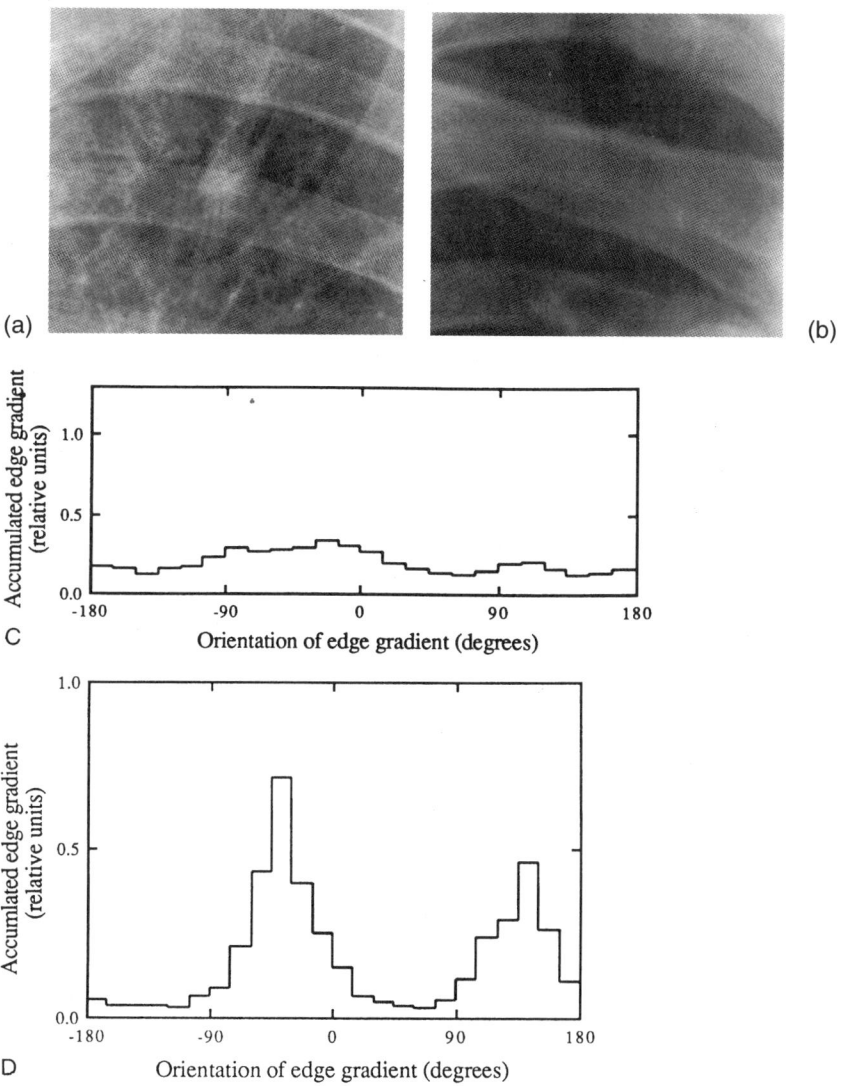

Fig. 10 (a) A region from an original digitized chest radiograph containing an actual nodule and (c) its corresponding gradient-orientation distribution. (b) A region from an original digitized chest radiograph containing a rib-clavicle crossing that was erroneously detected as a nodule (a false positive) by the computer and (d) its corresponding gradient-orientation distribution. Reprinted with permission from Ref. 81 (Figs. 1a, 8a, 4a, 8b).

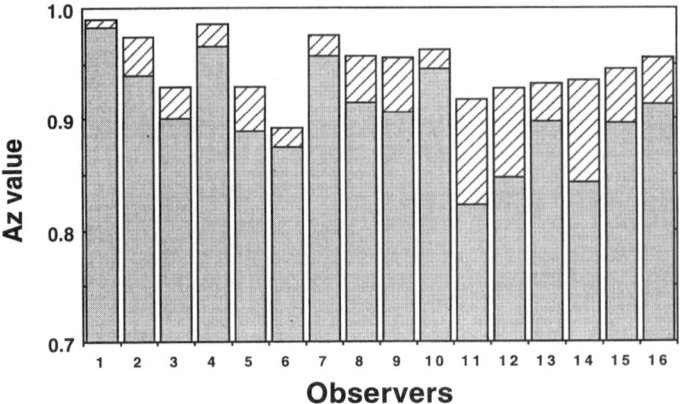

Fig. 11 Graphs showing comparison of A_z values for all observers in the nodule detection study. Gray shading represents A_z values when only the conventional chest radiographs were interpreted, and diagonal stripes correspond to the increase in A_z values achieved in conjunction with the CAD method. Observers 1,2 = Thoracic radiologists, 3–8 = general radiologist, 9–16 = residents in radiology. Reprinted with permission from Ref. 19 (Fig. 5).

based on a client-server model. The results are available for the radiologist on the workstation during the reading session. Pilot studies have indicated that such a workstation is user-friendly and provides beneficial information to the radiologist in a timely and efficient manner (84).

It should be noted that although these CAD methods have been developed specifically for PA chest radiographs, important diagnostic information is also

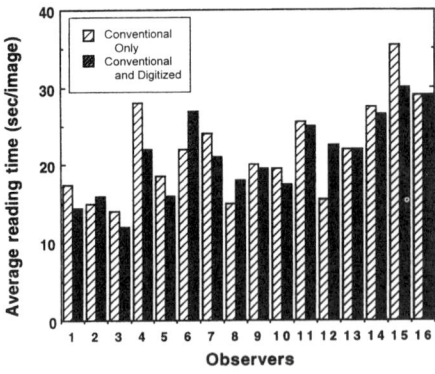

Fig. 12 Graph showing comparison of average interpretation time for all observers participating in the nodule detection study. Average interpretation time was reduced, for most observers, when CAD was used. Reprinted with permission from Ref. 19 (Fig. 6).

demonstrated in lateral radiographs. The lateral view is a routine component of a standard radiographic chest examination and provides a perspective of pulmonary anatomy and pathology that complements the PA view. In a study of missed bronchogenic carcinoma at chest radiography, for example, the lateral projection was judged to demonstrate the missed lesion better than the PA projection in 4 of 23 cases, including 1 case in which the PA radiograph did not show the lesion (10). The missed lesion did not appear in the lateral radiograph in only 2 of the 23 cases. It is possible that future development of lung nodule detection schemes for lateral radiographs will improve on the performance of current PA-image–based CAD methods.

C. CT Images of the Thorax

It is widely recognized that the sensitivity of thoracic computed tomography (CT) scans for the visualization of lung nodules is superior to that of plain chest radiographs (86–88). For this reason, the CT scan is generally regarded as the "gold standard" by which the presence of nodules is confirmed for the purpose of evaluating truth in studies involving PA radiographs. The most important advantage that CT offers over plain radiography is its ability to distinctly represent anatomical structures that would otherwise radiographically project in superposition. The practical consequence of this fundamental difference in imaging approaches is that the average size of peripheral cancers on CT scans missed by radiologists is 3 mm compared with 13 mm at radiography (89–90).

A potential disadvantage of conventional CT is the risk that differences in patient respiration between acquisitions of contiguous sections could result in a scan that fails to image portions of the anatomy (91). Conventional CT uses a "step-and-shoot" protocol in which each CT section image is successively obtained after the patient table is indexed to the next position within the scanner, and the patient is asked to maintain a breath hold. Consequently, the patient table is motionless during the acquisition of each section image, and the patient breathes between sections. The development of helical (or spiral) CT scanning procedures (92) allows for the recording of volumetric data in a single breath hold through simultaneous data acquisition and patient translation. These data are then reconstructed to yield section images, and the planes of reconstruction may be specified after data acquisition (93). This ability to retrospectively define the planes of reconstruction in helical CT has been shown to improve the detectability of lung nodules (94). Accordingly, helical CT may provide the most reliable method for detecting pulmonary nodules (95).

Increased sensitivity of helical CT over conventional CT with regard to identification of lung nodules has been observed (95–97). Remy-Jardin et al. (95) reported a significantly higher mean number of nodules seen per patient with helical versus conventional CT and a corresponding significantly higher mean number of nodules less than 5 mm in diameter. Costello et al. (97) reported four additional nodules detected on helical CT than were detected on conventional CT for 20 patients who underwent both procedures. On the basis of both phantom and clinical studies, Milla et al. (96) found that CT demonstrated a sensitivity for the detection of nodules less than 5 mm that was higher than conventional screen-film chest radiography, advanced multiple beam equalization radiography (AMBER), and CR.

A secondary benefit of helical CT is increased patient throughput resulting from the decreased scanning time. This aspect of helical CT, along with the increased detectability of lung nodules, has resulted in the implementation of helical CT as a modality for lung cancer screening (98). Scans acquired with lower x-ray exposure reduce the radiation risk to screened individuals. Trials to validate mass lung cancer screening with low-dose helical CT are currently underway in Japan, Germany, and the U.S.A. In one lung cancer screening study, a malignant nodule was identified in 2.7% of screened individuals in the prevalence phase of the study (107).

Although the potential camouflaging effect of overlapping anatomical structures is mostly eliminated in CT scans, identification of lung nodules is confounded by the prominence of blood vessels in CT images. Croisille et al. demonstrated a significant improvement in radiologists' detection of pulmonary nodules when vessels were removed from the volumetric data using a three-dimensional region-growing algorithm (99). Distinguishing between nodules and vessels typically requires visual comparison among several CT sections, which necessitates the radiologist to mentally construct a three-dimensional representation of patient anatomy. This task, although tedious for radiologists in view of complex anatomical structures, may be efficiently handled by a computerized method.

Efforts to develop automated nodule detection methods for CT scans have gained momentum in recent years. Ryan et al. (100) modeled nodules and vessels as spherical and cylindrical volumes, respectively. A comparison between soft tissue and air densities on the surface and within the volume of a bounding cube was then used to differentiate between nodules and vessels. Kanazawa et al. (101) used a fuzzy clustering algorithm to identify vessels and potential nodules within the lung fields. A rule-based approach incorporating distance from the lung boundary and circularity information was used to distinguish nodules from vessels on a section-by-section basis. The reported results indicate that this algorithm attained a sensitivity of 86% with 11 false-positive cases on a database of 224 helical CT cases. This work was expanded by Toshioka et al. (102), who included a comparison of immediately adjacent sections. On a database of 450 helical CT scans, sensitivities of 76% to 100% were attained, depending on radiologist-assigned tumor probability ratings. Okumura et al. (103) used spatial filtering, including a three-dimensional morphological filter, to automatically detect pulmonary nodules. In a database of 82 cases, all 21 nodules were detected along with 301 false-positive regions.

Fiebich *et al.* (104) reported on a computerized method for the detection of lung nodules in low-dose helical CT scans from a lung cancer screening program. The method attained an overall nodule detection sensitivity of 95.6% with approximately 15 false-positive detections per study and is being evaluated with clinical experience (105). Ko and Betke (106) developed a nodule detection method based on gray-level thresholding. When applied to 16 CT scans (eight different patients with two CT scans each), they achieved anodule detection sensitivity of 86% with an unspecified number of false-positive detections. Other investigators have also contributed to the important task of computerized lung nodule detection in CT images (107–109).

Giger et al. (110) in 1994 reported on an automated detection scheme that was trained and tested on a database of eight thoracic CT scans. In this scheme, gray-level thresholding was used to isolate the thorax and to segment the lung regions in each CT section. To distinguish nodules from vessels within the lung regions, geometrical feature analysis was implemented in conjunction with multiple gray-level thresholding. The final classification was made on the basis of a comparison of suspected regions in each section with suspected regions in adjacent sections. The method performed at a level of 94% sensitivity with an average of 1.25 false-positive detections per case. Armato et al. (111,112) have developed a nodule detection method that makes use of the volumetric nature of CT image data. Gray-level thresholding techniques were applied to identify three-dimensional structures in CT scans. A maximum-volume criterion was imposed on these structures to identify an initial set of nodule candidates, for which two- and three-dimensional morphologic and gray-level features were computed. Linear discriminant analysis was used to merge the features and reduce the number of candidates that correspond to nonnodules (Fig. 13). The method was improved and applied to a database of 43 standard-dose (diagnostic) CT scans and a database of 13 low-dose CT scans (113,114). With the exception of the training of the final-stage classifier, the computerized detection algorithm was kept constant. The method attained comparable performance levels when applied to these separate databases: 71% sensitivity (121 out of 171 nodules) with an average of 1.5 false-positive detections per section on the 43-case standard-dose database and 71% sensitivity (180 out of 255 nodules) with an average of 1.2 false-positive detections per section on the 13-case low-dose database.

IV. SUMMARY

The future of image processing and CAD in diagnostic radiology is more promising now than ever, with encouraging results being reported from observer performance studies. Clinical trials in years to come will help optimize the accuracy of the computerized methods and determine the actual contribution of CAD to the interpretation process; however, a physician will still make the final decision regarding diagnosis and patient management. Nonetheless, studies have indicated that computer output need not have greater overall accuracy than a given radiologist to improve his or her performance.

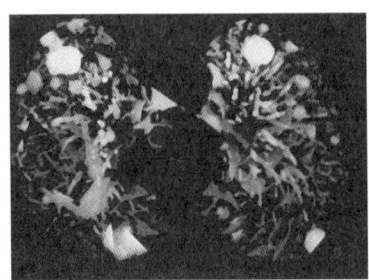
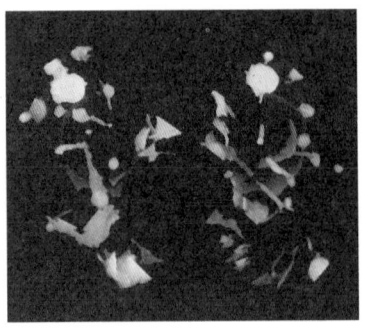

Fig. 13 Maximum intensity projection image representing the set of three-dimensional nodule candidates (a) before and (b) after merging of morphological and gray-level features through linear discriminant analysis. Reprinted with permission from Ref. 105 (Figs. 15, 18).

The computer should not be considered a "black box" that renders judgment on an image in a consistent but arbitrary manner. Indeed, the computerized methods that exist have been developed over the span of many years by scientific and medical researchers who have incorporated the various facets of image acquisition and interpretation into computer algorithms. Within these algorithms, concepts from physics, anatomy, pathology, statistics, and computer science are integrated to provide a metric for computer vision based on the imaging parameters and visual cues that serve as the foundation for human-vision interpretation of medical images by radiologists.

A systematic and gradual introduction of CAD into radiology departments will be necessary, so that radiologists may become familiar with the strengths and weaknesses of each CAD program, thereby avoiding either excessive reliance on or a dismissive attitude toward the computer output. This approach should ensure the acceptance of CAD and facilitate optimal diagnostic performance by the radiologist. In practice, each radiologist will individually define, according to personal training and observational skills, an appropriate role for the various CAD programs in his or her diagnostic decision-making process. Consequently, intraobserver variations may be reduced, and diagnostic performance may be optimized. It is expected that routine use of CAD methods will eventually be accepted as a viable means of improving patient care.

ACKNOWLEDGMENT

This work was supported in parts by the USPHS grants CA48985, CA24806, CA83908, and CA64370-02.

REFERENCES

1. RT Greenlee, MB Hill-Harmon, T Murray, M Thun. Cancer statistics, 2001. CA: Cancer J Clin 51:15–36, 2001.
2. PA Wingo, T Tong, S Bolden. Cancer statistics, 1995. CA: Cancer J Clin 45:8–30, 1995.
3. M Remy-Jardin, J Remy, F Giraud, C-H Marquette. Pulmonary nodules: Detection with thick-section spiral CT versus conventional CT. Radiology 187:513–520, 1993.
4. BJ Flehinger, M Kimmel, MR Melamed. The effect of surgical treatment on survival from early lung cancer: Implications for screening. Chest 101:1013–1018, 1992.
5. CJ Vyborny. The AAPM/RSNA physics tutorial for residents: Image quality and the clinical radiographic examination. RadioGraphics 17:479–498, 1997.
6. H MacMahon, K Doi. Digital chest radiography. Clin Chest Med 12:19–32, 1991.
7. J Muhm, W Miller, R Fontana, D Sanderson, M Uhlenhopp. Lung cancer detected during a screening program using four-month chest radiographs. Radiology 148:609–615, 1983.
8. W Tuddenham. Visual search, image organization and reader error in roentgen diagnosis. Radiology 78:694–704, 1962.
9. H Kundel. Peripheral vision, structured noise and film reader error. Radiology 114:269–273, 1975.
10. JHM Austin, BM Romney, LS Goldsmith. Missed bronchogenic carcinoma: Radiographic findings in 27 patients with a potentially resectable lesion evident in retrospect. Radiology 182:115–122, 1992.
11. J Forrest, P Friedman. Radiologic errors in patients with lung cancer. West J Med 134:485–490, 1981.
12. HL Kundel, CF Nodine, D Carmody. Visual scanning, pattern recognition and decision-making in pulmonary nodule detection. Investigative Radiology 13:175–181, 1978.
13. H Kundel, C Nodine, E Krupinski. Searching for lung nodules: visual dwell indicates locations of false-positive and false-negative decisions. Investigative Radiology 24:472–478, 1989.
14. C Nodine, H Kundel, J Polikoff, L Toto. Using eye movements to study decision making of radiologists. In: G Luer, U Lass, J Shallo-Hoffman, eds. Eye Movement Research: Physiological and Psychological Aspects. Gottigen, Germany: Hogrefe, 1988, pp 349–363.
15. C Nodine, H Kundel. A visual dwell algorithm can aid search and recognition of missed lung nodules in chest radiographs. In: Brogan D, eds. First International Conference on Visual Search. London, England: Taylor & Francis, 1990, pp 399–406.
16. H Kundel, C Nodine, E Krupinski. Computer-displayed eye position as a visual aid to pulmonary nodule interpretation. Investigative Radiology 25:••, 1990.
17. EJ Potchen, JHM Austin. Problems and pitfalls in the diagnosis of early lung cancer. In: EJ Potchen, RG Grainger, R Greene, eds. Pulmonary Radiology. Philadelphia: WB Saunders 1993, pp 315–328.
18. RH Sherrier, C Chiles, WE Wilkinson, GA Johnson, CE Ravin. Effects of image processing on nodule detection rates in digitized chest radiographs: ROC study of observer performance. Radiology 166:447–450, 1988.

19. T Kobayashi, X-W Xu, H MacMahon, C Metz, K Doi. Effect of a computer-aided diagnosis scheme on radiologists' performance in detection of lung nodules on radiographs. Radiology 199:843–848, 1996.
20. H Chan, K Doi, C Vyborny, et al. Improvement in radiologists' detection of clustered microcalcifications on mammograms: The potential of computer-aided diagnosis. Invest Radiol 25:1102–1110, 1990.
21. W Kegelmeyer, J Pruneda, P Bourland, A Hillis, M Riggs, M Nipper. Computer-aided mammographic screening for spiculated lesions. Radiology 191:331–337, 1994.
22. HL Kundel, G Revesz. Lesion conspicuity, structured noise, and film reader error. Am J Roentgenol 126:1233–1238, 1976.
23. K Hoffmann, K Doi, H MacMahon, et al. Development of a digital duplication system for portable chest radiographs. J Digital Imag 7:146–153, 1994.
24. H MacMahon, X-W Xu, K Hoffman, M Giger, H Yoshimura, K Doi. Clinical experience with an advanced laser digitizer for cost effective digital radiography. RadioGraphics 13:635–645, 1993.
25. H Yoshimura, X-W Xu, K Doi, et al. Development of a high quality film duplication system using a laser digitizer: comparison with computed radiography. Med Physics 20:51–58, 1993.
26. M Sonoda, M Takano, J Miyahara, H Kato. Computed radiography utilizing scanning laser stimulated luminescence. Radiology 148:833–838, 1983.
27. J Seibert, D Shelton, E Moore. Computed radiography x-ray exposure trends. Acad Radiol 3:313–318, 1996.
28. L Antonuk, J Boudry, Y El-Mohri, W Huang, J Siewerdsen, J Yorkston. A high-resolution, high frame rate, flat-panel TFT array for digital x-ray imaging. Proc SPIE 2163:118–128, 1994.
29. C Floyd Jr., H Chotas, C Ravin. Evaluation of a selenium-based digital chest radiography system. Proc SPIE 2163:110–116, 1994.
30. D Lee, L Cheung, L Jeromin. A new digital detector for projection radiography. Proc SPIE 2432:237–249, 1995.
31. M Ishida, P Frank, K Doi, J Lehr. High-quality radiographic images: improved detection of low-contrast objects and preliminary clinical studies. RadioGraphics 3:325–338, 1983.
32. M Ishida, K Doi, L Loo, C Metz, J Lehr. Digital image processing: effect on detectability of simulated low-contrast radiographic patterns. Radiology 150:569–575, 1984.
33. P Vuylsteke, E Schoeters. Multiscale image contrast amplification (MUSICA). Proc SPIE 2167:551–560, 1994.
34. M Ishida. Fuji Computed Radiography Technical Review No. 1 Digital Image Processing. Tokyo, Japan: Fuji Photo Film Co., Ltd., 1993.
35. JH Woodring. Pitfalls in the radiologic diagnosis of lung cancer. Am J Roentgenol 154:1165–1175, 1990.
36. R Lillestrand, R Hoyt. The design of advanced digital image processing systems. Photogramm Eng 40:1201–1217, 1974.
37. A Kano, K Doi, H MacMahon, D Hassell, M Giger. Digital image subtraction of temporally sequential chest images for detection of interval change. Med Phys 21:453–461, 1994.

38. J Kinsey, B Vannelli. Application of digital image change detection to diagnosis and follow-up of cancer involving the lungs. Proc SPIE 70:99–112, 1975.
39. C Metz. ROC methodology in radiologic imaging. Investigative Radiology 21: 720–733, 1986.
40. M Difazio, H MacMahon, X-W Xu, et al. Digital chest radiography: effect of temporal subtraction images on detection accuracy. Radiology 202:447–452, 1997.
41. D Ergun, C Mistretta, D Brown, et al. Single-exposure dual-energy computed radiography: improved detection and processing. Radiology 174:243–249, 1990.
42. L Lehmann, R Alvarez, A Macovski, W Brody, N Pelc, S Riederer. Generalized image combinations in dual kVp digital radiography. Med Phy 8:659–667, 1981.
43. F Kelcz, F Zink, W Peppler, D Kruger, D Ergun, C Mistretta. Conventional chest radiography vs dual-energy computed radiography in the detection and characterization of pulmonary nodules. Am J Roentgenol 162:271–278, 1994.
44. D Kruger, F Zink, W Peppler, D Ergun, C Mistretta. A regional convolution kernel algorithm for scatter correction in dual-energy images: comparison to single-kernel algorithms. Med Phys 21:175–184, 1994.
45. D Ergun, W Peppler, J Dobbins, et al. Dual-energy computed radiography: improvements in processing. Proc SPIE 2167:663–671, 1994.
46. J Ho, R Kruger. Comparison of dual-energy and conventional chest radiography for nodule detection. Invest Radiol 24:861–868, 1989.
47. D Ballard, C Brown. Computer Vision. Englewood Cliffs, NJ: Prentice-Hall Inc, 1982.
48. A Hasegawa, S Lo, M Freedman, S Mun. Convolution neural network based detection of lung structures. Proc SPIE 2167:654–662, 1994.
49. D Cheng, M Goldberg. An algorithm for segmenting chest radiographs. Proc SPIE 1001:261–268, 1988.
50. J Duryea, J Boone. A fully automated algorithm for the segmentation of lung fields on digital chest radiographic images. Med Phys 22:183–191, 1995.
51. M McNitt-Gray, H Huang, J Sayre. Feature selection in the pattern classification problem of digital chest radiograph segmentation. IEEE Trans Med Imag 14: 537–547, 1995.
52. E Pietka. Lung segmentation in digital radiographs. J Digital Imag 7:79–84, 1994.
53. R Sherrier, G Johnson. Regionally adaptive histogram equalization of the chest. IEEE Trans Med Imag MI-6:1–7, 1987.
54. M Sezan, A Tekalp, R Schaetzing. Automatic anatomically selective image enhancement in digital chest radiography. IEEE Trans Med Imag 8:154–162, 1989.
55. X-W Xu, K Doi. Image feature analysis for computer-aided diagnosis: accurate determination of ribcage boundary in chest radiographs. Med Phys 22:617–626, 1995.
56. X-W Xu, K Doi. Image feature analysis for computer-aided diagnosis: detection of right and left hemidiaphragm edges and delineation of lung field in chest radiographs. Med Phys 23:1613–1624, 1996.
57. O Tsujii, M Freedman, S Mun. Automated segmentation of anatomic regions in chest radiographs using an adaptive-sized hybrid neural network. Proc SPIE 3034:802–811, 1997.
58. S Armato III, M Giger, H MacMahon. Automated lung segmentation in digitized posteroanterior chest radiographs. Acad Radiol 5:245–255, 1998.

59. NF Vittitoe, R Vargas-Voracek, CE Floyd Jr. Identification of lung regions in chest radiographs using Markov random field modeling. Med Phys 25:976–985, 1998.
60. S Armato III, M Giger, K Ashizawa, H MacMahon. Automated lung segmentation in digital lateral chest radiographs. Med Phys 25:1507–1520, 1998.
61. FM Carrascal, JM Carreira, M Souto, PG Tahoces, L Gomez, JJ Vidal. Automatic calculation of total lung capacity from automatically traced lung boundaries in poster-anterior and lateral digital chest radiographs. Med Phys 25:1118–1131, 1998.
62. A Kahveci, S Dwyer III. Automated lesion detection in lung cancer. Proceedings of the 25th Annual Conference for Engineering in Medicine and Biology. 1972, p 46.
63. J Toriwaki, Y Suenaga, T Negoro, T Fukumara. Pattern recognition of chest x-ray images. Comp Graphics Image Proc 2:252–271, 1973.
64. D Ballard, J Sklansky. Tumor detection in radiographs. Comput Biomed Res 6:299–321, 1973.
65. D Ballard, J Sklansky. A ladder-structured decision tree for recognizing tumors in chest radiographs. IEEE Trans Comput 25:503–513, 1976.
66. M Giger, N Ahn, K Doi, H MacMahon, C Metz. Computerized detection of pulmonary nodules in digital chest images: use of morphological filters in reducing false positive detections. Med Phys 17:861–865, 1990.
67. H Yoshimura, M Giger, K Doi, H MacMahon, S Montner. Computerized scheme for the detection of pulmonary nodules: a nonlinear filtering technique. Invest Radiol 27:124–129, 1992.
68. N Vittitoe, J Baker, C Floyd Jr. Fractal texture analysis in computer-aided diagnosis of solitary pulmonary nodules. Acad Radiol 4:96–101, 1997.
69. J Lin, S Lo, M Freedman, S Mun. Application of artificial neural networks for reducing false positives in lung nodule detection on digital chest radiographs. Proc SPIE 2434:563–570, 1995.
70. Y Wu, K Doi, M Giger. Detection of lung nodules in digital chest radiographs using artificial neural networks: a pilot study. J Digital Imag 8:88–94, 1995.
71. Y Chiou, Y Lure. Hybrid lung nodule detection (HLND) system. Cancer Lett 77:119–126, 1994.
72. S Lo, J Lin, M Freedman, S Mun. Computer-aided diagnosis of lung nodule detection using artificial convolution neural network. Proc SPIE 1898:859–869, 1993.
73. X-W Xu, K Doi, T Kobayashi, H MacMahon, ML Giger. Development of an improved CAD scheme for automated detection of lung nodules in digital chest images. Med Phys 24:1395–1403, 1997.
74. H Suzuki, N Inaoka, H Takabatake, et al. Development of a computer-aided detection system for lung cancer diagnosis. Proc SPIE 1652:567–571, 1992.
75. H Yoshida, X-W Xu, T Kobayashi, M Giger, K Doi. Computer-aided diagnosis scheme for detecting pulmonary nodules using wavelet transform. Proc SPIE 2434:621–626, 1995.
76. F Mao, W Qian, J Gaviria, L Clarke. Fragmentary window filtering for multiscale lung nodule detection: preliminary study. Acad Radiol 5:306–311, 1998.
77. H Yoshida, S Katsuragawa, Y Amit, K Doi. Wavelet-based deformable contour and its application to detection of pulmonary nodules on chest radiographs. Proc SPIE 3169:328–336, 1997.

78. M Hashimoto, P Sankar, J Sklansky. Detecting the edges of lung tumors by classification techniques. Proc IEEE International Conference on Pattern Recognition. CH-1801:276–279, 1982.
79. M Giger, K Doi, H MacMahon. Image feature analysis and computer-aided diagnosis in digital radiography. III. Automated detection of nodules in peripheral lung fields. Med Phys 15:158–166, 1988.
80. M Giger, K Doi, H MacMahon, C Metz, F Yin. Pulmonary nodules: computer-aided detection in digital chest images. RadioGraphics 10:41–51, 1990.
81. T Matsumoto, H Yoshimura, K Doi, et al. Image feature analysis of false-positive diagnoses produced by automated detection of lung nodules. Invest Radiol 27:587–597, 1992.
82. Z Huo, M Giger, C Vyborny, et al. Analysis of spiculation in the computerized classification of mammographic masses. Med Phys 22:1569–1579, 1995.
83. X-W Xu, S Katsuragawa, K Ashizawa, H MacMahon, K Doi. Analysis of image features of histograms of edge gradient for false positive reduction in lung nodule detection in chest radiographs. Proc SPIE 3338:318–326, 1998.
84. KR Hoffmann, R Engelmann, H MacMahon, T Ishida, X-W Xu, K Doi. Development of a prototype intelligent workstation for chest CAD. In: HU Lemke, MW Vannier, K Inamura, eds. Proceedings Computer Assisted Radiology. New York: Elsevier, 1997, pp 337–341.
85. M Giger, K Doi, H MacMahon, R Nishikawa, K Hoffmann. An "intelligent" workstation for computer-aided diagnosis. RadioGraphics 13:647–656, 1993.
86. J Muhm, L Brown, J Crowe. Detection of pulmonary nodules by computed tomography. Am J Roentgenol 128:267–270, 1977.
87. R Pugatch, L Faling. Computed tomography of the thorax: a status report. Chest 80:618–626, 1981.
88. W Webb. Advances in computed tomography of the thorax. Radiol Clin North Am 21:723–739, 1983.
89. DP Naidich, H Rusinek, G McGuinness, B Leitman, DI McCauley, CI Henschke. Variables affecting pulmonary nodule detection with computed tomography: Evaluation with three-dimensional computer simulation. J Thorac Imaging 8:291–299, 1993.
90. J Gurney. Missed lung cancer at CT: imaging findings in nine patients. Radiology 199:117–122, 1996.
91. D Naidich, E Zerhouni, S Siegelman. Computed Tomography of the Thorax. New York: Raven Press, 1984.
92. C Crawford, K King. Computed tomography scanning with simultaneous patient translation. Med Phys 17:967–982, 1990.
93. WA Kalender, W Seissler, E Klotz, P Vock. Spiral volumetric CT with single-breath-hold technique, continuous transport, and continuous scanner rotation. Radiology 176:181–183, 1990.
94. J Buckley, W Scott Jr., S Siegelman, et al. Pulmonary nodules: effect of increased data sampling on detection with spiral CT and confidence in diagnosis. Radiology 196:395–400, 1995.
95. M Remy-Jardin, J Remy, F Giraud, C-H Marquette. Pulmonary nodules: detection with thick-section spiral CT versus conventional CT. Radiology 187:513–520, 1993.

96. N Milla, K Ito, M Ikeda, K Nakamura, M Hirose, T Ishigaki. Fundamental and clinical evaluation of chest computed tomography imaging in detectability of pulmonary nodules. Nagoya J Med Sci 57:127–132, 1994.
97. P Costello, W Anderson, D Blume. Pulmonary nodule: evaluation with spiral volumetric CT. Radiology 179:875–876, 1991.
98. M Kaneko, K Eguchi, H Ohmatsu, et al. Peripheral lung cancer: screening and detection with low-dose spiral CT versus radiography. Radiology 201:798–802, 1996.
99. P Croisille, M Souto, M Cova, et al. Pulmonary nodules: improved detection with vascular segmentation and extraction with spiral CT. Radiology 197:397–401, 1995.
100. W Ryan, J Reed, S Swensen, P Sheedy Jr. Automatic detection of pulmonary nodules in CT. Proceedings Computer Assisted Radiology. 1996, pp 385–389.
101. K Kanazawa, M Kubo, N Niki, et al. Computer assisted lung cancer diagnosis based on helical images. In: RT Chin, HHS Ip, AC Naiman, T-C Pong, eds. Image Analysis Applications and Computer Graphics: Proceedings of the Third International Computer Science Conference. Berlin: Springer-Verlag, 1995, pp 323–330.
102. S Toshioka, K Kanazawa, N Niki, et al. Computer-aided diagnosis system for lung cancer based on helical CT images. SPIE Proc 3034:975–984, 1997.
103. T Okumura, T Miwa, J Kako, et al. Image processing for computer-aided diagnosis of lung cancer screening system by CT (LSCT). SPIE Proc 3338:1314–1322, 1998.
104. Fiebich M, Wietholt C, Renger BC, Armato SG, III, Hoffmann KR, Wormanns D, Diederich S. Automatic detection of pulmonary nodules in low-dose screening thoracic CT examinations. *SPIE Proceedings* 3661:1434–1439, 1999.
105. Wormanns D, Fiebich M, Wietholt C, Diederich S, Heindel W. Automatic detection of pulmonary nodules at spiral CT—first clinical experience with a computer-aided diagnosis system. *SPIE Proceedings* 3979:129–135, 2000.
106. Ko JP, Betke M. Chest CT: Automated nodule detection and assessment of change over time—preliminary experience. *Radiology* 218:267–273, 2001.
107. Satoh H, Ukai Y, Niki N, Eguchi K, Mori K, Ohmatsu H, Kakinuma R, Kaneko M, Moriyama N. Computer aided diagnosis system for lung cancer based on retrospective helical CT image. *SPIE Proceedings* 3661:1324–1335, 1999.
108. Taguchi H, Kawata Y, Niki N, Satoh H, Ohmatsu H, Kakinuma R, Eguchi K, Kaneko M, Moriyama N. Lung cancer detection based on helical CT images using curved surface morphology analysis. *SPIE Proceedings* 3661:1307–1314, 1999.
109. Lou S-L, Chang C-L, Lin K-P, Chen T-S. Object-based deformation technique for 3-D CT lung nodule detection. *SPIE Proceedings* 3661:1544–1552, 1999.
110. M Giger, K Bae, H MacMahon. Computerized detection of pulmonary nodules in computed tomography images. Invest Radiol 29:459–465, 1994.
111. SG Armato III, ML Giger, CJ Moran, JT Blackburn, K Doi, H MacMahon. Computerized detection of pulmonary nodules in CT scans. RadioGraphics 19:1303–1311, 1999.
112. SG Armato III, ML Giger, JT Blackburn, K Doi, H MacMahon. Three-dimensional approach to lung nodule detection in helical CT. SPIE Proc 3661:553–559, 1999.
113. Armato SG, III, Giger ML, MacMahon H: Automated detection of lung nodules in CT scans: Preliminary results. Med Phys 28:1552–1561, 2001.
114. Armato SG, III, Giger ML, Doi K, MacMahon H. Computerized lung nodule detection: Comparison of performance for low-dose and standard-dose helical CT scans. *SPIE Proceedings* 4322:(in press), 2001.

11
Lung: X-Ray and CT

Michael F. McNitt-Gray and Matthew S. Brown
UCLA School of Medicine, Los Angeles, California

I. INTRODUCTION

With the advent of spiral scanning, computed tomography (CT) imaging is expected to take on a significant role in the detection of lung nodules both in a screening role for asymptomatic patients and in an evaluation role for patients who are known to have lung cancer. In spiral CT, volumetric data sets are acquired rather than incremental axial images. Data sets are obtained during a single suspended breath hold, eliminating potential sampling errors that result from respiratory variation between axial scans. In addition, because spiral data can be reconstructed at any incrementation, images can be overlapped to yield better resolution along the axis of the patient (z-axis). These factors taken together have been shown to improve lesion detection in the lungs by radiologists (1–4). This improved resolution comes at the cost of an increased number of images to read. This creates a significant burden for the radiologist to review each of these images.

Thus, image processing and pattern classification techniques are being investigated to assist radiologists in detection and quantification tasks. For the screening of lung cancer, image-processing techniques are being used to detect tumors in the lung at the earliest possible stage. For the evaluation of lung cancer patients and their response to treatment, image-segmentation techniques are being used to first detect lesions and then to measure tumor volumes that are being tracked over time.

II. CLINICAL SETTING

A. Lung Cancer

According to statistics from the American Cancer Society (5), lung cancer is the leading cause of cancer death among both men and women. In 1997, an estimated 178,000 new cases of lung cancer accounted for about 13% of all new cancers in the United States and about 29% of deaths from cancer. There were an estimated 160,400 deaths from lung cancer in 1997. For those whose cancer is found and treated early, before it has spread to lymph nodes or the other organs, the average survival rate is 48%. However, using present techniques, only 15% of lung cancers are found at this early, localized stage.

B. Lung Cancer Screening

A screening examination is one performed on a patient with little or no symptoms of lung cancer for the purposes of detecting early signs of the disease. Currently, it is generally accepted that screening for the early detection of lung cancer using chest radiography–based methods does not provide a significant benefit (6). Several large-scale randomized control trials (7–10), which included some combination of chest radiography and histological sputum analysis, concluded that these screening activities did not reduce lung cancer–specific mortality. However, conventional projectional radiography suffers from the inherent limitations that bones and organs overlap in the images, and this may obscure small lesions representing lung cancers at an early stage. The fact that survival rate is reasonably good when the cancer is detected at an early stage has motivated research into screening techniques that can detect lung cancer at an earlier stage. The National Cancer Institute is undertaking another large-scale study to investigate the efficacy of screening in lung, prostate, colon, and ovarian cancers. For lung cancer, the projectional chest radiograph in conjunction with sputum cytology techniques is being used in this study.

In Japan, there has recently been interest in using CT as a screening tool (11–13). Spiral CT yields volumetric image data sets that do not suffer from the overlap of anatomical structures that limits projectional radiography nor the breathing misregistration between slices that occurs in conventional CT. Low-dose scanning techniques have been developed and clinically deployed in Japan. Preliminary trials have shown spiral CT to provide a greater detection rate than the sputum cytology and miniature fluoroscopy techniques currently used for screening in Japan (.47% for CT compared with .03% to .05% for the latter) (11).

C. Evaluating Response to Therapy for Lung Cancer Patients

For patients in whom the lung cancer diagnosis has been established, CT has been used to determine their response to therapy (14–18). Typically using axial, incremental CT image data, radiologists make a series of cross-sectional diameter measurements for a few indicator lesions and then compare them with measurements made from previous scans to indicate response to therapy (tumor progression/regression/stability). However, these measurements of lesion diameter, although widely used, may not provide an accurate assessment of tumor size because of a number of factors, including (a) irregular lesions, lesions that do not grow spherically may not be adequately represented by a change in diameters; (b) interobserver and intraobserver measurement differences, involving selection of the image used for the measurement and where the lesion boundary is located; (c) differences in scanning levels from one examination to another, lesions may not be imaged at the exact same location from one examination to another, which affects how the lesion appears and makes comparisons between examinations difficult. Spiral CT and its ability to provide single breath-hold scans and its simultaneous ability to provide overlapping reconstructions improves the ability to image lesions at reproducible levels from different examinations. However, the measurement of these lesions is still a subjective task, subject to the variability described in (a) and (b) previously.

III. IMAGE PROCESSING METHODS USED IN PULMONARY NODULE DETECTION ON CT

A. Goals and General Problems

In either a screening or evaluation situation, one of the primary tasks of the radiologist is nodule detection. When spiral CT is used in either of these situations, the number of images to be examined by a radiologist for potential lesions could be very large. This is because (a) covering the entire thorax typically requires 30 to 40 cm of table movement (to cover from the thoracic inlet to the lung bases); (b) images are typically acquired using a collimation (slice thickness) of between 5 and 10 mm; and (b) spiral CT allows the ability to reconstruct overlapping images at small intervals. Using axial CT, a 40-cm long patient imaged using only 10-mm collimation would result in 40 images but would have required 5 or 10 different breath holds because of slower scan times and interscan delays. With a spiral scanner, this same 40-cm long patient would require one breath hold of 40 sec (or two 20-sec breath holds) and, if images were reconstructed at 5-mm intervals, would now result in 80 images.

The exact imaging protocol used can have a significant impact on the ability to detect nodules. In spiral CT, each image has an effective slice thickness associated with it. The thicker the slice, the greater the volume of tissue contributing to that image and the greater the volume averaging problem. Thus, a 5-mm spherical nodule in a 10-mm thick slice is averaged with approximately 5-mm thickness of other tissues (Fig. 1), whatever those tissues happen to be. When these tissues are low-attenuating lung tissues (mostly air), then the resulting pixel

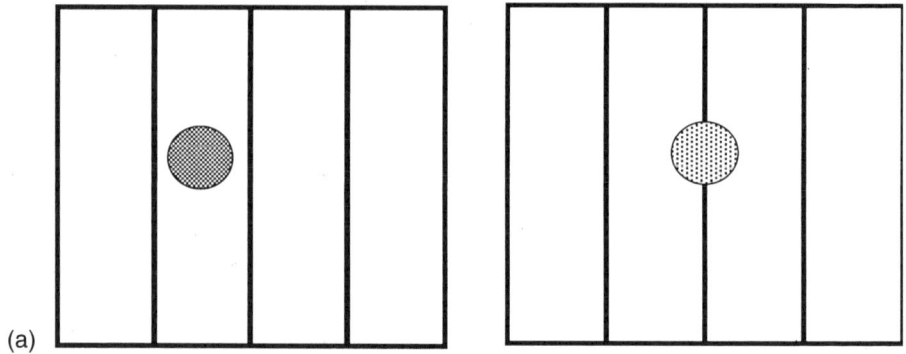

Fig. 1 Diagram illustrating 5-mm spherical nodule in a 10-mm thick slice. (a) With the best possible alignment between object and image. At its widest point, the sphere does not occupy the full slice width and is averaged with whatever tissues are adjacent to it. (b) With bad alignment between object and image. The signal from the nodule is now split between two images and in each image the nodule is further averaged with whatever tissues are adjacent to it.

shows an attenuation value lower than that of the nodule itself, which reduces the signal from the nodule and the radiologists' ability to detect it.

The factors that determine the effective slice thickness in spiral CT are collimation, pitch (table speed), and spiral interpolation algorithm (19–25). Collimation is set by the operator and determines the physical thickness of the detected x-ray beam. Pitch is the ratio of (table speed per rotation)/(collimation) and determines how far the table travels per rotation. The higher the pitch, the further the table moves per rotation and, because spiral CT uses interpolation to form its images, the larger the longitudinal range of data used in that interpolation. This results in greater effective slice thickness (and more volume averaging). Thus, greater patient coverage comes at a price of thicker effective slices and greater volume averaging. The spiral interpolation algorithm determines what that range of longitudinal data is used to form the image. Most CT manufacturers use either the 180LI method or the 360LI method (19–21). The 180LI method uses a smaller range of longitudinal data and results in a smaller increase in effective slice thickness than the 360LI (though the noise performance of the 360LI is better).

One other spiral CT technical parameter of note is the reconstruction interval. Because a volumetric data set is acquired in spiral CT, the exact location where images are reconstructed is arbitrary, as is the interval between images. Thus, overlapping images can be obtained without additional radiation to the patient but by merely reconstructing images from the original volumetric data set. Because the orientation of lesions with the images is not known a priori, it is very

Lung X-Ray and CT

likely that a nodule could be poorly aligned with an image as shown in Fig. 1b, exacerbating the volume averaging problem. Overlapping images (illustrated in Fig. 2) have been shown to improve the alignment between lesion and image and to minimize the volume averaging that is due to splitting the nodule signal between two images (26).

The image-processing task is to search a volumetric image data set to detect only lesions (tumors) and to avoid the false positives created by normal anatomical structures such as bronchial walls and blood vessels. Tumors and blood vessels have similar x-ray attenuation and may appear similar when viewed on cross-sectional images. Therefore, identification, and removal, of vascular structures is useful in lesion detection. However, removing vascular structures is not a complete solution, because nodules can be in contact with those vessels, the chest wall,

Contiguous Reconstruction - No Overlap

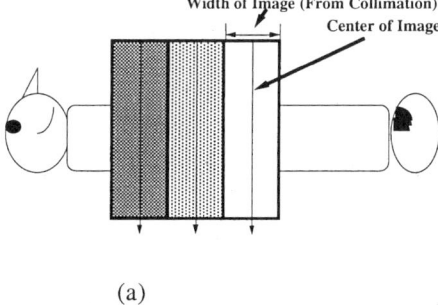

(a)

Overlapping Reconstruction - 50% Overlap

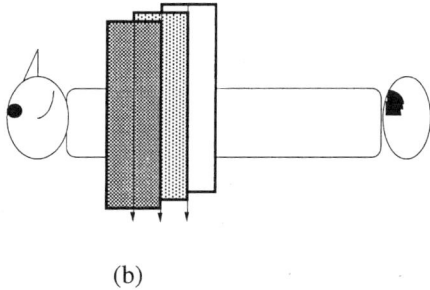

(b)

Fig. 2 Diagram illustrating the difference between (a) contiguous reconstruction, in which slice thickness and slice spacing are equal, and (b) overlapped reconstruction, in which slice spacing is less than slice thickness, in spiral CT. Overlapped reconstructions yield increased sampling in the longitudinal direction of the patient and can create better nodule-image alignment, which in turn reduces volume averaging as shown in Fig. 1.

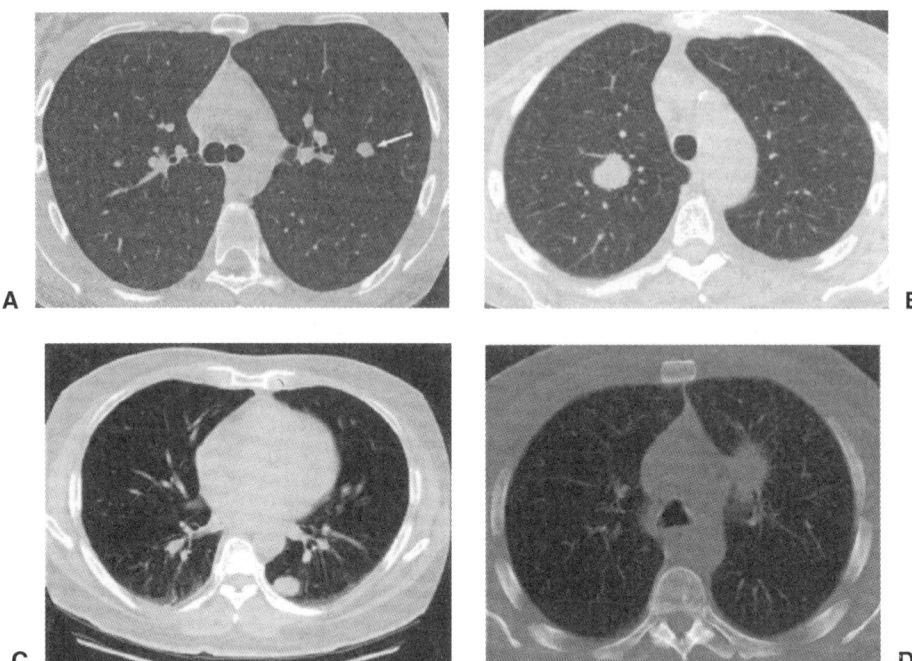

Fig. 3 Examples of (a) an isolated lesion identified by the arrow; (b) a lesion with a contacting vessel; (c) a lesion in contact with the chest wall pleural interface; and (d) a lesion contacting the mediastinum.

and/or the mediastinum. Examples of each of these are shown in Fig. 3. For the evaluation task, accurate (or at least reproducible) identification of lesion boundaries will give more consistent results in tumor measurement.

What follows is a summary of several approaches to the problems involved in nodule detection. We have broken these into groups of methods that (a) detect the pulmonary vasculature to assist in the detection of pulmonary nodules (if vasculature is removed, then only nodules should remain); (b) automatically detect objects in the CT image volume and attempt to distinguish between nodules and other structures such as vessels or the chest wall, etc.; and (c) automatically detect endobronchial lesions (those within the tracheobronchial tree).

B. Segmentation of Vascular Structures to Assist Nodule Detection

A three-dimensional analysis to detect and remove the pulmonary vasculature was used by Croisille et al. (27) to make detection of remaining pulmonary nodules easier for the radiologist. In this approach, sequential CT images were first put together to form an image volume. The heart was then manually removed before the extraction of the vascular tree. The vessels were extracted from the remaining volumetric data by using a three-dimensional seeded region growing algorithm. The seed point was selected by the user from the vascular lumen; all voxels within the user-specified gray level (or Hounsfield Unit (HU)—the normalized measure of attenuation used in CT) range that were six-connected (that is, x, y, or z connected) to the seed point were added recursively until the entire vascular tree was segmented. This should identify both the pulmonary arterial and venous trees. Once identified, the voxels belonging to the vascular tree were removed from the volumetric data set. The voxels remaining in the data set were then examined for pulmonary nodules by a radiologist. Fig. 4 shows an original CT image, with the segmented image showing only pulmonary nodules. With the vascularity removed, the nodules are much more conspicuous.

This approach was then applied to simulated and clinical image data sets that were read and scored by radiologists for nodule detection. All nodules included in the study (simulated and real) were less than 5 mm in diameter and were acquired with 8-mm collimation, 8 mm/sec table speed, and 4-mm reconstruction interval. The results were very encouraging, because the readers performed significantly better when using the images with the vascular tree removed. Thus, extracting the vascular tree from the CT images improves the ability of radiologists to detect small pulmonary nodules. However, some pulmonary nodules that were in close contact with the vascular tree were removed along with the vasculature, and some nodules in contact with the chest wall (pleural surface) were removed along with the pleural surface itself, resulting in several false negatives (missed nodules). The authors suggest that the latter may not be a significant problem, because many nodules at the pleural surface are easily detected in the original image data.

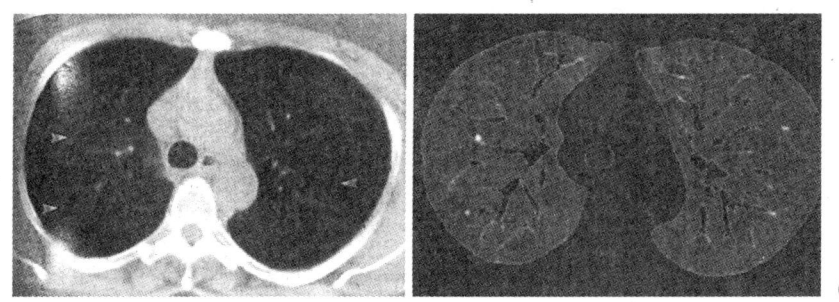

Fig. 4 CT scan showing pulmonary nodules (arrowheads in a) in a patient (a) before and (b) after the segmentation. (*Source:* Ref. 27; reprinted with permission.)

Further segmentation of the vascular tree into its arterial and venous components was explored by Tozaki (28). In this method, anatomical knowledge about the characteristics of the tracheobronchial tree and the accompanying pulmonary vascular tree was exploited, namely, that the pulmonary arteries generally run adjacent to the bronchial tree. Thus, proximity to a bronchial structure serves as a distinguishing characteristic of the pulmonary arteries. This may prove to be important in both detecting pulmonary nodules and, as Tozaki suggests, in distinguishing benign from malignant disease.

In Tozaki's approach, the lung region was extracted using thresholding and skeletonization techniques. From the lung region, a second threshold was applied to extract the combined bronchial and arterial trees. The next step was to find the bronchial tree and then, using anatomical information, to separate the arterial tree from the venous tree. The bronchial tree was extracted by thresholding to find the air-containing portion of the tree, and then region growing based on edge values was applied. Once the bronchial tree was identified, the remainder of the tree—the vascular portion—was thinned to determine the centerline of each branch. The distance between each vascular branch and the nearest bronchial branch was calculated, as well as the direction of each branch. If the distance was smaller than some threshold and the direction of the two branches was similar enough (i.e. if the inner product is below some threshold), then the branch was classified as a pulmonary artery. Otherwise, it was classified as a pulmonary vein. Some promising preliminary results obtained from thin-section images using 2-mm collimation, 2 mm/sec table speed, and 1-mm reconstruction interval are shown in Fig. 5. This figure shows the potential of image processing techniques to assist in the determination of connectivity of lesions to either pulmonary veins or arteries, which may be useful in determining the malignancy of lesions.

C. Automated Segmentation of Pulmonary Nodules

In these methods, the focus was on nodule detection, rather than the pulmonary vasculature tree. Even though the vascular tree is not explicitly segmented in these methods, a primary concern remains the ability to distinguish nodules from vessels. One method for automated detection of pulmonary nodules on CT using a combination of segmentation and morphological techniques was reported by Giger (29). This approach analyzed each two-dimensional (2-D) slice individually and then compared candidate nodules in neighboring slices. For each 2-D slice, the first step was to detect the thoracic boundary in the image. This was done by obtaining a profile from the center of the image to the edge of the image; this profile was used to determine a section-specific threshold from which the boundaries of connected regions are obtained. In the case of multiple regions, each region was analyzed in terms of its location, area, and circularity to determine whether it is truly the thorax or another object (e.g., patient table).

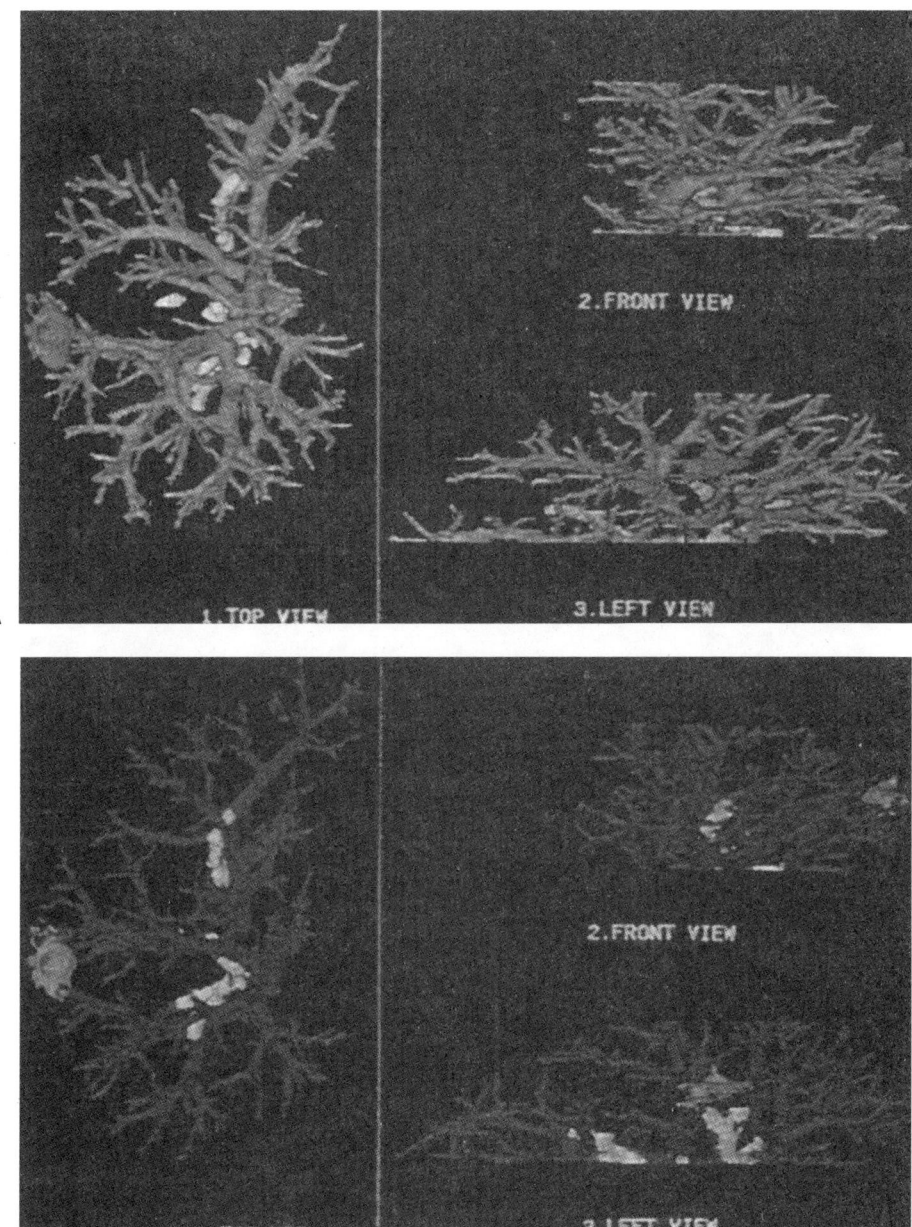

Fig. 5 (a) Segmented bronchus and pulmonary vein, (b) segmented bronchus and pulmonary artery; (c) segmented bronchus, pulmonary artery, and pulmonary vein; and (d) magnification images of segmented lesion, bronchus, artery, and vein using Tozaki's approach. (*Source:* Ref. 28; all reprinted with permission.) *(continued)*

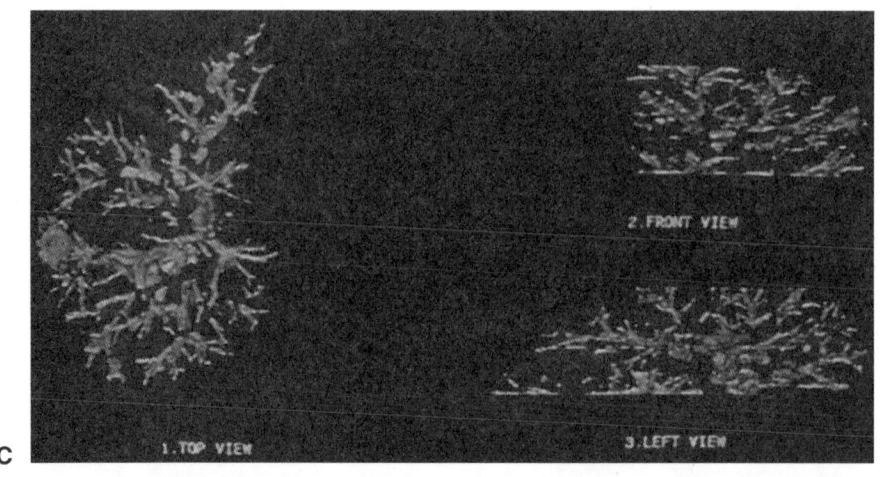

Fig. 5 Continued.

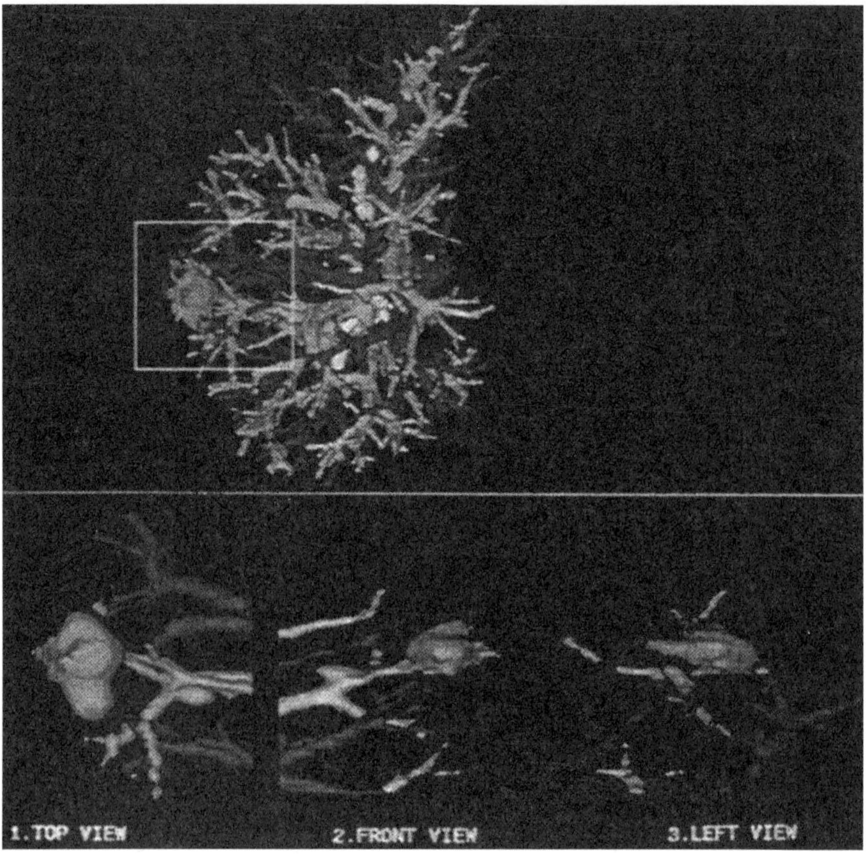

From within the thoracic boundary, the lung region was identified by using gray-level threshold techniques. A histogram of the thoracic region is obtained for each slice. This histogram contains a bimodal distribution (aerated lung vs soft tissue and bone). The gray level with the maximum separation between the groups is used as the threshold. From the thresholded image, connected regions within the thorax region are identified using an eight-point connectivity border tracker.

From within the lung regions, soft tissue objects were identified, which could be either nodules or vessels. This was accomplished by first thresholding objects within the lung boundaries at four different thresholds. At each threshold, a binary image was generated, and the location of objects above the threshold value was analyzed. As the threshold increased, the size of the candidate objects became smaller, and an object at one threshold sometimes separated into multiple objects at a higher threshold. Objects at one threshold were only analyzed if the center of the object was contained within an object that existed at a lower threshold. For each candidate object, morphological features were evaluated at each threshold. These features include the following:

- Perimeter
- Area
- Compactness = 4πArea/(perimeter)^2
- Elongation measure = Long axis/short axis
- Circularity = Compactness/elongation measure
- Distance measure = Distance from inner lung boundary/distance from outer lung boundary
- Total = Area $\times$ circularity $\times$ distance

From these measures a rule-based system was used to distinguish features describing nodules from those describing vessels. The initial classification was performed based on individual 2-D CT image sections. Ambiguities in the initial classification were resolved by comparisons with features in adjacent images. Comparisons to adjacent images allows vessels, especially those that travel perpendicular to the scan plane for several images, to be distinguished from nodules, which may appear strongly in one image and then more weakly in adjacent images because of the usually spherical nature of these objects.

The preliminary results from this approach were quite encouraging. When nodules with a "definitely a nodule" or "probably a nodule" score were counted, the system accurately detected 94% of the nodules from eight cases with an average of 1.25 false-positive detections per case.

Toshioka et al. (30) have also reported an automated 2-D method for detecting lung tumors from helical CT images. The first step is segmentation of the lung field using thresholding, followed by smoothing of the lung boundary. Tumors contacting the chest wall cause irregularities in the lung boundary and thus are included in the lung field after the smoothing operation. Fuzzy clustering (31) is applied within the lung field to separate pixels into two classes: "air part" or "blood vessels and tumors." The blood vessels and tumors are considered "candidate regions."

Feature analysis is used to identify the tumors separate from the blood vessels, because they cannot be reliably distinguished on the basis of CT number (i.e., by thresholding). The following features were calculated for each candidate region:

- *Area:* number of pixels in the candidate region
- *Thickness:* maximum gray-weighted distance in the candidate region
- *Circularity:* percentage of occupation inside the candidate region's circumscribed circle
- *Gray-level:* average CT number of pixels in the candidate region
- *Variance:* variance of CT numbers of pixels in the candidate region
- *Position:* minimum distance between the center of the candidate region's circumscribed circle and the lung boundary

Tumors are recognized using rules derived from the following pieces of "medical knowledge," which include (a) the shape of tumors is assumed to be spherical in a 2-D cross-sectional images, whereas vessels running in the scan plane appear oblong; (b) the thickness of blood vessels decrease as their position approaches the chest wall, whereas tumors are larger; (c) shadows contacting the chest wall are usually tumors, because blood vessels at the periphery are too small to be seen in the CT image; (d) the CT numbers of the blood vessels are usually higher than tumors when the vessels run perpendicular to the scan plane, and (e) the CT numbers within lung tumors are relatively uniform.

From this knowledge, heuristic rules were created and applied to 450 image data sets acquired using 10-mm collimation, table speed 20 mm/sec, with 10-mm reconstruction interval. Classification results were compared against three experts. Of the 225 lesions classified as "sure malignant lesion" or "probably malignant lesion" by at least one expert, the system correctly identified 11 of 11 lesions that were classified by all three experts; 35 of 40 lesions that were classified by two experts, and 141 of 174 lesions that were classified by one expert. There was an average of 9.6 false positives per case. Most of the false negatives were small tumors (< 5 mm). The false positives were caused by blood vessels being misidentified as tumors.

The systems described to this point have demonstrated the need for incorporating anatomical knowledge, in addition to CT number, to identify lung tumors separate from blood vessels and the chest wall. Typically, the knowledge has been incorporated in an ad hoc fashion using feature-based rules. In addition, these systems have demonstrated that segmentation of small tumors and tumors that contact or lie within the mediastinum requires more extensive and complex anatomical knowledge. To facilitate this, Brown et al. have described an architecture for

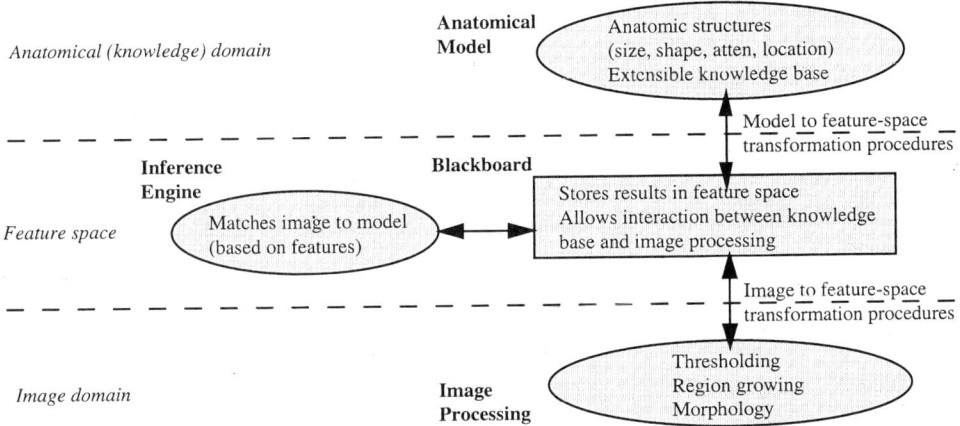

Fig. 6 Basic architecture for knowledge-based segmentation system showing separation of model and image processing routines and how they communicate through the blackboard.

knowledge-based segmentation (32), where knowledge is stored in the form of an explicit anatomical model, which can be extended in terms of the anatomy included and the features used to model the anatomy (33,34). This approach contrasts with methods that include heuristics or rules directly, or implicitly, in a pixel-based segmentation algorithm.

The method uses a modular architecture consisting of (see Fig. 6) an anatomical model, image-processing routines, and an inference engine, the interactions of which occur via a blackboard (35). This modular architecture represents a general-purpose framework for knowledge-based medical image analysis and interpretation (36–38). System components interact strictly by reading data from, and writing results to, the blackboard. This promotes independence between the modules and, in particular, between the anatomical model and image-processing routines.

Labeling the anatomical structures in the image data set involves matching image primitives to corresponding objects in the model. Matching is done by transforming data from the image and the model into a common, parametric feature-space for comparison. The inference engine compares features of image primitives with the predictions from the model and chooses the best match for each object.

The model contains information about specific anatomical parts, including expected size, shape, x-ray attenuation range, and location relative to other structures. These data are stored in a frame-based semantic network (39,40) as shown in Fig. 7.

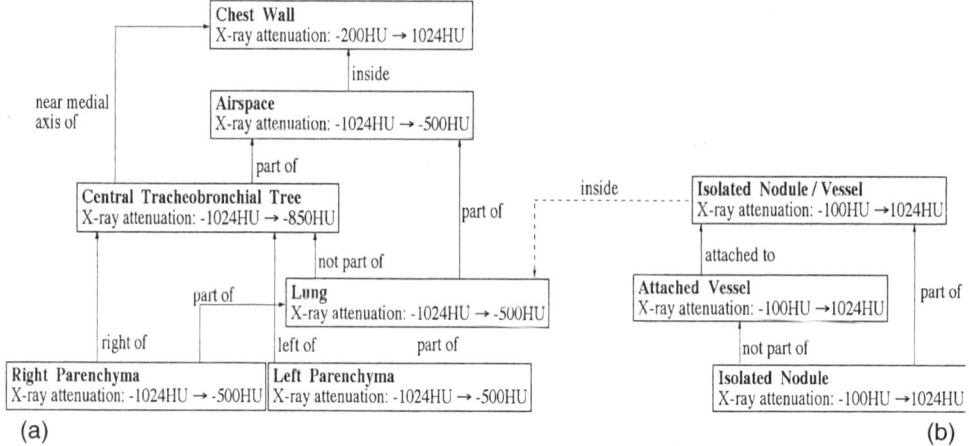

Fig. 7 (a) Semantic network description of lung including attenuation and positional relationships. (b) Extension of semantic network to include model of isolated nodule and attached vessel.

Image segmentation is done by means of a combination of gray-level thresholding, 3-D region growing, and mathematical morphology. These conventional algorithms are constrained using information from the anatomical model. The thresholding process is constrained by spatial relationships; for example, because the trachea is "part of" the airspace, only those voxels that have previously been labeled as airspace are considered when thresholding for the trachea. Morphological processing is used to extract shape properties of identified objects and to separate objects that are connected but of different size and shape.

The image-processing routines typically produce multiple candidates for a single anatomical structure. For a given candidate, confidence scores are generated, using fuzzy sets (41), for all individual constraints imposed by the model (e.g., size, shape). These confidence scores are used by the inference engine to quantify how well a candidate satisfies the given constraints. The inference engine selects the candidate with the highest score, effectively matching image structures to the model.

The control system is initialized by transferring information about the structures to be segmented from the model to the blackboard, complete with all of the knowledge used to constrain the segmentation. Each frame in the model is translated to a frame on the blackboard, including links for the various interdependencies (such as "inside of" or "part of"). Once the blackboard frames have been created, the control system must decide which frame to segment next. Scheduling is determined primarily by the dependency between frames; those having less dependencies are scheduled first. After image-processing routines are called to extract candidates, the inference engine identifies the candidate with the highest confidence score and stores it in the "best candidate" slot of the blackboard frame.

The system was developed originally to segment the lung parenchyma (32) (see Fig. 7a) and was then extended by adding nodule and vessel frames to the model, including expected shape and volume information (Fig. 7b). For candidate objects in the image that are within or exceed the volume constraint, 3-D binary morphological opening is applied. Contiguous sets of voxels remaining after the opening operation form a new set of candidates. The difference between the original and opened binary images is taken, and contiguous sets of voxels in the difference image (removed during opening) are also included as candidates. Thus, the original candidate is "split" into multiple smaller candidates. For nodules in contact with vessels, the morphological opening generates a candidate for the nodule with the vessels removed.

For these isolated lung lesions, simple measures of shape were used to distinguish lesions from vessels using a measure of compactness:

Compactness estimate $= 3v/(4\pi r^3)$.
Where d = maximum dimension (x, y, or z) of object's bounding box,
$r = d/2$,
v = volume of the object.

As the shape approaches spherical, as may be the case for a nodule, the compactness estimate approaches 1; whereas, a long thin vessel will yield a value closer to 0.

Fig. 8 shows results from an automated segmentation of an lung nodule with contiguous vessels, as well as the original images. This figure shows that, using the knowledge-based methods described earlier, the vessels and nodule are individually segmented. A seeded region-growing approach without knowledge guidance (a) requires manual interaction to place a seed point within the tumor and (b) is not able to differentiate the nodule from the vessel, because they have similar

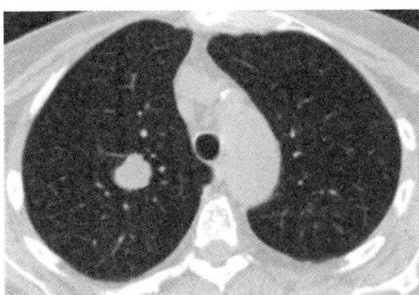 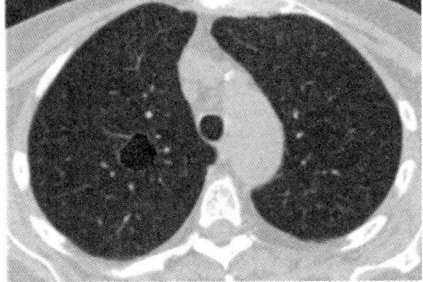

Fig. 8 (a) Original thoracic CT image showing nodule in contact with vessel, (b) pulmonary nodule (black) segmented separate from contacting vessel.

attenuation and are anatomically contiguous or at least appear so because of volume averaging or noise effects. In such cases, the region-growing algorithm "leaks" from one structure to the other, incorrectly combining them into a single set of contiguous voxels.

The system has also been extended to identify lung nodules that contact the lung-chest wall interface. In this case, the morphological operation removes the nodules from the otherwise smooth chest wall, so that the difference operation produces candidates for the nodule. Fig. 9 shows a lung mass contacting the chest wall pleural interface, which was successfully segmented. This figure shows that the chest wall, spine, anterior junction line, and mediastinum were approximately segmented to guide the isolation of the lesion. The results from this approach are promising but still preliminary. The ability to add knowledge to the system has been shown to be important for approaching the difficult problems in nodule detection described previously.

D. Segmentation of Endobronchial Lesions

Image processing techniques have also been applied to the detection of lesions that appear within the tracheobronchial tree (42) rather than in the lung parenchyma. In this approach, Summers suggested the use of surface curvature in conjunction with virtual reality techniques to automatically detect these lesions. First, a volumetric CT scan is analyzed using a 3-D seeded region growing technique to identify the walls of the airways. In one detection approach (the "patch" method), the airway surface is smoothed, and an overlapping bicubic parameter B-spline patch was fit to each point of the surface. The local curvature at each vertex was computed using first- and second-order derivatives of the B-spline patch (43,44). The calculated curvatures were analyzed, so that potential lesions were identified as those having elliptical curvature of the peak subtype (based on the signs of the principal curvatures). In a second detection method (the "gray-scale"

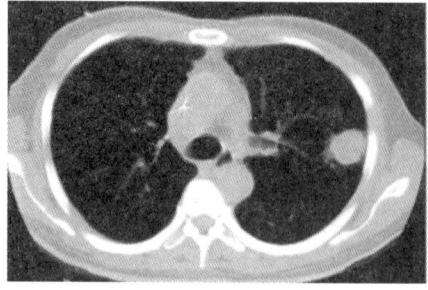 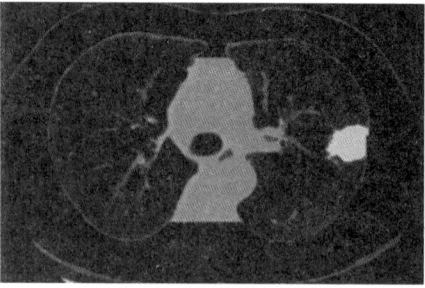

(a) (b)

Fig. 9 (a) Original thoracic CT image, (b) segmented chest wall (black), mediastinum (gray), and lesion (white) contacting the chest wall.

method), 3-D filters were applied to compute the partial derivatives directly from the image data (45,46). These partial derivatives were used to compute the gaussian (K), mean (H), and principal curvatures (κ_{min}, κ_{max}) at each vertex on the airway surface. These curvature values were then used to identify potential lesion sites.

For either approach, potential lesion sites were then evaluated using a 3-D surface geometry viewer and airway navigation software tools (47). The preliminary results showed that, when applied to patient scan data, the patch method was more sensitive (94%) than the gray-scale method (53%–65%), while yielding similar specificities (63%–78%), and that both methods performed reasonably well for lesions that were 5 mm in diameter or larger. This early work demonstrates some promise for the difficult problem of early detection of lesions that do not lie in the lung parenchyma but exist within the tracheobronchial tree.

IV. FUTURE WORK

A. Contributions of Automated Segmentation

For pulmonary nodule detection, the automatic identification (segmentation) of both normal anatomy and lesions in the lungs remains a fundamental limitation. For lung cancer screening, segmentation of anatomy will facilitate the identification of lesions that need to be reviewed by radiologists; for evaluation of lung cancer patients, segmentation will identify not just indicator lesions but potentially all of the lesions within the lung, so that their volumes can be calculated and compared across examinations. In each case, the ability to segment isolated lesions and those that contact other soft tissue structures (vessels, the chest wall as well as the mediastinum) is required for these approaches to be successful. To perform the required segmentation will require the addition of anatomical knowledge in one form or another. The methods described here hold some promise but require further testing to determine their reliability in detecting nodules and the number of false positives per image.

B. Image Processing Methods to Diagnose Solitary Pulmonary Nodules from CT

In addition to the nodule detection tasks described earlier, CT is commonly used as a follow-up and evaluation examination for solitary pulmonary nodules, especially those identified on a prior chest radiograph. These nodules present a common and difficult diagnostic problem (48–50), because they usually appear as a small, roughly circular object in the lungs of unknown origin, as shown earlier in Fig. 3. These nodules arise because of many different underlying processes ranging from a simple infection to a cancerous (malignant) lesion. The follow-up options are, obviously, quite different, depending on whether the nodule is thought to be benign or malignant and range from simple radiographic follow-up to needle biopsy of the tissue or, even more aggressively, surgical removal of the nodule. Interest in performing less-invasive tests has led to current research into the use of contrast-enhanced CT studies for diagnosis (51–53) and approaches that seek to quantify various properties of the nodule (e.g. size, shape, texture, rate of growth) that may aid in the diagnosis of the solitary lesion (54–59).

Several approaches have been described that use image-processing methods to quantify many of the properties currently described subjectively by a radiologist in an attempt to predict the nodule's diagnosis. Cavouras demonstrated promising results by using quantitative measures of nodule density and texture, extracted directly from the image data, in a classifier scheme to characterize SPNs (54). The features extracted included density measures (RCT, etc.); density histogram measures; and 12 texture measures from a spatial gray-level dependency (co-occurrence) matrix. A least squares minimum distance (LSMD) classifier was used to classify nodules and was very successful, because it correctly diagnosed 90.2% (46 of 51) of nodules. The authors concluded that although their method was successful, additional information may be provided by including the nodule's contour shape and size in the analysis.

McNitt-Gray (55,56) extended this approach to include quantitative measures from the following categories: (a) voxel intensity measures; (b) intensity histogram measures; (c) spatial distribution of intensity; (d) size; (e) shape; and (f) various texture measures (co-occurrence matrix measures and Laws' microtexture masks and various fractal based measures). For each nodule, all of the measures in each category were calculated. A feature selection step was performed to identify which features provided the most discriminatory power between the benign and malignant classes of nodules. The selected features were then used to train and test a pattern classifier to predict an individual nodule's diagnosis. Preliminary results yielded 28 of 31 (90.3%) correct with 2 false positives and 1 false negative.

In addition, because of the complex nature of the solitary nodules and our ability to image them in three dimensions with spiral CT, several groups have begun investigating the 3-D properties of the nodules. The 3-D nature of the nodule is demonstrated in Figs. 10 and 11. Fig. 10 shows a solitary nodule with calcium, whose distribution varies in location from slice to slice. Fig. 11 shows a 3-D rendering of the calcium distribution. This complex distribution of the nodule's density requires that it be analyzed with methods that take into account the 3-D nature of the object. These methods include techniques to assess the surface shape of the nodule (57) [similar to the methods used in (42)]. In addition, Reeves (58) and Yankelevitz (59) are investigating the morphological properties of nodules in three dimensions to detect changes over time, which may also be indicative of a lesion's diagnosis.

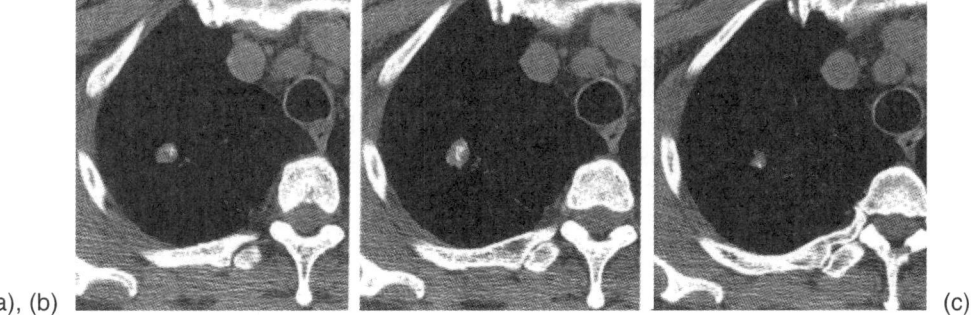

(a), (b), (c)

Fig. 10 CT images from an overlapped spiral acquisition (3-mm collimation, reconstructed every 1.5 mm) through a solitary pulmonary nodule viewed under "soft tissue" window and level settings (L = 40 HU, W = 400). Note the change in calcium distribution within the nodule from image to image.

In the near future, combinations of contrast-enhanced scanning with image processing methods that analyze both 2-D and 3-D properties will be evaluated to determine the efficacy of CT imaging in the diagnosis of solitary pulmonary nodules.

C. Technological Advances in Spiral CT Scanners

Technical developments in spiral CT continue to improve the ability to acquire images rapidly. In the late 1990s, commercial manufacturers introduced subsec-

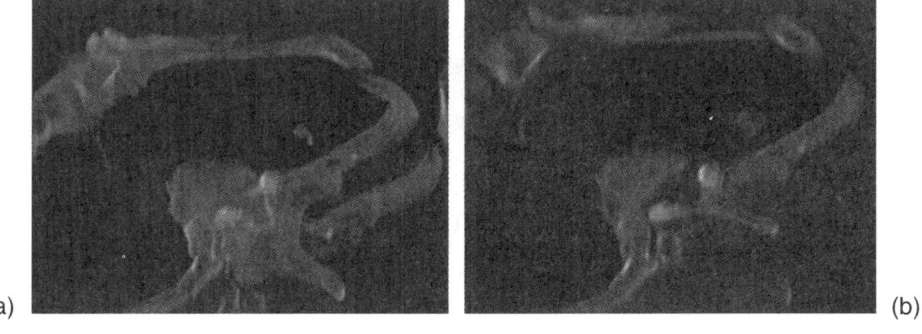

(a), (b)

Fig. 11 Volume rendered images of volumetric image data set through the solitary nodule imaged in Fig. 6 (a) opacity table set so that soft tissue is transparent, emphasizing the complex three-dimensional shape of the solitary nodule; and (b) opacity table set so that soft tissue is more opaque, showing the relationship of the calcium to the soft tissue of the nodule.

ond spiral scanning (complete 360-degree tube rotation in less than a second) and multiple detectors. By the fall of 1998, commercially available scanners could perform a complete rotation in .5 second; systems with two and four detectors were also commercially available with significant increases in the number of detectors on the near horizon. These developments allow the coverage of a volume of data in a very rapid fashion using very thin slices. Using a four-detector system with a .5 second rotation time, it would be possible to cover a 40-cm long thorax using 5-mm collimation in 20 seconds—a reasonable breath hold for most patients. If overlapping reconstructions were used (every 2.5 mm), this results in approximately 160 images. These developments result in (a) thinner effective slices, which reduce volume-averaging problems and increase the ability to detect smaller and smaller lesions; (b) increased longitudinal sampling for better nodule-image alignment; and (c) yet another significant increase in the number of images for radiologists to review. All three of these aspects further motivate the need for intelligent image-processing techniques to assist in lung tumor detection when spiral CT imaging is used.

REFERENCES

1. M Remy-Jardin, J Remy, F Giraud, CH Marquette. Pulmonary nodules: detection with thick-section spiral CT versus conventional CT. Radiology 187(2):513–20, 1993.
2. P Vock, M Soucek, M Daepp, W Kalendar. Lung: Spiral volumetric CT with single-breath-hold technique. Radiology 176:864–867, 1990.
3. K Mori, Y Saito, K Tominaga, K Yokoi, N Miyazawa, Y Kouda, A Okuyama, M Sasagawa, N Moriyama. Three-dimensional computed tomography image of small pulmonary lesions. Jpn J Clin Oncol 22:159–163, 1992.
4. P Costello, W Anderson, D Blume. Pulmonary nodule: evaluation with spiral volumetric CT. Radiology 179(3):875–876, 1991.
5. American Cancer Society. Cancer Facts and Figures 1998. Atlanta, GA: American Cancer Society, 1998.
6. D Eddy. Screening for lung cancer. Ann Intern Med 111:232–237, 1989.
7. BJ Flehinger, MR Melamed, MB Zaman, RT Heelan, WB Perchick, N Matini. Early lung cancer detection: Results of the initial (prevalence) radiologic and cytologic screening in the Memorial Sloan-Kettering study. Am Rev Respir Dis 130:555–560, 1984.
8. R Fontana, DR Sanderson, LB Woolner, et al. Lung cancer screening: The Mayo Program. J Occup Med 28:746–750, 1986.
9. M Tockman. Survival and mortality from lung cancer in a screend population: The Johns Hopkins study. Chest 57:44–53, 1986.
10. A Kubik, J Polak. Lung cancer detection: Results of a randomized prospective study in Czechoslovokia. Cancer 57:2427–2437, 1986.

11. S Sone, S Takashima, T Honda, T Yamanda, Y Maruyama, K Kanazawa, Y Kawata, N Niki, H Satoh. Screening for lung cancer using spiral CT. Radiology 205(P):689, 1997.
12. N Nitta, M Takahashi, K Murata, M Mori, R Morita. Ultra low-dose spiral CT for the lung cancer screening. Radiology 205(P):676, 1997.
13. R Kakinuma, H Ohmatsu, M Kaneko, K Eguchi, N Niki, N Moriyama, et al. Computer-assisted diagnosis system for lung cancer based on helical CT images. Radiology 205(P):739, 1997.
14. World Health Organization. WHO Handbook for Reporting the Results of Cancer Treatment. Geneva: WHO Offset Publication No. 48, 1979.
15. BD Fornage. Measuring masses on cross-sectional images. Radiology 187(1):289, 1993.
16. GH Guyatt, M Lefcoe, S Walter, D Cook, S Troyan, et al. Interobserver variability in the computed tomographic evaluation of mediastinal lymph node size in patients with potentially resectable lung cancer. Chest 107:116–119, 1995.
17. KD Hopper, JA Jozefiak, CJ Kasales, MA Van Slyke, TR Ten Have. Variation among readers in measuring tumor bulk in patients with metastatic chest and/or abdominal malignancy. Radiology 197(P):446, 1995.
18. DR Aberle, JDN Dionisio, MF McNitt-Gray, RK Taira, AF Cardenas, JG Goldin, K Brown, RF Figlin, WW Chu. An integrated multimedia timeline for medical images and data in thoracic oncology patients. Radiographics 16:669–681, 1996.
19. WA Kalender, A Polacin. Physical performance characteristics of spiral CT scanning. Med Physics 18(5):910–5, 1991.
20. A Polacin, WA Kalender, J Brink, MA Vannier. Measurement of slice sensitivity profiles in spiral CT. Med Physics 21(1):133–40, 1994.
21. A Polacin, WA Kalender. Evaluation of section sensitivity profiles and image noise in spiral CT. Radiology 185(1):29–35, 1992.
22. M McNitt-Gray, C Cagnon, T Solberg. Tradeoffs in helical CT: The effects of collimation and pitch on dose, noise and slice sensitivity profiles. In: RL Metter, J Beutel, eds. Proceedings SPIE 2708:427–437. Medical Imaging 1996: Physics of Medical Imaging.
23. G Wang, MW Vannier. Low-contrast resolution in volumetric x-ray CT—analytical comparison between conventional and spiral CT. Med Physics 24(3):373–376, 1997.
24. H Hu, SH Fox. The effect of helical pitch and beam collimation on the lesion contrast and slice profile in helical CT imaging. Med Physics 23(12):1943–1954, 1996.
25. G Wang, MW Vannier. Optimal pitch in spiral computed tomography. Med Physics 24(10):1635–1639, 1997.
26. G Wang, MW Vannier. Longitudinal resolution in volumetric x-ray computerized tomography—analytical comparison between conventional and helical computerized tomography. Med Physics 21(3):429–433, 1994.
27. C Croisille, M Souto, M Cova, S Wood, Y Afework, JE Kuhlman, EA Zerhouni. Pulmonary nodules: Improved detection with vascular segmentation and extraction with spiral CT. Radiology 197:397–401, 1995.
28. T Tozaki, Y Kawata, N Noki, H Ohmatsu, K Eguchi, N Moriyama. Three-dimensional analysis of lung area using thin slice CT images. Medical Imaging Proc SPIE 2709:2–11, 1996.

29. ML Giger, KT Bae, H MacMahon. Computerized detection of pulmonary nodules in computed tomography images. Invest Radiol 29(4):459–465, 1994.
30. S Toshioka, K Kanazawa, N Niki, H Satoh, H Ohmatsu, K Eguchi, N Moriyama. Computer aided diagnosis system for lung cancer based on helical CT images, image processing: KM Hanson, ed. Proc SPIE 3034:975–984, 1997.
31. J Toriwaki, A Fukumura, T Maruse. Fundamental properties of the gray weighted distance transformation, Trans IEICE Japan, J60-D(12):1101–1108, 1977.
32. MS Brown, MF McNitt-Gray, NJ Mankovich, JG Goldin, J Hiller, DP Tashkin, DR Aberle. Method for segmenting chest CT image data using an anatomic model: Preliminary results. IEEE Trans Med Imag 16(6):828–839, 1997.
33. MS Brown, MF McNitt-Gray, JG Goldin, DR Aberle. An extensible knowledge-based architecture for segmenting computed tomography images. IEEE Int Con Image Proc 3:516–519, 1997.
34. MS Brown, MF McNitt-Gray, JG Goldin, DR Aberle. An extensible knowledge-based architecture for segmenting CT data. Proc SPIE Med Imag 3338, in press, 1998.
35. HP Nii. Blackboard systems: the blackboard model of problem solving and the evolution of blackboard architectures. The AI Magazine pp 38–53, 1986.
36. MS Brown, RW Gill, T Loupas, HE Talhami, LS Wilson, BD Doust, LM Bischof, EJ Breen, Y Jiang, C Sun. Model-based interpretation of chest x-rays. Proc S/CAR 94: 344–349, 1994.
37. LS Wilson, MS Brown, HE Talhami, RW Gill, C Sun, BD Doust. Medical Image Understanding using anatomical models: application to chest X-rays. In: Y Bizais, ed. Information Processing in Medical Imaging 1995. Kluwer, 1995.
38. MS Brown, RW Gill, HE Talhami, LS Wilson, BD Doust. Model-based assessment of lung structures: Inferencing and control system. Proc SPIE Med Imag 2433: 167–178, 1995.
39. M Minksy. A framework for representing knowledge. In: PH Winston, ed. The Psychology of Computer Vision. New York: McGraw-Hill Book Company, 1975, pp 211–277.
40. MR Quillian. Semantic memory. In: MM Minsky, ed. Semantic Information Processing. Cambridge: M.I.T. Press, 1968.
41. LA Zadeh. Fuzzy sets. Inform Control 8:338–353, 1965.
42. RM Summers, LM Pusanik, JD Malley. Automatic detection of endobronchial lesions with virtual bronchoscopy: comparison of two methods. Proc SPIE Med Imag 3338, in press, 1998.
43. PJ Besl, RC Jain. Segmentation through variable-order surface fitting. IEEE Trans Pattern Anal Machine Intell 10:167–192, 1988.
44. P Dierckx. Curve and Surface Fitting with Splines. Oxford: Clarendon, 1993.
45. O Monga, S Benayoun. Using partial derivatives of 3D images to extract typical surface features. Comput Vision Image Understand 61:171–189, 1995.
46. J-P Thirion, A Gourdon. Computing the differential characteristics of isointensity surfaces. Comput Vision Image Understand 61:190–202, 1995.
47. Summers RM, Feng DF, Holland SM, Sneller MC, Shelhamer JH. Virtual bronchoscopy: segmentation methods for real time display. Radiology 200:857–862, 1996.

48. SS Siegelman, EA Zerhouni, FP Leo, NF Khouri, FP Stitik. CT of the solitary pulmonary nodule. AJR 135:1–13, 1980.
49. SS Siegelman, NF Khouri, FP Leo, EK Fishman, RM Braverman, EA Zerhouni. Solitary pulmonary nodules: CT assessment. Radiology 160:307–312, 1986.
50. AV Proto, SR Thomas. Pulmonary nodules studied by computed tomography. Radiology 156(1):149–153, 1985.
51. SJ Swensen, RL Morin, BA Schueler, LR Brown, DA Cortese, PC Pairolero, WM Brutinel. Solitary pulmonary nodule: CT evaluation of enhancement with iodinated contrast material—a preliminary report. Radiology 182(2):343–347, 1992.
52. SJ Swensen, LR Brown, TV Colby, AL Weaver. Pulmonary nodules: CT evaluation on enhancement with iodinated contrast material. Radiology 194:393–398, 1995.
53. K Yamashita, S Matsunobe, T Tsuda, T Nemoto, K Matsumoto, H Miki, J Konishi. Solitary pulmonary nodule: preliminary study of evaluation with incremental dynamic CT. Radiology 194:399–405, 1995.
54. D Cavouras, P Prassopoulos, N Pantelidis. Image analysis methods for the solitary pulmonary nodule characterization by computed tomography. Eur J Radiol 14:169–172, 1992.
55. MF McNitt-Gray, EM Hart, N Wyckoff, JW Sayre, JG Goldin, DR Aberle. Characterization of solitary pulmonary nodules using features extracted from high resolution CT images. Radiology 205(P):395, 1997.
56. MF McNitt-Gray, EM Hart, N Wyckoff, JW Sayre, JG Goldin, D. Aberle. The application of image analysis techniques to distinguish benign from malignant solitary pulmonary nodules imaged on CT. Proc SPIE Med Imag 3338, in press, 1998.
57. Y Kawata, N Niki, H Ohmatsu, R Kakinuma. Classification of pulmonary nodules in thin section CT images based on shape characterization. IEEE Int Conf Image Proc 3:528–531, 1997.
58. AP Reeves, B Zhao, DF Yankelevitz, CI Henschke. Characterization of three-dimensional shape and size changes of pulmonary nodules over time from helical CT images. Radiology 205(P):396.
59. DF Yankelevitz, ER Peters, B Zhao, D Shaham, T Gade, CI Henschke. Can computer-aided morphologic analysis of solitary pulmonary nodules predict pathology? Radiology 205(P):529, 1997.

12
Optimal Processing of Brain MRI

Hamid Soltanian-Zadeh
Henry Ford Health System, Detroit, Michigan; University of Tehran, Tehran, Iran; and Case Western Reserve University, Cleveland, Ohio

Joe P. Windham
Henry Ford Health System, Detroit, Michigan

I. INTRODUCTION

The ultimate goal of medical image analysis in general, and brain magnetic resonance imaging (MRI) analysis in particular, is to extract important clinical information that would improve diagnosis and treatment of disease. In the past few years, MRI has drawn considerable attention for its possible role in tissue characterization. The image gray levels in MRI depend on several tissue parameters, including proton density (PD); spin-lattice (T1) and spin-spin (T2) relaxation times; flow velocity (v); and chemical shift (δ). A sequence of MRI images of the same anatomical site (an MRI scene sequence) contains information pertaining to the tissue parameters. This implicit information is used for image analysis.

In brain tumor studies, existence of abnormal tissues is easily detectable most of the time. However, accurate and reproducible segmentation and characterization of abnormalities are not straightforward. For instance, a major problem in tumor treatment planning and evaluation is determination of the tumor extent. Clinically, T2-weighted and gadolinium (Gd)-enhanced T1-weighted MRI have been used to indicate regions of tumor growth and infiltration (1,2). Conventionally, simple thresholding or region growing techniques have been used on each image individually to segment the tissue or volume of interest for diagnosis, treatment planning, and follow-up of the patients. These methods are unable to exploit all the information provided by MRI. Advanced image analysis techniques have been and still are being developed to optimally use MRI data and solve the problems associated with the previous techniques.

Image analysis is performed by comparative and composite analysis of three-dimensional (3-D) brain MRI data. The aim of comparative analysis is to measure changes in the normal and tumorous tissue over time. The aim of composite analysis is to combine complementary information about the brain tissues from multiple MRI protocols to perform tissue segmentation and characterization. A given cerebral tumor may be composed of confluent areas of coagulation necrosis, compact areas of anaplastic cells, and areas of adjacent brain parenchyma infiltrated by tumor cells. This tumor may then be surrounded by reactive astrocytes and a rim of edema (3,4). Without considering all of the information obtained from different MRI protocols, segmentation and characterization of the tumor compartments are not feasible.

In an image analysis system designed for brain studies, the input image is first preprocessed. Preprocessing consists of (a) registration of multiple MRI studies; (b) segmentation of intracranial cavity from skull, scalp, and background; (c) correction of image nonuniformities; and (d) noise suppression. The resulting images may be combined to enhance the image contrast (5); the contrast-enhanced images may then be used to improve visual inspection of the scene. They may also be combined to generate a composite image in which a desired object (tumor) is segmented from its surrounding tissue (normal tissue) (6–12). In addition, it is possible to extract certain features from the images and use these features to segment the image into its components (13). The segmented image may be used for clinical studies, such as guided biopsy procedures, or it may be passed to an image classifier, which assigns the segmented regions to one of several objects. The results may be used for 3-D visualization, or they may be analyzed by an image-understanding system, which determines the relationships between different objects to form a scene description. These image analysis steps are shown in Fig. 1.

In the field of MRI, Vannier et al. (14) presented the first work in which the multiparametric (multispectral) nature of the MRI data was used for tissue characterization. Clarke et al. (15) have reviewed some of the MRI segmentation work in recent years. They conclude that feature extraction is a crucial step for MRI segmentation. Rather than using all the information in the images at once, feature extraction and selection breaks down the problem of segmentation to the grouping of feature vectors (16–19). Features can be pixel intensities themselves, features calculated from the pixel intensities, or edge and texture features (15).

Over the past 10 years, several approaches have been proposed for the analysis of multiparameter MRI data (5). These approaches include the maximum contrast method (20), artificial neural networks (21–24), a variety of clustering techniques (25–34), eigenimage filtering (6–12), and an optimal feature space method (13), all of which have been applied to tissue segmentation and characterization. Before getting into the details of the techniques, let us intro-

Processing of Brain MRI

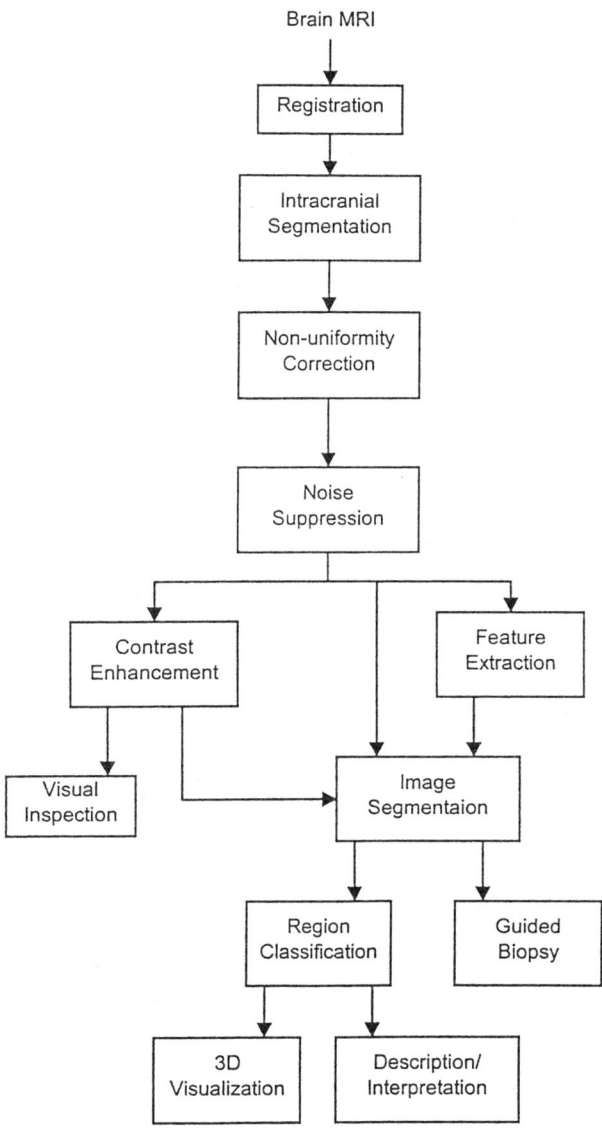

Fig. 1 A flowchart of image-processing steps for analysis of brain MRI studies.

duce the concepts related to spatial and feature domain representations of brain MRI.

A. Spatial and Feature Domain Representation

An MRI scene sequence shows spatial locations of different tissues, with a different contrast in each image. It can therefore be considered as a *spatial domain* representation of the tissues in a slice. In a spatial domain representation, pixels corresponding to a specific tissue are locally connected but may be distributed over different sections of the image. A *feature space* (*domain*) representation of tissues can be generated from an MRI scene sequence. In a feature space representation, pixels corresponding to a specific tissue are connected as clusters, even though their spatial locations in the image domain may be far apart. For an MRI scene sequence consisting of n images, a feature space representation is generated by defining an n-dimensional pixel vector for each pixel in the image (spatial) domain, using pixel gray levels of the same location from different images in the sequence as elements of this vector.

Image analysis can be accomplished using an appropriate feature space method. Feature space methods can be useful for all three steps of image analysis: (a) identification of objects; (b) segmentation of objects; and (c) quantitative measurements on objects, to obtain information that can be used in decision making (diagnosis, treatment planning, and evaluation of treatment). Basics of image processing and the interrelationship of the preceding three steps in image analysis are discussed in Refs. 35–38.

In this chapter, we present a supervised segmentation method that is based on visualization of the generated feature space (i.e., visualization of the multidimensional histogram of the data), which we call a cluster plot. This constrains the dimensionality of the feature space. As the dimensionality of the feature space increases, its visualization becomes more difficult. One- and two-dimensional (1-D and 2-D) feature spaces can be easily visualized with a conventional histogram and an image whose pixel intensity is proportional to the number of data points in a certain range (i.e., a 2-D cluster plot). With a little bit more effort, we may generate a 3-D cluster plot, by drawing three axes of an orthogonal coordinate system in an image, for 3-D perception, and making image pixel gray levels proportional to the number of data points in certain ranges. Furthermore, we may generate a 4-D feature space, by creating 3-D feature spaces and showing them in a loop (i.e., using time as the fourth axis). This visualization will, however, be limited in that the operator cannot easily draw regions of interest (ROIs) on it and find the corresponding pixels in the image domain. More difficulties will be involved with visualizing feature spaces of dimensions higher than four. Therefore, we restrict our attention to feature spaces with dimensions not larger than three.

Considering pixel intensity features and those extracted from them by applying a transformation, methods of preparing data for an MRI feature space representation can be partitioned into three categories: (a) tissue-parameter-weighted images [e.g., (14,39)]; (b) explicit calculation of tissue parameters [e.g., (40,41)]; and (c) linear transformations [e.g., generation of color composite images (42,43) or principal component analysis (PCA) (44)] and nonlinear transformations [e.g., angle images (45)].

Both categories (a) and (b) require acquisition of multiple images using specific MRI protocols. A difficulty with category (b) is that it requires protocols that are usually different from those routinely used in clinical studies. In addition, noise propagation, through the required nonlinear calculations, combines with the model inaccuracies and yields unsatisfactory results (46–48). As illustrated in Ref. 49, because of the nonlinearity of the transformation from pixel intensity space to tissue parameter space, optimal linear decision functions in the intensity space translate to nonlinear decision functions in the tissue parameter space. Thus, unless these nonlinear decision functions are used, the decision is not optimal.

Category (c) can be applied to any MRI scene sequence and can improve the clustering properties of the data for the feature space representation while reducing its dimensionality. However, general purpose transformations found in the literature are not appropriate for MRI. For instance, a difficulty with the feature space generated by principal component images is its limitation related to the size of the objects in the scene. Small objects make slight contributions to the covariance matrix and thus are not enhanced and visualized in the first few principal component images. The first few principal component images are normally used for the feature space representation, because they have the best signal/noise ratios (SNRs). A concern with angle images is the nonlinearity of the transformation that generates curves, rather than lines, for partial volume regions in the cluster plot; this complicates the distinction between clusters for partial volume regions and those for heterogeneous tissues.

Soltanian-Zadeh, et al. (13) have devoted a significant effort toward derivation of an *optimal linear* transformation to prepare MRI data for feature space analysis. It should be noted that an important distinction for feature extraction methods is whether they need class information or not. PCA does not; hence it is widely used in other fields as a general purpose approach. The method presented in this chapter, which is related to discriminant analysis (DA) (50), needs some class information (signature vectors for normal tissues); hence it has specific compatibility to MRI and is most appropriate for this field. The features extracted from the image define clusters in the feature space. A correspondence exists between these clusters and the tissue types in the image. We explain how this correspondence is explored, and the scene is segmented using the information present in the cluster plot. Visualization of the feature space (cluster plot) is therefore critical to the optimal method.

Several general purpose unsupervised methods have also been proposed for segmentation of normal and abnormal tissues from brain MRI. They include clustering approaches such as K-means and fuzzy C-means and neural networks such as multilayer perceptron, which are general purpose segmentation and classification techniques. In this chapter, we present methods that have been *specifically developed* for MRI and thus are *optimal* for MRI. Wherever necessary, these methods use intraframe and interframe information to achieve best performance. In developing these methods, vector space notations and methods were used. We present these notations in the next section.

B. Notations

For presenting mathematical bases of the techniques, we use an n-dimensional vector space $(\mathcal{R}^n, \mathcal{R})$, where n is the number of images in the MRI scene sequence. For example, when dealing with an MRI scene sequence consisting of a T1-weighted and four T2-weighted spin-echo images for each anatomical location, we use a five-dimensional vector space. Using the vector space concept, the following representations are introduced. The MRI scene sequence is represented by *pixel vectors*. A pixel vector $\mathbf{P}_{jk} = [P_{jk1}\ P_{jk2}\ \cdots\ P_{jkn}]^T$ is a vector whose elements are the corresponding gray levels of the (j, k)-th pixels in the MR images (see Fig. 2). The image size determines the number of these pixel vectors (e.g., for

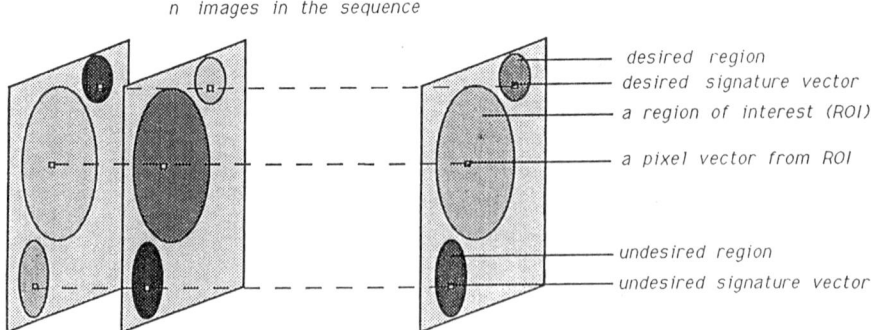

Fig. 2 A schematic representation of a sequence of images of a specific anatomical site consisting of different materials. As an example, the upper region is considered as the desired region, and a pixel vector is chosen from that region as the desired signature vector. Similarly, the lower region is considered as the undesired region, and a pixel vector is selected from that region as the undesired signature vector. The large region in the middle is assumed to be a region of interest, which might be a combination of the desired and undesired tissues or something else. A pixel vector is also shown from the region of interest. (*Source:* Ref. 7.)

256 × 256 images there are 65,536 pixel vectors). The MRI characteristics of tissue types are represented by *signature vectors*. For image analysis, one is normally interested in clearly visualizing one of the tissue types (referred to as desired tissue), whereas other tissue types (referred to as undesired or interfering tissues) interfere with its visualization. A *desired signature vector* $\mathbf{d} = [d_1\ d_2\ \cdots\ d_n]^T$ is defined as a vector whose i-th element is the average gray level of the desired tissue in the i-th image. *Undesired (interfering) signature vectors* $\mathbf{u}_i = [u_{1i}\ u_{2i}\ \cdots\ u_{ni}]^T$, $1 \leq i \leq m$, are similarly defined for the interfering tissues. Finally, vectors $\mathbf{P}_{jk}^d$ and $\mathbf{P}_{lm}^u$ are pixel vectors from the desired tissue at location (j, k) and the undesired tissue at location (l, m), respectively. These notations and those defined later are summarized in a list that follows the following list of abbreviations.

1. List of Abbreviations

   AVG: Average
   CNR, SNR: Contrast/noise ratio and signal/noise ratio, respectively
   CSF: Cerebrospinal fluid
   ROI: Region of interest
   DROI: Desired tissue ROI
   UROI (IROI): Undesired (interfering) tissue ROI
   EPV, OPV: Estimated and original partial volumes, respectively
   LS: Least squares
   MLE: Maximum likelihood estimate
   MR, MRI: Magnetic resonance and magnetic resonance imaging/images, respectively
   NS: Neighborhood size
   P_D, P_F: Probabilities of detection and false alarm, respectively
   PD, N(H): Proton density
   IED, IAD: Interset and intraset euclidean distances, respectively
   MMAC: Maximized minimum absolute contrast/noise ratio
   MAC: Minimum absolute contrast/noise ratio

2. List of Mathematical Notations

   CNR_i: The CNR between desired tissue and i-th interfering tissue
   $\mathbf{d}$: The desired tissue signature vector
   $\mathbf{e}$: The weighting vector for the eigenimage filter
   $E[\cdot]$: The expected value operator
   $\hat{E}[\cdot]$: An expected value estimator (here, the sample mean)
   EI_{jk}: The gray level of the (j, k)-th pixel in the eigenimage
   m: The number of interfering tissues in the scene
   n: The number of images in the MRI scene sequence
   N: The number of pixels in the DROI

P_{jk}: The gray level of the (j, k)-th pixel in an image
P_{jki}: The gray level of the (j, k)-th pixel in the i-th image
$\mathbf{P}_{jk}$: A pixel vector (i.e., an n-dimensional vector whose i-th element is P_{jki})
P_{jk}^d: The gray level of the (j, k)-th pixel in the DROI of an image
$\mathbf{P}_{jk}^d$: A pixel vector in the DROI
P_{jk}^u: The gray level of the (j, k)-th pixel in an UROI of an image
P_{jk}^{ui}: The gray level of the (j, k)-th pixel in the i-th UROI of an image
$\mathbf{P}_{jk}^{ui}$: A pixel vector in the i-th UROI
σ: The standard deviation of white noise
SNR_d: The SNR of the desired tissue
S_i: The MRI signal from the i-th tissue
$\mathbf{u}$: An undesired tissue signature vector
$\mathbf{u}_i$: The i-th undesired tissue signature vector
$Var(\cdot)$: The variance operator
$\widehat{Var}(\cdot)$: A variance estimator (here, the sample variance)
V_l: The partial volume of the l-th tissue in a voxel
V_{ljk}: The partial volume of the l-th tissue in the (j, k)-th voxel
V: The total volume of a voxel
$\mathbf{w}$: The weighting vector for a linear filter
w_{jk}: The zero-mean white noise at the (j, k)-th pixel of an image
w_{jki}: The zero-mean white noise at the (j, k)-th pixel of the i-th image

II. PREPROCESSING

Preprocessing consists of (a) registration of multiple MRI studies; (b) segmentation of intracranial cavity from skull, scalp, and background; (c) correction of image nonuniformities; and (d) noise suppression. Methods specifically designed for these tasks are explained in the following sections.

A. Registration

To follow sequential changes that may occur over time, it is necessary to register the image sets obtained at different times. Also, if the patient moves between different scans, images should be registered before multispectral image processing and analysis are applied (see Fig. 3).

Several methods have been proposed for medical image registration [e.g., (12,15,51–55)]. These techniques can be partitioned into three categories: (a) landmark based (point matching); (b) surface based (surface matching); and (c) intensity based (volume matching). Compared with landmark-based methods, surface-based methods do not need landmarks, and compared with intensity-based methods, they are faster. Most of the surface-based methods use the head surface,

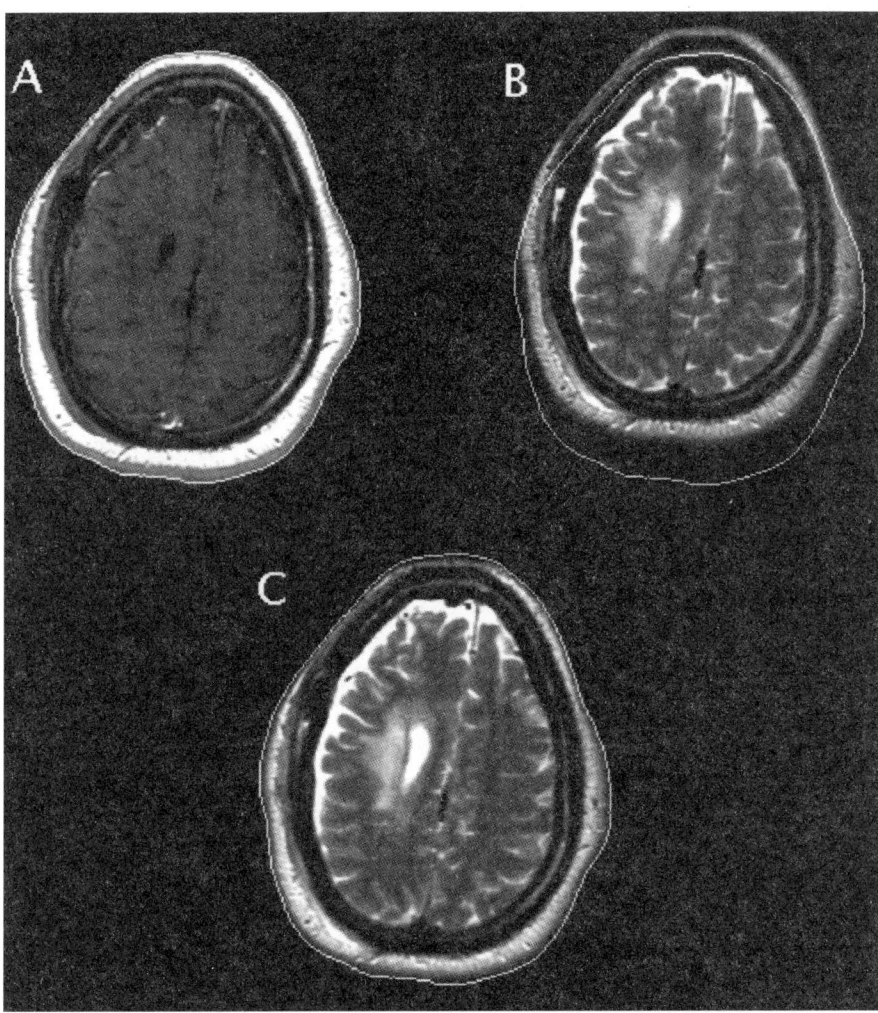

Fig. 3 An illustration of image registration. A, An axial T1-weighted MRI of a tumor patient, with skin edges (contour) overlaid. B, Corresponding axial T2-weighted MRI, with contour of the T1-weighted image overlaid to show the need for registration. C, The T2-weighted image after being registered to the T1-weighted image, with the contour of the T1-weighted image overlaid to illustrate the match generated by the image registration method.

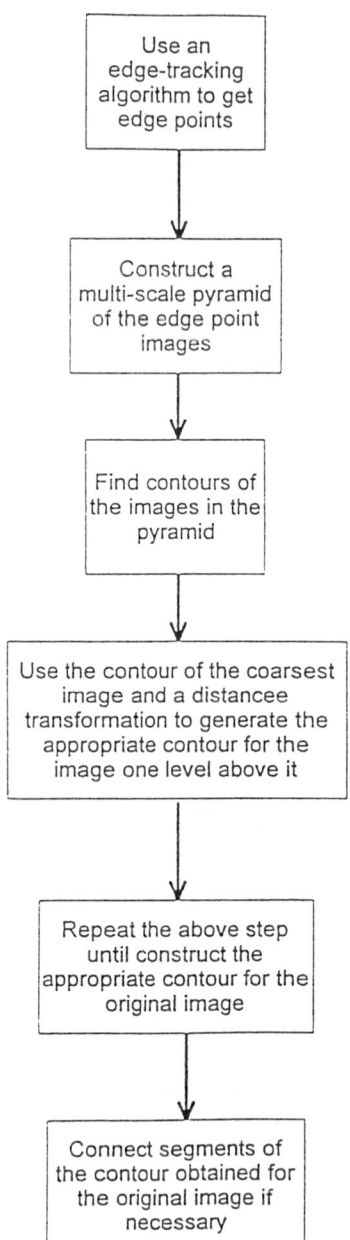

Fig. 4 Steps of the multiresolution approach for automatic contour extraction. (*Source:* Ref. 62.)

brain surface, or inner/outer surface of the skull to estimate rotation and translation parameters [see (12,51–53) for details]. The surface is usually characterized by a set of edge or contour points extracted from cross-sectional images. Manual drawing of the contours is very time consuming. Automatic extraction of the contour points by standard edge-based, region-based, or classification-based algorithms has shown problems (56). Both region-based and classification-based algorithms are affected by inhomogeneity artifacts. Edge-based techniques are affected by the partial volume effects creating wide transition zones between tissue types. Researchers have developed a variety of complex and heuristic systems to overcome these difficulties and to automate the contour extraction procedure for specific applications (56–60). A thorough survey of the recent work in the area of contour extraction for intracranial cavity segmentation is given in Ref. (56).

Because of its simplicity and its capability to follow an appropriate path in the middle of the partial volume regions, an edge-tracking algorithm similar to the one proposed by Henrich et al. (61) can be used. In using this algorithm, it was found that this method has difficulties caused by discontinuity of edges in the back of the eyes and ears and sometimes by edge discontinuities resulted from a previous surgery (see Fig. 5) or an inadequate field of view. To solve this problem, Soltanian-Zadeh and Windham (62) developed an automated method that uses a multiresolution pyramid to connect edge discontinuities. A flowchart of the algorithm is presented in Fig. 4, and an example is shown in Figs. 5 and 6.

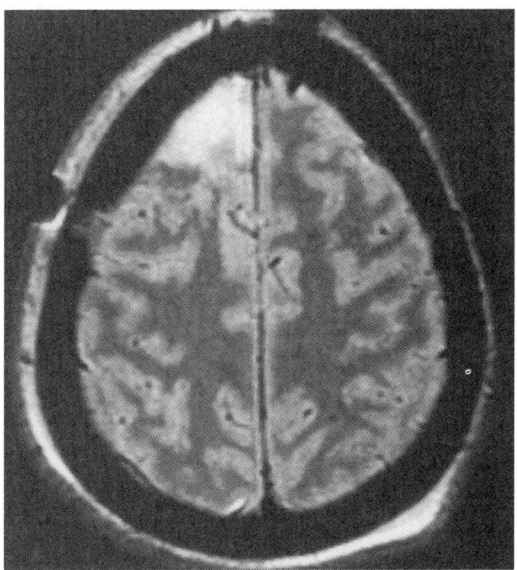

Fig. 5 A T2-weighted MRI of a tumor patient in which the edge-tracking algorithm does not find correct edges because of soft tissue discontinuity. (*Source:* Ref. 62.)

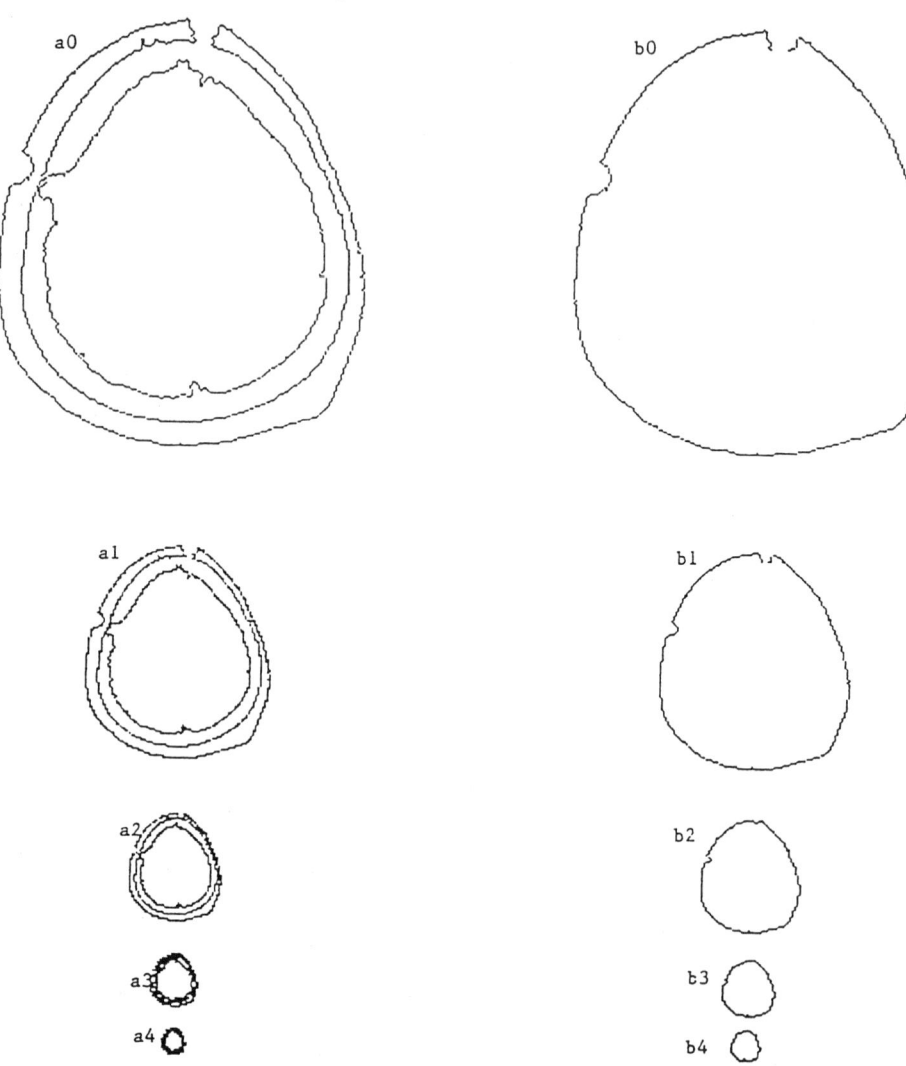

Fig. 6 Steps of the multiresolution approach for connecting gaps in MR images. **a0–a4,** Skin edges extracted from the MR image shown in Fig. 5 and four lower-resolution versions of it, respectively. **b4,** *Exterior* edge of **a4. b3,** Points on the *exterior* edge of **a3,** found by selecting edge points in **a3** that are less than 2 units of chessboard distance from a blowup of **b4.** Similarly, **b2** is found using **b3** and **a2; b1** is found using **b2** and **a1;** and **b0** is found using **b1** and **a0.** (*Source:* Ref. 62.)

B. Intracranial Segmentation

The image background does not usually contain any useful information but complicates the image restoration and tissue segmentation/classification and increases the processing time. It is therefore beneficial to remove the image background before image restoration and analysis begins. In addition, in brain studies, tissues such as scalp, eyes, and others that are outside of the intracranial cavity are not of interest. Hence, it is preferred to segment the intracranial cavity volume from scalp and background. This segmentation is usually straightforward for brain MRI studies. Thresholding and morphological operators (35–38) have been used to do this segmentation.

C. Nonuniformity Correction

MRI brain images acquired using standard head coils suffer from several possible sources of nonuniformity, including (a) main field (B_0) nonuniformity; (b) the time domain filter applied before Fourier transformation in the frequency encoding direction; (c) nonuniformity caused by uncompensated gradient eddy currents; (d) transmitted and received radiofrequency (RF) field nonuniformity; (e) RF penetration depth effects; and (f) RF standing wave effects. Simmons et al. (63,64) have investigated the magnitude of these effects on clustering properties of MRI data acquired using a GE Signa system. The first effect is usually corrected by using a multiple spin-echo sequence. Condon et al. (65) have discussed methods for correcting the second effect. However, because most of the current scanners use digital filters whose effect on the image is limited to two or three pixels at the edge of the image, this correction is usually unnecessary. The third effect on modern MRI systems, such as GE Signa, that are equipped with shielded gradients is small for spin-echo sequences at long repetition times used in tumor studies. The fourth effect needs to be estimated and used to correct MRI scans (66). Approaches for estimating this nonuniformity are explained in the next paragraph. The fifth and sixth effects are normally negligible in tumor patient studies; thus, no correction is necessary for them.

Ignoring the random noise, the measured MRI pixel gray level P_{ij} can be related to the true MRI signal by the relation $P_{ij} = A_{ij}I_{ij}$, where A_{ij} is the nonuniformity factor at location (i, j) in the image and I_{ij} is the artifact-free intensity value at the same location. A number of approaches to the correction of RF-induced intensity variations have been proposed [e.g., (67–73)]. All of these methods rely on the division of the acquired image by a reference image that approximates the nonuniformity profile A_{ij} but differ in the way the reference image is obtained.

One approach is to use a water or oil phantom. These phantoms are cylinder shaped plastic containers of about the same size as an average human head (about 20 cm in diameter and 25 cm in height) filled with water or solid oil. Using an oil phantom compared with a water phantom has the advantage of avoiding spurious RF penetration depth and standing wave effects. Both of these phantoms have limitations associated with changing nonuniformity pattern over time and loading of the coil. Therefore, approaches such as those explained in the following that estimate the nonuniformity pattern from the acquired images (in a reasonable amount of time) are more appropriate.

1. Assuming that the inhomogeneity in the RF coil sensitivity manifests itself as a low-frequency component, A_{ij} is estimated by smoothing the image using a 33 × 33 kernel of 1's (69). We have modified this approach by not averaging the background pixels to avoid the artifacts generated around the outside of the brain. Also, cerebrospinal fluid (CSF) and other high-contrast regions are replaced by the average of white and gray matter values to avoid other edge artifacts.
2. Making the assumptions that T1, T2, and proton density (PD) values for a single tissue type do not vary significantly across a particular slice and that reference points for at least one tissue type can be identified across the image, an intensity surface is fitted to the reference points to estimate the nonuniformity profile. Two methods (direct and indirect) have been proposed (70). In the direct method, the user selects multiple points to define a tissue type across the field of view. In the indirect method, the user selects an initial point, and the reference points are selected automatically throughout the image using a similarity criterion. Then, using the basis functions, $F_i = d_i^2 \ln(d_i)$, where d_i is the euclidean distance, an intensity pattern is fitted to the reference points by a least squares fit. This method has also been used by researchers such as Nocera and Gee (74).

D. Tissue Inhomogeneities

A tissue type may have biological variations throughout the imaged volume. For example, biological properties of white matter in the anterior and posterior of the brain are slightly different. A tissue type may also have biological heterogeneity in it; many brain lesions are heterogeneous in nature. These cause variations of signal intensity for a single tissue in the imaged volume. The feature space representation of the entire volume may therefore be spread out (i.e., clusters for different tissues may overlap). Sources of this variation include the difference in the proton density and T1 and T2 relaxation times from voxel to voxel. These differences generate a different multiplicative factor in image gray levels from voxel to voxel, and application of a ratio filter seems appropriate (5). However, in general, because of these effects, feature space analysis is not recommended for the entire 3-D volume in one stage; superior results may be obtained using a slice-by-slice analysis approach.

E. Noise Suppression

Noise limits the performance of both human observers and computer vision systems. As such, noise should be suppressed before inputting data to image segmentation and classification algorithms. To reduce the computation time, noise suppression is performed after *intracranial* volume segmentation. General purpose filters such as low-pass, Weiner, median, or anisotropic diffusion filters may be used. However, an optimal filter specifically designed for MRI (75) generates superior results. We explain this filter next.

The filter is a multidimensional nonlinear edge-preserving filter. It has been specifically developed for *multiparameter* (multispectral) MR image restoration (noise suppression) in which multiple images of the same section are processed together. The filter uses both intraframe (spatial) and interframe (temporal) information by considering a neighborhood around each pixel and calculating the euclidean distance of each pixel vector in this neighborhood from the pixel vector in the center and comparing the result with a preset threshold value. The threshold value is found by calculating probabilities of detection (P_D) and false alarm (P_F). In applications for which a good model exists for interframe information (e.g., the exponential model for multiple spin-echo images), the filter uses the model. It also uses the widely used zero-mean white gaussian noise model for the statistical noise. Details of the method for multiple spin-echo sequences are explained below.

For a multiple spin-echo sequence with n echoes, the signal S_i, arising from a region with tissue-specific parameters N(H) and T1 and T2 relaxation times in the ith image is given by

$$S_i = N(H)\left[1 - (-1)^n\left[2\sum_{l=1}^{n}(-1)^l e^{\frac{(2l-1)TE-2TR}{2T1}} + e^{\frac{-TR}{T1}}\right]\right] \times e^{\frac{-iTE}{T2}}, \quad 1 \le i \le n \quad (1)$$

where TR = *repetition time* and TE = *echo time* are pulse sequence parameters.

Considering the additive white noise, the intensity of the jk-th pixel in the ith image (P_{jki}) can be represented by

$$P_{jki} = M_{jk} e^{\frac{-iTE}{T2_{jk}}} + w_{jki}, \quad 1 \le i \le n \quad (2)$$

where M_{jk} is a function of $T1$ and $N(H)$ of the tissue at position (j, k) and TR of the pulse sequence, and w_{jki} is a white gaussian noise. The model in Eq. (2) provides a means for obtaining a least-square (LS) or maximum-likelihood (ML) estimate of the pixel intensities, because it shows the relationship between corresponding pixels from different images in the sequence that we refer to as interframe (temporal) information. It should be noted that for the gaussian model in Eq. (2), the ML estimate coincides with the LS estimate (76). Intraframe (spatial) information refers to the relationship between pixels from a particular tissue within the same image in the sequence. This information is provided by the anatomical structures visualized in the image.

The filter works as follows. A neighborhood around each pixel is considered. The euclidean distance of each pixel vector in the neighborhood from the pixel vector in the center is found. If this distance is smaller than a specific threshold value, η, the pixel vector is considered in the LS or ML estimation, otherwise it is not. The threshold η is selected on the basis of the noise standard deviation σ in the images, the contrast between adjacent tissues, and partial volume averaging effects that are reflected in the sharpness of edges in each image. In practice, η is calculated on the basis of the probabilities of detection and false alarm. An approximate LS or ML estimate for the average of the contributing pixel vectors is determined and saved for all of the contributing pixel vectors, using the model in Eq. (2). Then, the neighborhood is moved, and the procedure is repeated. Finally, the average of several estimates obtained for a particular pixel vector is calculated to obtain the filter output for the pixel vector.

In the derivation of the filter, we have considered an approximate LS or ML estimate, because the exact estimate requires solving a nonlinear system of equations, which is computationally intense. To do the approximation, we factor the signal $M_{jk} \exp\left[\frac{-iTE}{T2_{jk}}\right]$ out of Eq. (2) and take its natural logarithm. Using a Taylor series expansion for $\ln(1 + x)$ and neglecting x^2 and higher order terms, because $M_{jk} \exp\left[\frac{-iTE}{T2_{jk}}\right]/w_{jki} \gg 1$ thus $x = w_{jki}/M_{jk} \exp\left[\frac{-iTE}{T2_{jk}}\right] \ll 1$, we get

$$\ln(P_{jki}) = \ln\left(M_{jk} e^{\frac{-iTE}{T2_{jk}}}\right) + \ln\left(1 + \frac{w_{jki}}{M_{jk} e^{\frac{-iTE}{T2_{jk}}}}\right)$$

$$\simeq \ln\left(M_{jk} e^{\frac{-iTE}{T2_{jk}}}\right) + \frac{w_{jki}}{M_{jk} e^{\frac{-iTE}{T2_{jk}}}} \quad (3)$$

$$= \ln(M_{jk}) - \frac{iTE}{T2_{jk}} + ws_{jki} = a_{jk} + b_{jk}i + ws_{jki}$$

Note that ws_{jki} is also zero-mean and gaussian distributed, because it is a scaled version of w_{jki}. So, the maximum likelihood estimate of $\ln(P_{jki})$ is identical to a weighted least-squares estimate for the line $a_{jk} + b_{jk}i$. Weights for the least squares estimate are $\left[M_{jk} \exp\left[\frac{-iTE}{T2_{jk}}\right]\right]^{-1}$, which we approximate by $(P_{jki})^{-1}$ [See Eq. (2)].

Processing of Brain MRI

In the selection of the threshold η, we consider the probabilities of detection P_D and false alarm P_F. It is ideal to have a P_D equal to 1.0 and a P_F equal to 0.0. The probability of detection P_D is the chance of correctly identifying a pixel vector $\mathbf{P}_{jk}^d$ in the neighborhood that represents the same tissue type as the pixel vector $\mathbf{P}_{lm}^d$ in the center. These pixel vectors are assumed to be uncorrelated and gaussian distributed, with mean vector $\mathbf{d}$ and covariance matrix $\sigma^2 \mathbf{I}$. The difference vector $\mathbf{D}_{jk}^d = \mathbf{P}_{lm}^d - \mathbf{P}_{jk}^d$ is therefore gaussian distributed, with mean vector $\mathbf{0}$ and covariance matrix $2^2_\sigma \mathbf{I}$. The square of the euclidean distance $ED_{jk}^2 = \|\mathbf{D}_{jk}^d\|^2$ between these pixel vectors has a scaled chi-squared distribution with n degrees of freedom, a mean of $2n\sigma^2$, and a variance of $8n\sigma^4$ (77). Using the threshold value η for the euclidean distance, ED_{jk} yields the following probability of detection P_D:

$$P_D = \int_0^{\frac{\eta^2}{2\sigma^2}} f_X(x)dx = \frac{1}{2^{\frac{n}{2}}\Gamma(\frac{n}{2})} \int_0^{\frac{\eta^2}{2\sigma^2}} x^{\frac{n}{2}-1} e^{-\frac{x}{2}} dx \tag{4}$$

The probability of false alarm P_F is the chance of wrongly classifying a pixel vector in the neighborhood (i.e., the probability of misclassifying $\mathbf{P}_{jks}^u$ representing tissue u_s) into tissue class d corresponding to pixel vector $\mathbf{P}_{lm}^d$. As before, these pixel vectors are assumed to be uncorrelated and gaussian distributed, with identical covariance matrices $\sigma^2 \mathbf{I}$ but different mean vectors $\mathbf{u}$ and $\mathbf{d}$, respectively. The difference vector $\mathbf{D}_{jk}^u = \mathbf{P}_{lm}^d - \mathbf{P}_{jk}^u$ is then gaussian distributed with mean vector $\mathbf{m} = \mathbf{d} - \mathbf{u}$ and covariance matrix $2^2_\sigma \mathbf{I}$. The square of the euclidean distance between these pixel vectors $ED_{jk}^2 = \|\mathbf{D}_{jk}^u\|^2$ has a *noncentral* chi-squared distribution. Using standard techniques for deriving probability density functions (pdf) (78), the pdf for the square of the i-th component of the difference vector divided by $2\sigma^2$ is obtained as

$$f_{Y_i}(y) = \frac{1}{2\sqrt{2\pi y}} \left[e^{-\frac{(\sqrt{y}-m_i)^2}{2}} + e^{-\frac{(\sqrt{y}-m_i)^2}{2}} \right], \tag{5}$$

$$y > 0, \quad 1 \leq i \leq n$$

where m_i is the ith component of the difference vector $\mathbf{m}$ divided by $\sqrt{2}\sigma$. The pdf $f_Y(y)$ for the euclidean distance squared ED_{jk}^2 divided by $2\sigma^2$ is found by convolving n pdfs given in Eq. (5), i.e.

$$f_Y(\cdot) = f_{Y_1}(\cdot) * f_{Y_2}(\cdot) * \cdots * f_{Y_n}(\cdot) \tag{6}$$

Finally, the probability of false alarm P_F is

$$P_F = \int_0^{\frac{\eta^2}{2\sigma^2}} f_Y(y) dy \tag{7}$$

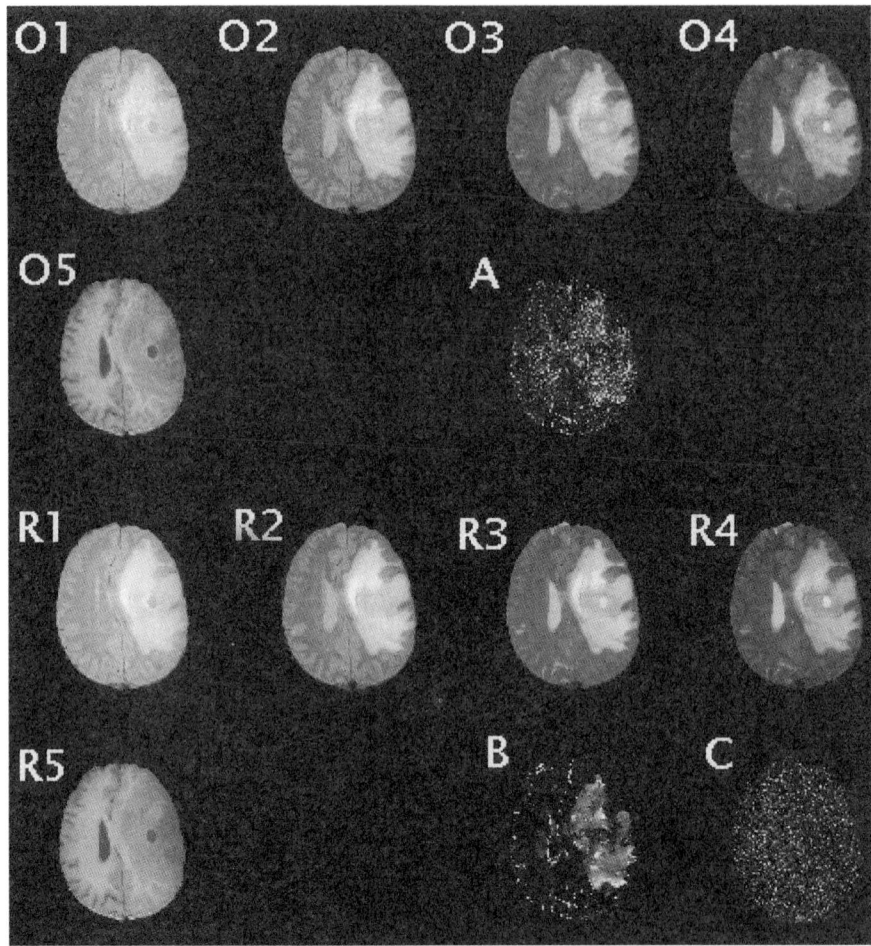

Fig. 7 **O1–O5,** Four T2-weighted multiple spin echo images (TE/TR = 25–100/2000 msec) and a T1-weighted image (TE/TR = 20/500 msec) of a tumor patient, respectively, after registration and intracranial segmentation. **A,** Transformed image (eigenimage) created for the lesion by applying the optimal transformation method explained in Sec. VB to images **O1–O5. R1–R5,** Noise-suppressed images generated using the filter described in Sec. IID. **B,** Transformed image (eigenimage) created for the lesion by applying the optimal transformation method to images **R1–R5. C,** Difference image generated by subtracting image **B** from image **A.** Note the quality improvement in the original images and the lesion eigenimage generated by the noise suppression filter. Image C illustrates that the filter has suppressed the noise without removing useful image information.

Processing of Brain MRI

Theoretical and experimental results have shown that when processing MRI scene sequences with four or five images per slice, a 9×9 neighborhood and a threshold value of $\eta = 4\sigma$ generates optimal results (75).

1. An Example

Fig. 7 shows a sequence of four T2-weighted and a T1-weighted MRI of a tumor patient after registration and intracranial segmentation. It also shows noise-suppressed images generated using the filter described earlier. Transformed images (eigenimages) created for the lesion by applying the optimal transformation method (explained in Sec. VB) to the original and noise-suppressed images and the corresponding difference image are also shown. Note the quality improvement in the original images and the lesion eigenimage generated by the noise-suppression filter. This figure illustrates the significance of noise suppression before eigenimage filtering.

III. CONTRAST ENHANCEMENT

Contrast/noise ratio is one of the standard measures of MR image quality. There are at least three approaches for improving the image CNR: (a) by injecting contrast agents to the patient; (b) by optimizing MRI protocols and pulse sequence parameters; and (c) by combining multiple MR images obtained in clinical studies. Image combination techniques can be applied to an existing set of MR images without any extra image acquisitions or contrast agent administration. Also, they are applied off line, thus do not take any extra time from the patient. Here, we explain an optimal *linear* method for MR image combination, which is traditionally named a "maximum CNR filter."

The maximum CNR filter has its roots in signal processing, where it was originally used for detecting one of two known signals in white gaussian noise (79). There is no unique extension of the filter to a general case of having more than two tissues in the scene (multiple interfering case). In many clinical applications there exist multiple interfering tissues. For example, in brain studies, considering pathology as the desired tissue and normal tissues (white matter, gray matter, and CSF as interfering, we have a scene with three interfering tissues.

A reasonable approach for extending the filter to the case of multiple interfering tissues is to define the maximum CNR filter as one that provides the largest value for the minimum absolute CNR (max.{min.{ $|CNR|$ }}) between a desired tissue and multiple interfering tissues (80). We refer to this filter as *maximized minimum absolute* CNR (MMAC) (20). This technique requires a search among several possibilities to find the optimal filter.

Brown et al. (80) used a parametric method to find the optimal weighting vector for the MMAC filter. They did not solve the problem for the case of having more than two interfering tissues (or CNRs of interest) in the scene. Note that if one is interested in CNRs between interfering tissues in addition to the CNRs between the desired and interfering tissues, then even for the case of two interfering tissues in the scene there are three CNRs to be considered. Their approach lacks an easy derivation of the analytical solution for the general case of multiple interfering tissues.

Soltanian-Zadeh and Windham (20) have developed a new approach that derives the analytical solution for the general case of multiple interfering tissues. Major contributions of Ref. 20 are: (a) a general formulation of the MMAC filter for an arbitrary number of interfering tissues, as *constrained optimization problems* and a formula for the number of candidate weighting vectors; and (b) a novel solution using the simple method of Gram-Schmidt orthogonalization.

Here, we present the theoretical basis for the MMAC filter. We then present a clinical application of the technique. We calculate theoretical CNRs of the composite images and compare them with those of the actual images. We show all 13 composite images for a representative study to illustrate possible use of these images for medical image analysis and interpretation.

A. Problem Formulation

Linearly transformed images (LTI_l, $l = 1, \cdots, M$, where M is the number of transformed images) are weighted sums (linear combinations) of original images in the sequence (P_t, $t = 1, \cdots, n$). Using the notations defined in Sec. IB, this is written as:

$$LTI_l = \sum_{t=1}^{n} W_{lt} P_t, \quad l = 1, \cdots, M \tag{8}$$

where $\{\mathbf{W}_l = (W_{l1}\ W_{l2}\ \cdots\ W_{ln})^T,\ l = 1, \cdots, M\}$ are the transform coefficients (weighting vectors).

The CNR between the desired tissue and i-th interfering (undesired) tissue (CNR_{dui}) is defined as (46)

$$CNR_{du_i} = \frac{E(P_{jk}^d) - E(P_{jk}^{u_i})}{\sqrt{\dfrac{Var(P_{jk}^d) + Var(P_{jk}^{u_i})}{2}}} \tag{9}$$

where $E(P_{jk}^d)$ and $Var(P_{jk}^d)$ are the mean and the variance of pixel values in the DROI, respectively. Similarly, $E(P_{jk}^{u_i})$ and $Var(P_{jk}^{u_i})$ are the mean and the variance of pixel values in the i-th interfering ROI (IROI_i), respectively.

We make the following assumptions that were also made in many articles [e.g., (46,81,82)] (a) statistical noise in tissue regions of an MRI scene sequence can be modeled as a multidimensional zero-mean white noise field with standard deviation σ; and (b) signature vectors are a priori known fairly well. Then, the standard formula for noise propagation (83,84) shows that the CNR_{du_i} in the l-th filtered image is expressed by

$$CNR_{du_i}^l = \frac{\mathbf{W}_l \cdot \mathbf{d} - \mathbf{W}_l \cdot \mathbf{u}_i}{\sigma(\mathbf{W}_l \cdot \mathbf{W}_l)^{\frac{1}{2}}} = \frac{\mathbf{W}_l \cdot (\mathbf{d} - \mathbf{u}_i)}{\sigma(\mathbf{W}_l \cdot \mathbf{W}_l)^{\frac{1}{2}}} \tag{10}$$

where $\cdot$ represents the usual inner product.

The ultimate goal is to find a weighting vector that maximizes the smallest of $\{|CNR_{du_i}^l|, i = 1, \cdots, m\}$. For each i, $CNR_{du_i}^l$ is a nonlinear functional of $\mathbf{W}_l$. Defining another nonlinear functional $\mathbf{MAC}(\mathbf{W}_l)$ as the minimum of $\{|CNR_{du_i}^l|, i = 1, \cdots, m\}$, the goal would be to find the global maximum of $\mathbf{MAC}$, which we refer to as the *objective functional*. Usually, this objective functional is not concave and has several local maxima. The possible weighting vectors corresponding to these maxima are from one of the following m classes.

- Class (1): At a $\mathbf{W}_l$, which gives the maximum value for a particular $|CNR_{du_k}^l|$. This occurs when $\mathbf{W}_l$ provides larger absolute values for all other $CNR_{du_i}^l$, $i \neq k$. There are $2^0 \binom{m}{1} = m$ possibilities for this situation. Here $\binom{p}{q}$ is the number of possible combinations for choosing q objects from p objects.
- Class (2): At a $\mathbf{W}_l$, which provides $|CNR_{du_k}^l| = |CNR_{du_{k'}}^l|$. This happens when $\mathbf{W}_l$ provides larger absolute values for all other $CNR_{du_i}^l$, $i \neq k$, and $i \neq k'$. There are $2^1 \binom{m}{1}$ possibilities for this class.
⋮
- Class (r): At a $\mathbf{W}_l$, which gives equal absolute values for r CNR^ls, i.e., $|CNR_{du_{k_1}}^l| = \cdots = |CNR_{du_{k_r}}^l|$, $1 \leq k_1, k_2, \cdots, k_r \leq m$. There are $2^{r-1}\binom{m}{r}$ possibilities for this situation.
⋮
- Class (m): At a $\mathbf{W}_l$, which provides equal absolute values for all CNR^ls (i.e., $|CNR_{du_1}^l| = |CNR_{du_k}^l|$ for all $2 \leq k \leq m$). There are $2^{m-1}\binom{m}{m} = 2^{m-1}$ possibilities for this class.

The total number of possible weighting vectors (M), corresponding to local maxima of the objective functional, is therefore

$$M = \sum_{i=1}^{m} 2^{i-1} \binom{m}{i} = \frac{3^m - 1}{2} \tag{11}$$

B. Solution

To find the weighting vector corresponding to the global maximum, all of the weighting vectors for the possible local maxima are found, and the corresponding CNR's are calculated and compared. To find the candidate (possible) weighting vectors, we note that the problems in class (1) are unconstrained optimization problems whose solutions are readily obtained by recalling the maximum CNR filter (46). All other classes specify constrained optimization problems, which are solved by use of the theorem given in Ref. 20.

As an example, we consider the first problem in class (r), which is

$$\max. \left\{ CNR_{12} = \frac{\mathbf{W}_{r1} \cdot (\mathbf{s}_1 - \mathbf{s}_2)}{\sigma(\mathbf{W}_{r1} \cdot \mathbf{W}_{r1})^{\frac{1}{2}}} \right\} \qquad (12)$$

subject to the constraint that

$$CNR_{12} = CNR_{13} = CNR_{14} = \cdots = CNR_{1r} \qquad (13)$$

Eq. (13) is equivalent to the following $(r - 2)$ constraints:

$$\begin{aligned}
\mathbf{W}_{r1} \cdot (\mathbf{s}_2 - \mathbf{s}_3) &= 0 \\
\mathbf{W}_{r1} \cdot (\mathbf{s}_2 - \mathbf{s}_4) &= 0 \\
&\vdots \\
\mathbf{W}_{r1} \cdot (\mathbf{s}_2 - \mathbf{s}_r) &= 0
\end{aligned} \qquad (14)$$

Hence, we have a constrained optimization problem with $(r - 2)$ constraints. By the theorem given in Ref. 20, the solution is

$$\mathbf{W}_{r1} = (\mathbf{s}_1 - \mathbf{s}_2) - (\mathbf{s}_1 - \mathbf{s}_2)^p \qquad (15)$$

Here $(\mathbf{s}_1 - \mathbf{s}_2)^p$ represents the projection of $(\mathbf{s}_1 - \mathbf{s}_2)$ onto the subspace defined by $\{(\mathbf{s}_2 - \mathbf{s}_3), (\mathbf{s}_2 - \mathbf{s}_4), \cdots, (\mathbf{s}_2 - \mathbf{s}_r)\}$ which is obtained using Gram-Schmidt orthogonalization.

1. An Example

Fig. 8 shows the best 3 original images and all of the 13 candidate images generated for the MMAC filter. It can be seen that in some of the composite images tumor compartments and their extents are visualized better than any of the original images. Comparison of CNRs of the original and composite images has shown that the MMAC filter improves the MAC value by about 30% on average.

IV. FEATURE EXTRACTION

Brain tumors are normally large, and detection of their existence is simple. They may be found by a symmetry analysis of the image gray levels in the axial images,

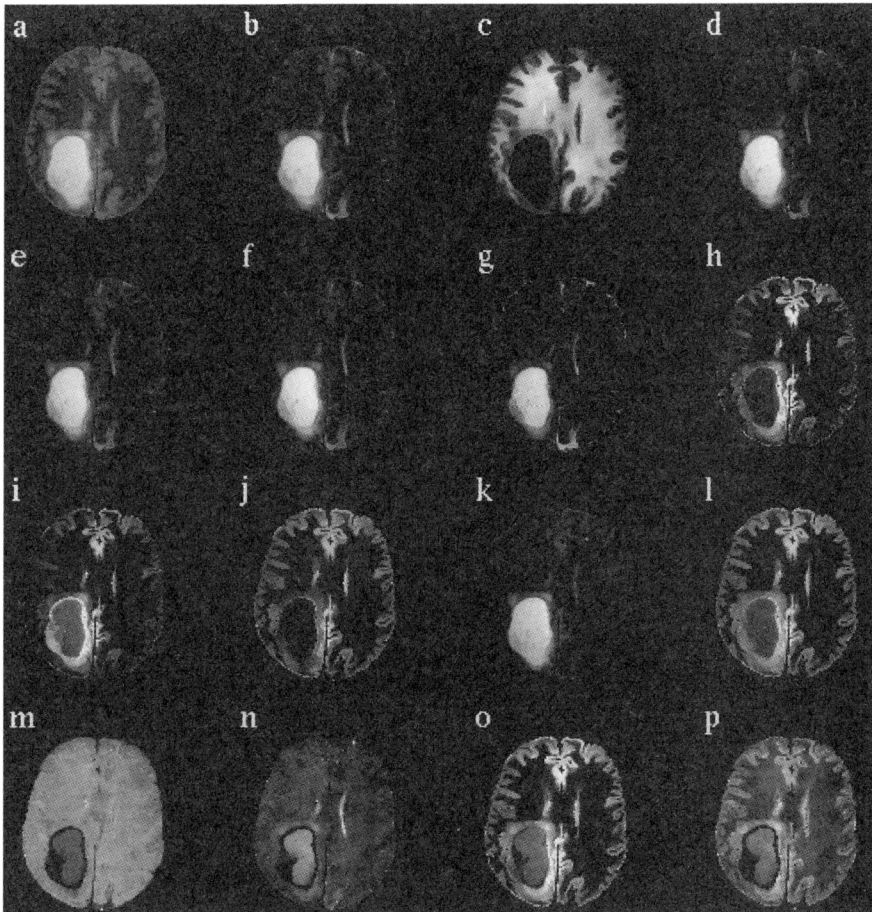

Fig. 8 MMAC filter applied to a tumor patient study. **a–c (best original images),** two spin-echo T2-weighted (TE/TR = 25,100/2500 ms) and one T1-weighted (TE/TR = 25/500 ms) MRI of a brain tumor patient, respectively. Here, the desired tissue is the tumor and the interfering tissues are white matter, gray matter, and CSF. **d–p (composite images),** Thirteen composite images obtained using the candidate weighting vectors for the MMAC filter.

because they generate significant gray level asymmetry in these images. Detection of multiple zones in the tumor and accurate estimation of the tumor extent are, however, difficult, and different image analysis approaches may be used for this purpose. We present the most relevant image analysis techniques and the issues related to this topic in the remainder of this chapter.

A critical step in this analysis is feature extraction. Conventional methods include explicit calculations of the tissue parameters (40,41); tissue parameter–weighted images (14,39); principal component images (44,47); and angle images (45). Explicit calculations of the tissue parameters is not usually recommended (and not explained in this chapter) because of the following reasons: (a) this approach requires data using several specific pulse sequences that are different from routine clinical protocols (40,41); (b) the results are prone to noise propagation through the nonlinear calculations involved (48); and (c) the optimal linear decision boundaries for the resulting feature space do not match with those of the original data (49). Clinically feasible techniques are described next.

A. Tissue Parameter-Weighted Images

Using a multiple spin-echo pulse sequence with a short echo time (e.g., TE = 25 ms) and a long repetition time (e.g., TR = 2500 ms), a sequence of four images (corresponding to TE = 25, 50, 75, 100 ms) can be acquired. The contrast in the first image is mainly due to the proton density difference between tissues, thus it is called proton density weighted. The contrast in the third and fourth images is mainly due to the T2 relaxation difference between tissues, thus it is called T2-weighted. Likewise, using a single spin-echo pulse sequence with a short echo time (e.g., TE = 20 ms) and a moderate repetition time (e.g., TR = 500 ms), a T1-weighted image can be acquired. These three images define a 3-D feature space representation of the tissues. Alternatively, a T1-weighted image can be acquired using an inversion recovery pulse sequence, with a short echo time (e.g., TE = 12 ms), moderate inversion time (e.g., TI = 500 ms), and long repetition time (e.g., TR = 1500 ms).

B. Principal Component Images

Principal component analysis is a linear transformation that has been applied in a variety of fields including MRI (44,47). It has been used in digital image processing as a technique for image coding, compression, enhancement, and feature extraction (85–88). For MRI feature space representation, PCA generates linear combinations of the acquired images that maximize the image variance. The weighting vectors for these linear combinations are the normalized eigenvectors of the sample covariance matrix estimated using all of the acquired images. The number of principal component images equals the number of acquired images, but the variance (equivalently, SNR) of the principal component images sharply decreases from the first image to the last. The first three principal component images contain most of the information and may be used to define a 3-D feature space representation of the tissues.

C. Angle Images

Angle images are defined by calculating a set of parameters for each pixel vector in an orthogonal subspace defined by the constant vector ($\mathbf{cv} = [1, 1, \cdots, 1]^T$) and the signature vectors for normal tissues ($\mathbf{s}_i, i = 1, \cdots, M$) that are encountered in a study, (e.g., white matter, gray matter, and CSF for the brain) (45). The orthogonal subspace is defined by inputing $\mathbf{cv}$ and $\mathbf{s}_i$ into a Gram-Schmidt orthogonalization procedure.

Among all the possibilities for a 3-D feature space, it has been found that the feature space generated by (a) the euclidean norm of each pixel vector (b) the angle between each pixel vector and the constant vector; and (3) the angle between each pixel vector and the orthogonal complement of white matter to the constant vector best separates normal and abnormal tissues in a brain study (45).

D. Optimally Transformed Images

Soltanian-Zadeh et al. (13) have recently developed an optimal feature space method for MRI. In this method, a multidimensional histogram (cluster plot) is generated, and clusters are found and marked on the result by visual inspection. Because of visualization limitations, a 3-D cluster plot is usually used. To generate such a cluster plot, three images need to be extracted for each slice from the original MRI study, which may have up to six images per slice. The proposed method for optimally extracting these features (images) is presented next.

1. Problem Formulation

In the derivation of the transformation, we use the following notation: (a) uppercase boldface letters, such as **V**, to refer to a vector space; (b) uppercase **sans serif** letters, such as V, to refer to a matrix each of whose columns is a point in **V**; and (c) lowercase boldface letters, such as **v**, to refer to the vector coordinates of a point in **V**.

Let **V** and **W** be n-dimensional and p-dimensional real vector spaces, respectively. Then points in **V** and **W** are vectors in $\Re^n$ and $\Re^p$, respectively. Further assume that a collection of data can be classified or categorized in terms of M predefined groups, with data points in a group more *similar* to other data points in the group than to the data points in other groups. Let each data category have a target position in **W**, about which transformed data are expected to be well clustered. Denote the number of data points in each category as $NS(j), j = 1, \cdots, M$. A linear transformation T is desired that maps points in **W** to points in **V** as follows:

$$\mathbf{c} = \mathsf{T}\mathbf{v} \tag{16}$$

The transformation matrix T is to be found such that the ratio of interset distance (IED) to intraset distance (IAD) is maximized. (The ratio of IED to IAD is

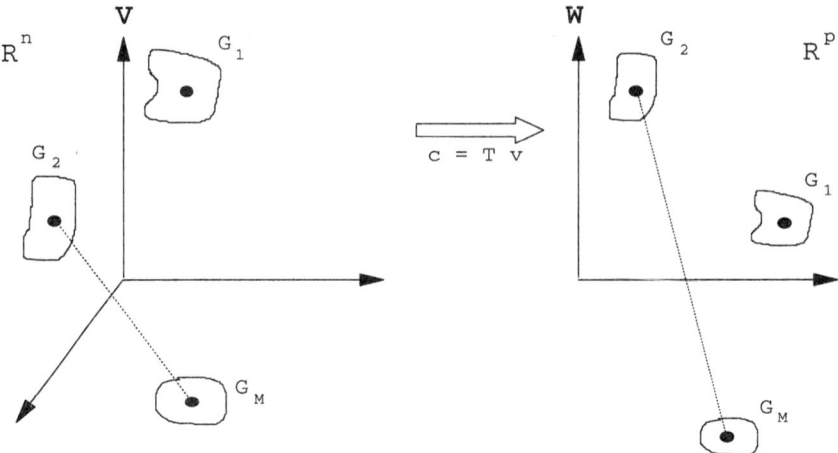

Fig. 9 Transformation of categorical data to target positions and improving its clustering properties by reducing its dimensionality. (*Source:* Ref. 13.)

a standard criterion for quantifying clustering properties of data (89)—see Fig. 9.) This problem can be formulated as the following constrained optimization problem

$$\text{Maximize} \quad \frac{IED}{IAD} \tag{17}$$

$$\text{Subject to} \quad \mathbf{c}_j = T\bar{\mathbf{v}}_j, \quad 1 \leq j \leq M \tag{18}$$

where $\mathbf{c}_j$ is the target position for the average vector of the jth group ($\bar{\mathbf{v}}_j$) defined by

$$\bar{\mathbf{v}}_j = \frac{1}{NS(j)} \sum_{l=1}^{NS(j)} \mathbf{v}_j^l \tag{19}$$

with $\mathbf{v}_j^l$ being the lth data point in the jth group.

The IED reflects the average distance between different data groups. It is defined as the average of distances between each pair of the average vectors from different groups (89) in the transformed domain:

$$IED^2 = \frac{2}{M(M-1)} \sum_{j=1}^{M} \sum_{i=j+1}^{M} \|T\bar{\mathbf{v}}_j - T\bar{\mathbf{v}}_i\|^2 \tag{20}$$

where $\bar{\mathbf{v}}_j$ and $\bar{\mathbf{v}}_i$ are the average vectors for the jth and ith groups, respectively, and $\|\cdot\|$ represents the euclidean distance. This definition makes the interset distance independent of the number of points in each data group. This is an important property in that it avoids dependency of the transformation to the object size in contrast to principal component analysis. The IAD reflects the average variance of the data points in each group. It is defined as the average of distances between each vector in a group and the average vector from the same group, again in the transformed domain:

$$IAD^2 = \frac{1}{\sum_{j=1}^{M} NS(j)} \sum_{j=1}^{M} \sum_{i=1}^{NS(j)} \|\mathbf{T}\mathbf{v}_j^i - \mathbf{T}\bar{\mathbf{v}}_j\|^2 \tag{21}$$

where $\mathbf{v}_j^i$ is the ith data point in the jth group.

2. Solution

To attain easy distinction between normal and abnormal tissues, we may project the average vectors of the normal tissues onto prespecified locations (e.g., on the axes of the new subspace). This is sometimes referred to as projection of categorical data to target positions. Once target positions are specified, IED is fixed. Therefore, maximizing the ratio of IED to IAD will be equivalent to minimizing IAD. Minimizing IAD, in turn, will be similar to minimizing the mean-square error between specified target positions in $\mathbf{W}$ and projections of the measurement data (90). The solution will be obtained by taking partial derivatives of IAD^2 with respect to elements of $\mathbf{T}$ and solving the resultant systems of equations.

3. Special Case

A special case, with an analytical solution, is defined if $M = p$, and we decide to assign the target positions for normal tissues to be on the axes of the new subspace, (i.e., $\mathbf{c}_i = [0, \cdots, 0, c_i, 0, \cdots, 0]^T$ with $c_i > 0$ in the ith row). This will require

$$\mathbf{t}_i \cdot \bar{\mathbf{v}}_j = 0, \quad 1 \leq j \leq M, j \neq i, \quad \text{and} \quad \mathbf{t}_i \cdot \bar{\mathbf{v}}_i = c_i \tag{22}$$

where $\mathbf{t}_i$ is the ith row of the $M \times n$ transformation matrix $\mathbf{T}$. For this case, it can be shown that IED^2 simplifies to

$$IED^2 = \sum_{i=1}^{M} \|\mathbf{c}_i\|^2 \tag{23}$$

Using the white noise gaussian model with standard deviation σ for MRI noise simplifies IAD^2 to

$$IAD^2 = \sigma^2 \left[\sum_{i=1}^{M} \|\mathbf{t}_i\|^2 \right] \tag{24}$$

With an additional constraint that $\|\mathbf{t}_i\| = 1$, $1 \leq i \leq M$, it can be shown that Eq. (17) and Eq. (18) may be equivalently formulated as

$$\text{Maximize} \quad \frac{\mathbf{t}_i \cdot \bar{\mathbf{v}}_i}{\sigma [\mathbf{t}_i \cdot \mathbf{t}_i]^{\frac{1}{2}}}, \quad 1 \leq i \leq M \quad (25)$$

$$\text{Subject to} \quad \mathbf{t}_i \cdot \bar{\mathbf{v}}_j = 0, \quad 1 \leq j \leq M, \quad j \neq i \quad (26)$$

In this formulation, $\{\|\mathbf{t}_i\| = 1, 1 \leq i \leq M\}$ is equivalently considered in the problem formulation by using $\|\mathbf{t}_i\| = [\mathbf{t}_i \cdot \mathbf{t}_i]^{\frac{1}{2}}$ in the denominator of the objective function Eq. (25). (See Ref. 91 for a mathematical proof of this equivalence.) Soltanian-Zadeh and Windham (20) have derived analytical solutions to a class of optimization problems, which are in the form given in Eq. (25) and Eq. (26).

E. Discriminant Analysis Images

For a $(p + 1)$-class problem, the natural generalization of Fisher's linear discriminant involves p discriminant functions. Similar to the optimal transformation described earlier, the projection is from n-dimensional space to a p-dimensional space. However, the objective function is defined using within ($\mathbf{S}_W$) and between ($\mathbf{S}_B$) scatter matrices [50]:

$$\mathbf{S}_W = \sum_{i=1}^{p+1} \mathbf{S}_i \quad (27)$$

where

$$\mathbf{S}_j = \sum_{i=1}^{NS(j)} (\mathbf{v}_j^i - \bar{\mathbf{v}}_j)(\mathbf{v}_j^i - \bar{\mathbf{v}}_j)^T \quad (28)$$

and

$$\mathbf{S}_B = \sum_{j=1}^{p+1} N S(j)(\bar{\mathbf{v}}_j - \bar{\mathbf{v}})(\bar{\mathbf{v}}_j - \bar{\mathbf{v}})^T \quad (29)$$

where

$$\bar{\mathbf{v}} = \frac{1}{\Sigma N S(j)} \sum_{i=1}^{p+1} N S(i) \bar{\mathbf{v}}_i \quad (30)$$

To find the transformation matrix $\mathbf{T}$, the following objective function is maximized.

$$J(\mathbf{T}) = \frac{|\mathbf{T} \mathbf{S}_B \mathbf{T}^T|}{|\mathbf{T} \mathbf{S}_W \mathbf{T}^T|} \quad (31)$$

It has been proved in Ref. 92 that the rows of T (i.e., t_i) can be found by numerically solving the following generalized eigenvalue problem:

$$S_B t_i = \lambda_i S_W t_i \tag{32}$$

Because the determinant is the product of the eigenvalues, it is the *product* of the variances in the principal directions, thereby measuring the square of the hyperellipsoidal scattering volume (50). Eq. (31) therefore represents the ratio of products of between-class variances to the products of within-class variances.

The interesting point is that if the within-class scatter is isotropic, the eigenvectors are the eigenvectors of S_B that span the subspace defined by the vectors $\bar{v}_i - \bar{v}$. The rows of T can be found by applying the Gram-Schmidt orthogonalization procedure to p vectors $\{\bar{v}_i - \bar{v}, i = 1, \cdots, p\}$ (50). This is similar to the "Special Case" explained earlier, except that instead of normal tissue signature vectors, linear combinations of them are used in the Gram-Schmidt orthogonalization procedure. Also, four tissues are needed instead of three. Because there are only three normal tissues in the brain, the DA transformation will depend on the pathology, and thus the resulting feature space and the location of the clusters changes from study to study.

Note that the solution is not unique, because rotations and scaling of the axes do not change the value of $J(T)$. However, for the optimal transformation derived in the previous section the solution is unique, because we fixed the location of normal tissue clusters. Also, note that instead of p known tissues needed by the proposed approach, discriminant analysis needs $p + 1$ known tissues.

1. Examples

The effectiveness of the preceding feature extraction techniques in brain tumor studies is demonstrated in Ref. 13. Here, using the analytical solution for the special case presented in Sec. IVD, cluster plots for a phantom and a human brain are generated and shown in Figs. 10–12 and 21, respectively. Note how well clusters corresponding to all of the solutions in the phantom have been visualized in the cluster plot and are segmented by the method. Also, in the human study it can be seen that clusters for normal tissues, their partial volume regions, and zones of the lesion are clearly visualized in the cluster plot and appropriately segmented by the method.

V. IMAGE SEGMENTATION

Tumor segmentation methods are mainly region based. They use MRI pixel intensities or features extracted from them as representatives of biological properties of tissue. Image pixels are classified into different regions on the basis of these features. Classification is done using a decision method such as those explained in the next section.

A. Decision Engine

Because the gaussian model has been widely used to characterize the MRI noise (46,49,80,82), and our own experience has also illustrated its validation (5,7,9,10), we have been using statistical pattern classification methods that have sound mathematical bases. These methods are presented next.

Three approximations to the optimal Bayes method (89) can be used: (a) minimum distance pattern classifier using standard euclidean distance; (b) minimum distance pattern classifier using generalized euclidean distance (each coordinate is normalized to the noise standard deviation in that direction); and (c) maximum likelihood classifier (MLC). These techniques are similar to those used in multispectral satellite data (14). Because the first and second methods can be considered special cases of the third method, we briefly review the latter.

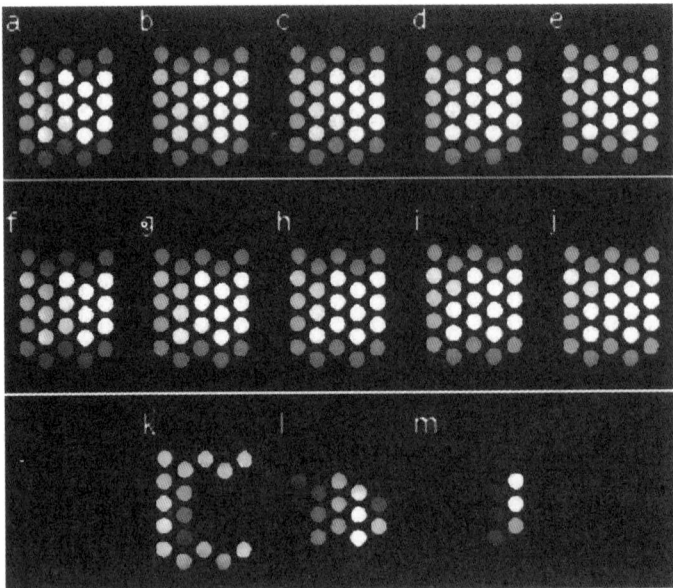

Fig. 10 **a–e,** Four T2-weighted multiple spin echo images (TE/TR = 25–100/2000 ms) and a T1-weighted image (TE/TR = 20/500 ms) of a solution phantom. **f–j,** Noise-suppressed images generated using the filter described in Sec. IID. **k–m,** Transformed images created by applying the optimal transformation explained in Sec. VB, using the signature vectors for water and solutions with maximum concentrations. (*Source:* Ref. 99.)

Processing of Brain MRI

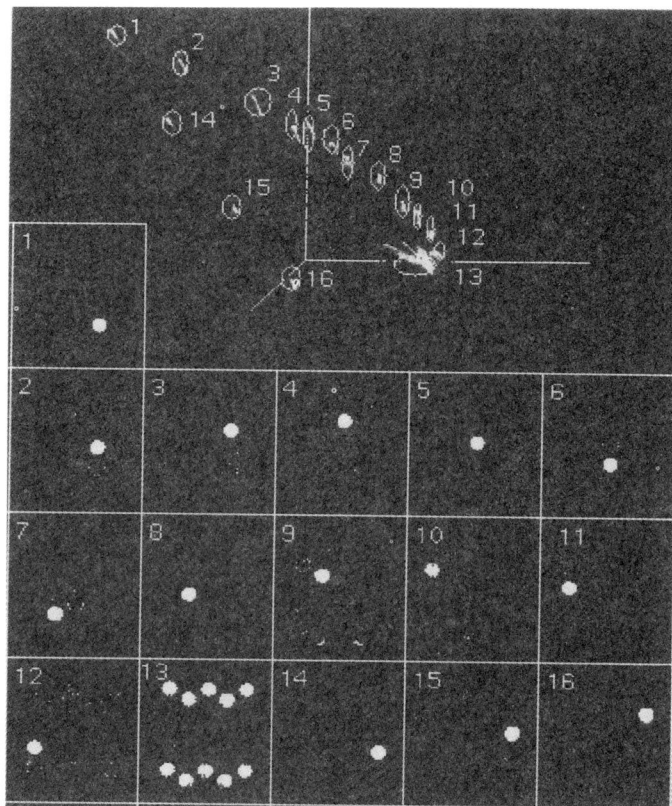

Fig. 11 Cluster plot generated by the optimal transformation explained in Sec. IVD. 1–16, Segmented objects (water, different concentrations of $CuSO_4$, and $CuSO_4$ plus creatine). (*Source:* Ref. 99.)

The MLC classifies multivariate vectors by evaluating the probability for each class membership using statistics of the training regions (93,94). The decision function for the classifier is

$$d_i(\mathbf{x}) = \frac{P(i)}{(2\pi)^{n/2}|\mathbf{K}_i|^{1/2}} \, exp\left[-\frac{1}{2}(\mathbf{x}-\overline{\mathbf{x}}_i)^T \mathbf{K}_i^{-1}(\mathbf{x}-\overline{\mathbf{x}}_i)\right] \quad (33)$$

where $\mathbf{x}$ is the multivariate sample that is being classified, $\overline{\mathbf{x}}_i$ is the sample mean vector for the ith tissue type calculated from the transformed images, $\mathbf{K}_i$ and $|\mathbf{K}_i|$ are the sample covariance matrix and its determinate, n is the number of images in the scene sequence, $P(i)$ is the a priori probability of class i, and ^{T} means transpose. The sample mean vectors and sample covariance matrix are estimated using

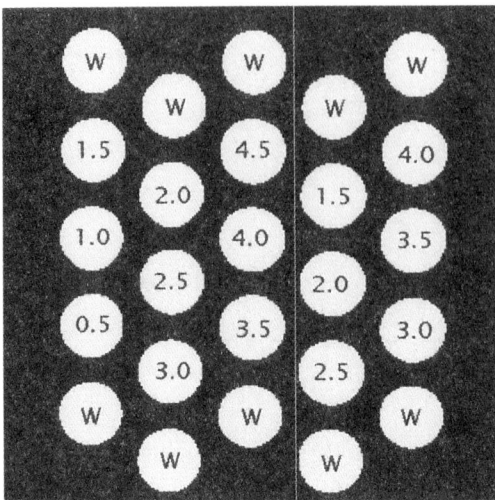

Fig. 12 Structure of the solution phantom shown in Figs. 10 and 11. W refers to water, and numbers are actual concentrations of $CuSO_4$ in millimole. On the right hand side, there exist $CuSO_4$ solutions, and on the left hand side, there exists $CuSO_4$ solutions plus 50 millimole of creatine. (*Source:* Ref. 99.)

the training data sets, and $P(i)$ is assumed to be equal for all classes. The tissue i for which $d_i(\mathbf{x})$ (equivalently $P(i\,|\,\mathbf{x})$) is the highest is assumed to be the most probable class. When K_i is a diagonal matrix or a scaled version of the identity matrix, the above approximate classifiers (b) or (a) are obtained, respectively. Also, because $P(i)/(2\pi)^{n/2}\,|K_i|^{1/2}$ is constant, the maximum of $d_i(\mathbf{x})$ coincides with the minimum of $(\mathbf{x} - \bar{\mathbf{x}}_i)^T K_i^{-1}(\mathbf{x} - \bar{\mathbf{x}}_i)$, which is called the Mahalanobis generalized distance (89).

B. Supervised Methods

In supervised methods, the operator has a significant interaction with the computer. He or she analyzes the data slice by slice. This has the advantage of having visual control on what is happening throughout the imaged volume and the disadvantage of being time consuming and operator dependent. Operator dependency can be minimized by designing a step-by-step protocol that is followed closely by the operator.

A variety of supervised methods can be designed for MRI segmentation. As an example, we present the method we have developed for brain studies based on the optimal transformation presented in Sec. IVD.

1. The operator draws a sample ROI for each of the normal tissues (white matter, gray matter, and CSF) over the slice that he or she wants to analyze. These ROIs may be small but should be carefully drawn to include pure pixels only (i.e., without any partial volume averaging).
2. The computer program finds the sample mean and standard deviation of the pixel gray levels in each ROI for every image in the sequence. It then defines signature vectors for the normal tissues, using the mean values.
3. The operator specifies target locations for each of the normal tissues. The computer program finds the minimum mean square error transformation to these target positions, applies it to the images of the slice under consideration, and then generates a multidimensional (3-D for the brain) feature space representation (i.e., a cluster plot).
4. The operator draws ROIs for any clusters he or she finds in the cluster plot. His or her a priori knowledge regarding the location of the clusters for normal tissues will help him or her in identifying clusters corresponding to partial volume pixels and abnormal tissues (see Figs. 11 and 21).
5. The computer program finds pixels in the image domain that correspond to each of the ROIs drawn over the clusters and generates the corresponding region in the image domain for each cluster.
6. The computer program uses the statistics (sample mean and covariance matrix) of the pixels corresponding to each region and using the euclidean, generalized euclidean, or Mahalanobis generalized distance, assigns each pixel in the image domain to one of the classes. It then assigns an integer number (equivalently, a color) to all pixels in each class. Segmentation results may be presented as multiple binary images each representing a segmented region (see Figs. 11 and 21). They may also be presented as a color image that is not shown here because of publication limitations.

1. Optimal Method for Partial Volume Estimation

To determine the tumor extent, the amount of tumorous tissue within each voxel needs to be found. In the following sections, we present MRI partial volume model and the optimal method for extracting partial volume information from MRI.

2. Partial Volume Model

The MR signal S from a voxel containing m different tissues is given by Ref. 95

$$S = \sum_{l=1}^{m} \left(\frac{V_l}{V}\right) S_l \tag{34}$$

where V_l is the volume of the l-th tissue within the voxel, V is the total volume of the voxel, and S_l is the signal from the l-th tissue. The gray level P_{jk} of the (j, k)-th pixel (corresponding to the (j, k)-th voxel) in an MR image is given by

$$P_{jk} = E[P_{jk}] + w_{jk} = \sum_{l=1}^{m} \left(\frac{V_{ljk}}{V}\right) S_l + w_{jk} \tag{35}$$

where V_{ljk} is the partial volume of the l-th tissue in the (j, k)-th voxel, and w_{jk} represents statistical noise that is assumed to be an additive zero-mean white gaussian noise field, uncorrelated between different scenes of the same MRI sequence, with standard deviation σ. Note that $E[P_{jk}]$ is deterministic but unknown, whereas the noise w_{jk} is stochastic, so that the pixel gray level P_{jk} is the sum of a deterministic value (to be estimated) and noise. We use the notation $E[P_{jk}]$ to denote the original, deterministic value of the pixel gray level, which contains information pertaining to partial volume averaging effects.

Extraction of partial volume averaging effects is necessary for robust interpretation and analysis of MR images, as well as for volume calculations (12,96,97). To extract partial volume information, we generate an image whose pixel gray levels, on average, are proportional to the percentages of a specific tissue in the corresponding voxels. Mathematically, this may be translated to generating a transformed image in which

$$E[TI_{jkd}] = \left(\frac{V_{djk}}{V}\right) E[\mathfrak{T}_d(\mathbf{P}^d_{lm})] \tag{36}$$

where $E[T I_{jkd}]$ is the mean value of the (j, k)-th pixel in the transformed image, V_{djk} is the partial volume of the desired tissue in the (j, k)-th voxel, and $E[\mathfrak{T}_d(\mathbf{P}^d_{lm})]$ is the mean value of the (l, m)-th pixel in a desired ROI (e.g., the ROI that was used for defining the desired signature vector) from the transformed image. The underlying reason for using the expected value operator in defining extraction of partial volume averaging by Eq. (36) is to *exclude* the additive noise, which contains no information pertaining to this effect. An alternative definition may therefore consist of using a noiseless image model (pixel vector) in Eq. (36) while dropping the expectation operator. Either definition may be used to test extraction of partial volume averaging information. The first definition is usually more appropriate for experimental work, whereas the second definition is sometimes more appropriate for theoretical development. To find optimal $\mathfrak{T}_d$, an analytical expression for the resulting image SNR is needed. This expression is described in the next section.

3. Signal/Noise Ratio

Linearly transformed images are linear combinations of the images in the sequence, using different transformation vectors. Because we have m signature vec-

Processing of Brain MRI

tors, each of which can be considered as the desired signature vector, there are a total of m different transformation vectors resulting in m different transformed images. The pixel gray levels of these linearly transformed images ($\{LTI_d, d = 1, \cdots, m\}$) are given by

$$LTI_{jkd} = \sum_{i=1}^{n} T_{id} P_{jki} = \mathbf{t}_d \cdot \mathbf{P}_{jk}, \qquad d = 1, \cdots, m \tag{37}$$

where LTI_{jkd} is the gray level of the (j, k)-th pixel in the d-th linearly transformed image, $\mathbf{t}_d = [T_{1d}\ T_{2d}\ \cdots\ T_{nd}]^T$ is the d-th transformation vector to be determined, and $\mathbf{T} = [\mathbf{t}_1, \mathbf{t}_2, \cdots, \mathbf{t}_m]$ is the transformation matrix. For a linear transformation with the transformation vector $\mathbf{t}_d$, and the presence of an additive zero-mean white noise field with standard deviation σ in the image sequence, the SNR of the desired tissue with the signature vector $\mathbf{s}_d$ is expressed by (5,9)

$$SNR_d = \frac{\mathbf{t}_d \cdot \mathbf{s}_d}{\sigma (\mathbf{t}_d \cdot \mathbf{t}_d)^{\frac{1}{2}}} \tag{38}$$

4. Problem Formulation

We seek a transformation that achieves the following objectives simultaneously:

- Extraction of partial volume averaging information
- Maximizing SNR of the desired tissue

Theorems 1 and 2 in (10) have established the relationship between extraction of partial volume averaging information, removal of the interfering tissues, and the linearity of the transformation. In the following section, we review the final solution.

5. Solution

The solution to the problem

$$\mathbf{max.} \left\{ SNR_d = \frac{\mathbf{t}_d \cdot \mathbf{s}_d}{\sigma (\mathbf{t}_d \cdot \mathbf{t}_d)^{\frac{1}{2}}} \right\} \tag{39}$$

subject to the constraint that

$$\mathbf{t}_d \cdot \mathbf{s}_k = 0, \qquad \text{for} \qquad k = 1, \cdots, m, k \neq d \tag{40}$$

is given by

$$\mathbf{t}_d = \mathbf{s}_d - \mathbf{s}_d^p \tag{41}$$

where $\mathbf{s}_d^p$ is the projection of $\mathbf{s}_d$ onto the subspace spanned by $\{\mathbf{s}_k, k = 1, \cdots, m, k \neq d\}$ (undesired subspace). In addition, $\mathbf{t}_d$ is computed using a Gram-Schmidt orthogonalization procedure. A composite image generated by the optimal trans-

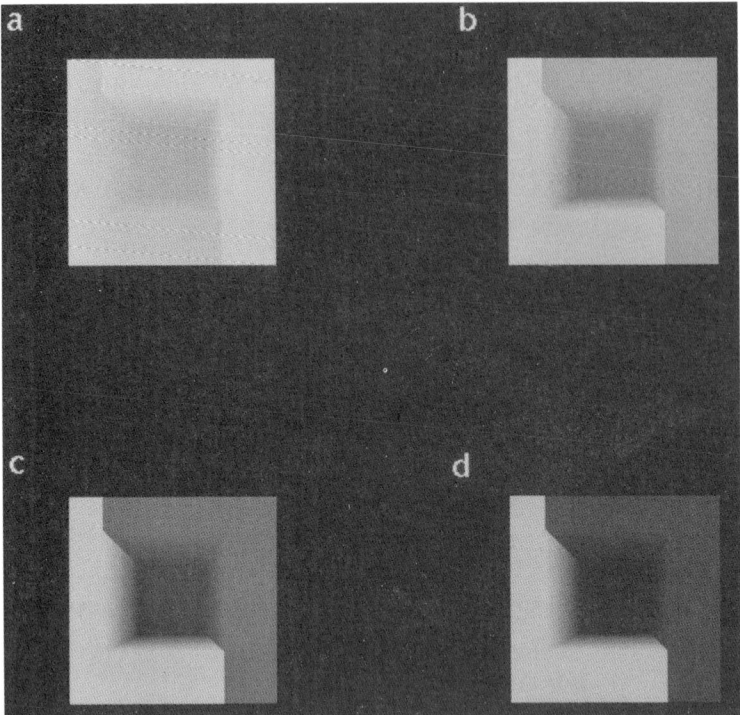

Fig. 13 Original images of a simulation study. **a–d,** Four multiple spin-echo images with TE/TR = 25, 50, 75, 100/2500 ms, respectively. (*Source:* Ref. 10.)

formation has been previously called an eigenimage (6). We continue to use this name, although for the case of multiple interfering tissues, the transformation is obtained using a different formulation.

6. Existence of the Solution

To guarantee the existence of the transformation vectors, the signature vectors should be linearly independent. This requires that the number of unique images in the sequence (n) be *greater* than or *equal* to the number of signature vectors (m). Here, a unique image is one that is not a linear combination of other images in the sequence.

7. Examples

Figs. 13 and 14 show the original images of a simulation and the resulting composite images in which partial volume information is extracted. Table 1 compares the original partial volumes with those estimated from the composite images. It illustrates a close agreement between the original and estimated values.

Processing of Brain MRI

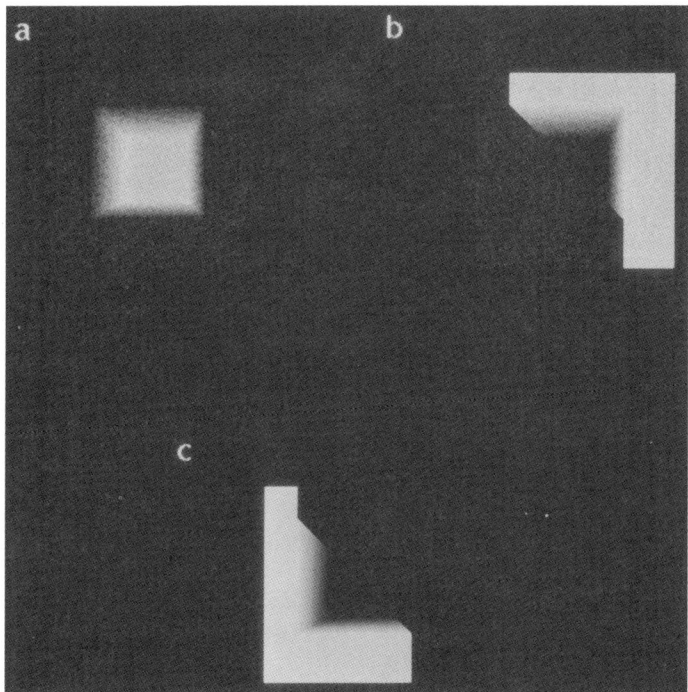

Fig. 14 Transformed images (eigenimages) of the simulation obtained by the optimal transformation described in Sec. VB. **a–c,** Transformed images for the central region, the region on the right, and the region on the left, respectively. Note how the partial volume information is extracted and visualized in these images. (*Source:* Ref. 10.)

Table 1 Original (org) and Estimated (est) Values of Partial Volumes in the Simulation Study Shown in Figs. 13 and 14.

Central region	org	10.00%	20.00%	40.00%	55.00%
	est	9.69%	19.81%	41.33%	54.06%
	org	65.00%	80.00%	95.00%	100.00%
	est	65.35%	79.66%	94.84%	100.08%
Left region	org	10.00%	20.00%	40.00%	60.00%
	est	10.01%	19.99%	40.23%	59.78%
	org	70.00%	85.00%	95.00%	100.00%
	est	70.05%	84.94%	95.13%	99.93%
Right region	org	10.00%	20.00%	30.00%	50.00%
	est	10.46%	20.92%	29.79%	49.65%
	org	60.00%	80.00%	90.00%	100.00%
	est	58.68%	80.30%	89.93%	99.98%

Source: Ref. 10.

The method has been applied to several tumor patient MRI studies, and segmentation results were compared with biopsy results (96). Figs. 15–18 illustrate the method by showing original and composite images for a representative clinical tumor study. In all of the studies conducted, it was found that the lesion extended into normal tissue at least to the location in which the biopsy sample was

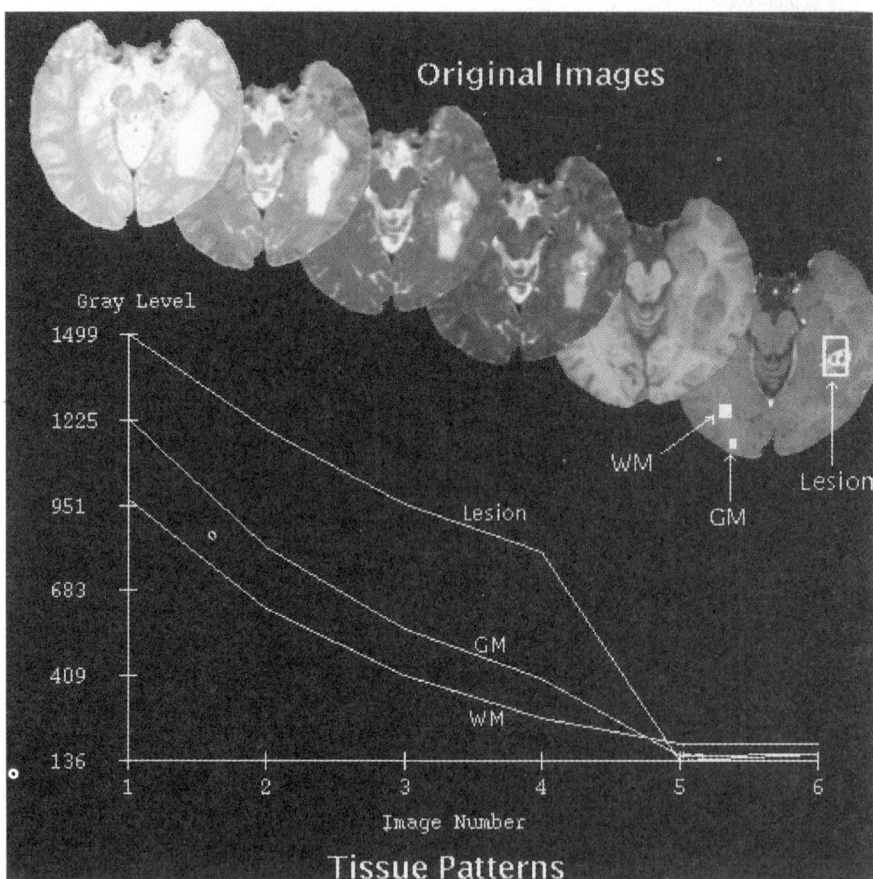

Fig. 15 Illustration of eigenimage filtering as applied to brain tumor studies. Original T2-weighted images (with four echos) and two T1-weighted spin echo images (before injection and after injection of Gd) from a tumor patient with a glioblastoma multiforme lesion. The images are windowed (histogram equalized) individually to optimize visualization of the tissues. The ROIs selected for white matter (WM), gray matter (GM), and the lesion are shown on the Gd-enhanced image. The tissue signature vectors (patterns) extracted from these ROIs are also shown. The elements of the tissue signature vectors are connected by straight lines to enhance visual distinction of them. (*Source:* Ref. 97.)

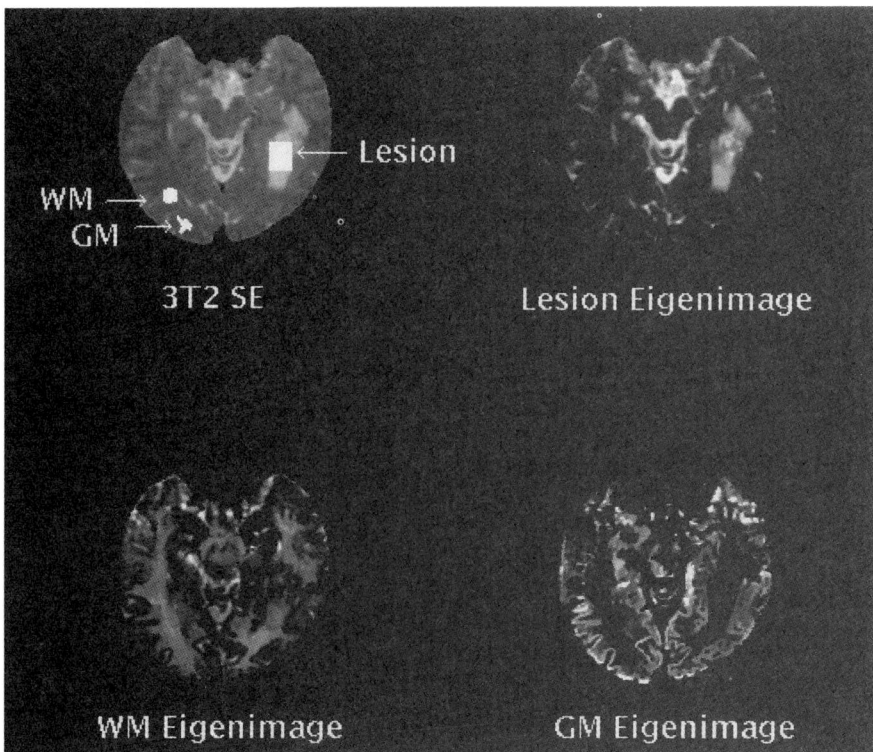

Fig. 16 Eigenimages generated in a clinical study of a tumor patient. The upper left image displays the ROIs selected for white matter (WM), gray matter (GM), and the lesion. The upper right is the eigenimage, created using the lesion as the desired tissue and WM and GM as undesired tissues. CSF is visualized in this image, because it was not chosen as an undesired tissue. In the bottom row, eigenimages created using the normal tissues as desired tissues are displayed. (*Source:* Ref. 97.)

taken. In most cases, the image analysis results suggested that the lesion extended several millimeters beyond the point in which the biopsy sample was taken. In some cases, the extent of the lesion into normal tissue was well beyond the boundary seen on T1- or T2-weighted images. An example of this is demonstrated in the representative case shown in Fig. 18. In this figure, the original images and the transformed image are shown with the biopsy location (indicated by the cross). This sample was chosen as the edge of the T2-weighted hyperintensity. Pathology results showed this sample to be diffusely infiltrated by poorly differentiated neoplastic cells. Note how the extent of the lesion posterior to the biopsy location is not visualized on the original images. From the combined image in Fig. 18 and the

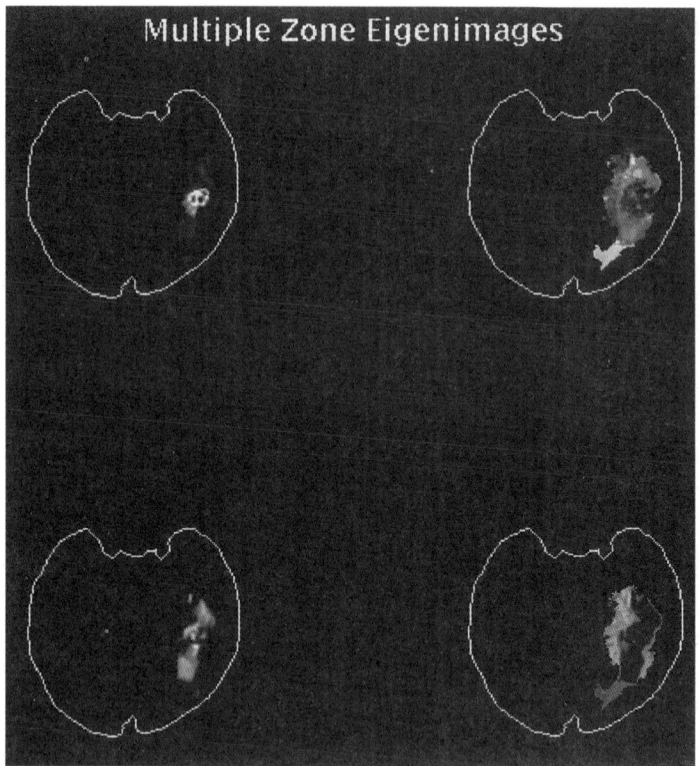

Fig. 17 Eigenimages generated for multiple zones found within a tumor lesion. Note how an area of infiltration is visualized in the left parieto-occipital region. This area is not seen in the original T2- or T1-weighted images. (*Source:* Ref. 97.)

multiple zone eigenimages in Fig. 17, it can be seen that the tumor extends well beyond this edge. In fact, this extension of the lesion corresponds to the white matter tract in this area of the brain. The white matter tract can be easily visualized in the WM eigenimage in Fig. 16. This infiltration along a white matter tract is a recognized pattern of spread for glioblastoma multiforme (2).

C. Unsupervised Methods

In these methods, the operator has minimal interaction with the computer. He or she specifies the image set that should be analyzed and a set of parameters that is used by the unsupervised method. A computer program, implementing a cluster search algorithm such as K-means (16,17), fuzzy C-means (15), or ISO-DATA (98), finds clusters for the selected data set. It defines signature vectors

Processing of Brain MRI

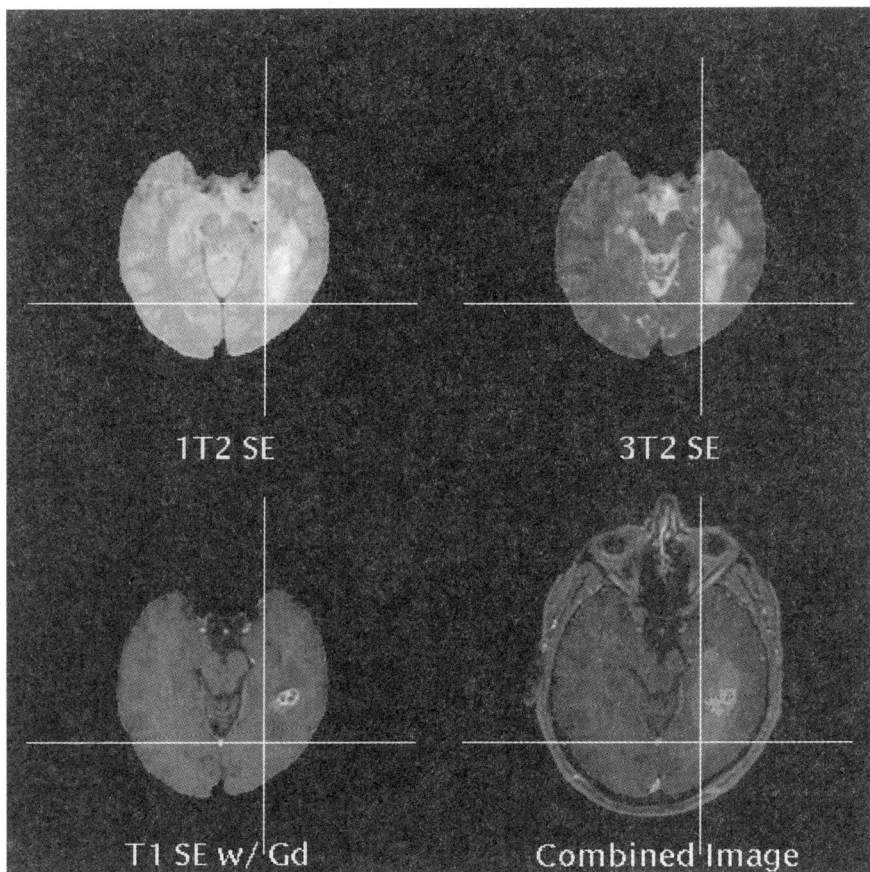

Fig. 18 Three original images and a combined image of a clinical tumor patient study displaying the location where a biopsy sample was taken. This region was sampled as the edge of the hyperintensity seen on the T2-weighted spin echo image. The pathological studies from his biopsy site show extensive tumor cell infiltration. (*Source:* Ref. 97.)

for each cluster and segments the image using a decision rule such as those explained in Sec. VA. Velthuizen et al. (30) have used fuzzy C-means and an iterative least squares clustering (ILSC) approach for this purpose. Soltanian-Zadeh et al. (34) have developed a variation of ISODATA algorithm. The approach is similar in principle to the K-means clustering in the sense that cluster centers are iteratively determined sample means; however, it includes a set of additional merging and splitting procedures. These steps have been incorporated into the algorithm as a result of experience gained through experimentation. A block diagram of the proposed approach is shown in Fig. 19, and details are given in the following section.

1. ISODATA Algorithm

The steps of the algorithm proposed in Ref. 34 are as follows.

1. Specify the following parameters:
    - K = Number of cluster centers desired

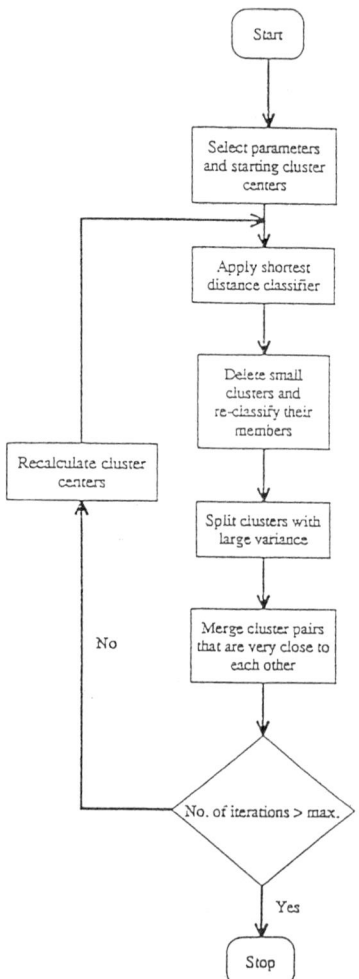

Fig. 19 A flowchart of the ISODATA algorithm explained in Sec. VC. (*Source:* Ref. 34.)

- θ_N = A parameter to which the number of samples in each cluster is compared
- θ_s = Standard deviation parameter
- θ_c = Lumping parameter
- L = Maximum number of pairs of clusters that can be lumped in one iteration
- I = Number of iterations allowed

2. Distribute the pixel vectors among the current cluster centers (Z_j) based on the smallest euclidean distance criterion.
3. Discard cluster centers with fewer than θ_N members, and reduce the number of clusters (N_c) by the number of clusters discarded.
4. Redistribute the pixel vectors associated with the cluster centers discarded in the previous step into the cluster centers remaining.
5. Calculate the average intraset euclidean distance (IAD_j) of pixel vectors in each cluster from their center:

$$IAD_j = \frac{1}{N_j} \sum_{i=1}^{N_j} \|Z_j^i - Z_j\| \tag{42}$$

where N_j is the number of samples and Z_j^i is the ith data point in the jth group.

6. Calculate the overall average distance of the pixel vectors (IAD) using the weighted average of the IAD_js found for the clusters in the previous step:

$$IAD = \frac{1}{N} \sum_{j=1}^{N_c} N_j IAD_j \tag{43}$$

where N is the total number of samples.

7. Do one of the following that applies:
   - If this is the last iteration, set $\theta_c = 0$ and go to Step 11
   - If $N_c \leq 0.5K$, go to Step 8
   - If this is an even-numbered iteration or if $N_c \geq 2K$, go to Step 11
   - If $0.5K < N_c < 2K$, go to Step 8
8. Find the standard deviation vectors for the clusters. This vector contains the standard deviations of individual elements of the pixel vectors in each cluster. Standard deviation is estimated using the sample standard deviation formula.
9. Find the maximum element of each standard deviation vector and denote it σ_{jmax}.
10. If $\sigma_{jmax} > \theta_s$ and
    - $IAD_j > IAD$ and $N_j > 2(\theta_N + 1)$ or

- $N_c \leq 0.5K$ then split Z_j into two new cluster centers Z_j^+ and Z_j^-, delete Z_j, and increase N_c by 1. The cluster center Z_j^+ is formed by adding a given quantity γ_j to the component of Z_j, which corresponds to σ_{jmax}. Similarly, Z_j^- is formed by subtracting γ_j from the same component of Z_j. If splitting took place in this step, go to Step 2, otherwise continue.
11. Calculate interset euclidean distance (IED) between cluster centers:

$$IED_{ij} = \|Z_i - Z_j\| \tag{44}$$

12. Find L cluster pairs that have smaller IED than the rest of the pairs and order them.
13. Starting with the pair that has the smallest IED, perform a pairwise lumping according to the following rule. If neither of the clusters has been used in lumping in this iteration and if the distance between the two cluster centers is less than θ_c, merge these two clusters and calculate the center of the resulting cluster; otherwise, go to the next pair. Once all of the L pairs are considered, go to the next step.
14. If this is the last iteration, the algorithm terminates; otherwise, go to Step 2.

2. Selection of Parameters

We use $K = 8$ (to ensure that we do not lose any clusters), $\theta_N = 500$, $\theta_s =$ twice of the average standard deviation of white matter in MR images being segmented, $\theta_c =$ euclidean distance between white and gray matter, which is usually the minimum distance between normal tissues in the brain, $L = 1$, $I = 60$, and $\gamma_j = 0.25\sigma_{jmax}$. The algorithm does not show severe sensitivity to these parameters, but for the best performance these parameters need to be optimized.

3. An Example

The ISODATA method has been applied to several tumor patient MRI studies. Fig. 20 shows original images and segmentation results obtained in a representative clinical tumor study. It can be seen that the method has segmented normal tissues and multiple zones of the lesion. Comparing the results with those shown in Fig. 21 for the optimal feature space method, it is noted that the results are similar to some extent. However, it can be seen that in the optimal feature space method, segmentation results make more sense. It can also be noted that in the optimal feature space method, one sees a correspondence between each segmented region and its location in the feature space compared with the normal tissue locations. This provides information regarding biological properties of the lesion zones.

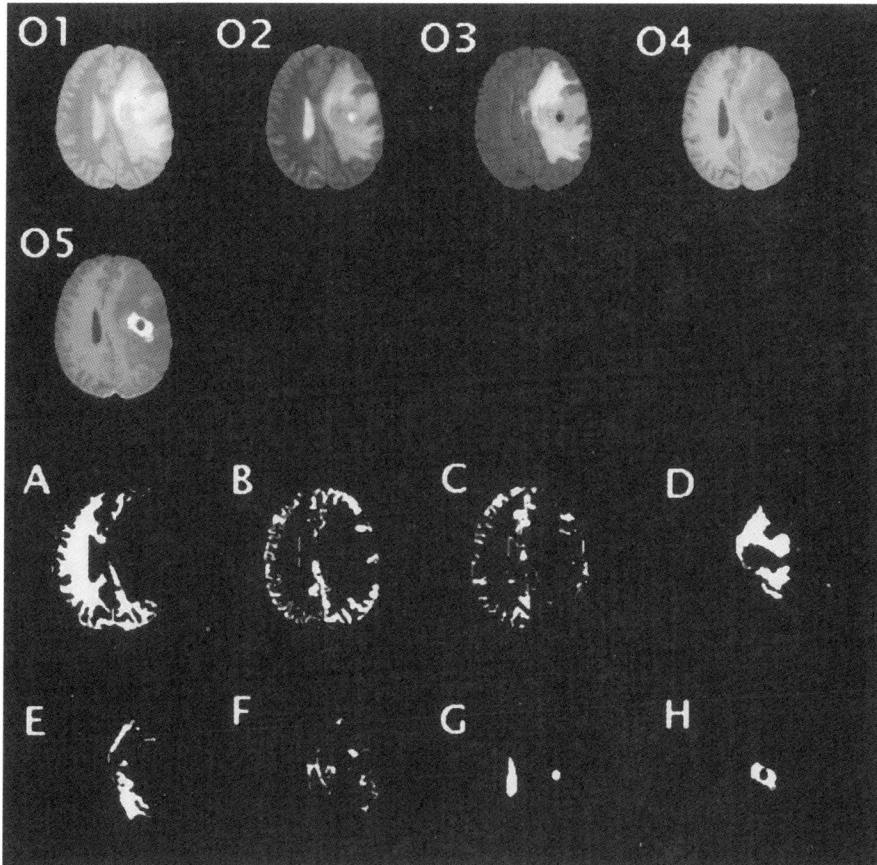

Fig. 20 O1–O5, Two T2-weighted fast spin echo images (TE/TR = 22,88/3500 ms), a FLAIR image (TE/TI/TR = 155/2200/10000 ms), two T1-weighted images—before and after gadolinium (TE/TR = 14/500 ms) of a tumor patient, respectively, after registration, intracranial segmentation, and noise suppression. **A–H,** Segmented regions generated by the ISODATA algorithm explained in Sec. VC.

VI. DISCUSSION

Detecting the existence of brain tumors from MRI is relatively simple. This detection is usually carried out automatically by a symmetry analysis. However, fast, accurate, and reproducible segmentation and characterization of brain tumors are complicated. As such, diagnostic classification of brain tumors, as well as that of other cerebral space-occupying lesions that need to be distinguished from brain tu-

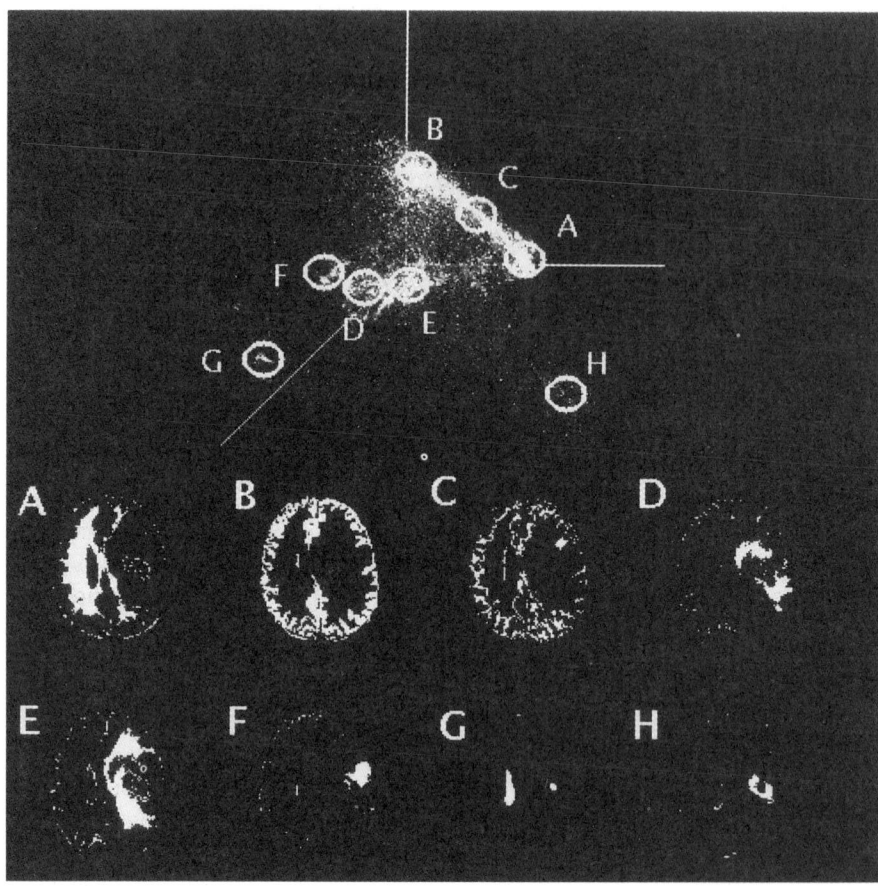

Fig. 21 **Top,** Optimal feature space (cluster plot) generated by the transformation described in Sec. IVD. Selected ROIs for the clusters are superimposed on the cluster plot. **A–H,** Segmented regions for white matter, gray matter, partial volume between white and gray matter, multiple zones of the nonenhancing lesion, CSF, and enhancing lesion, respectively.

mors, is still based on histological examination of tissue samples obtained by means of biopsy or excision. These examinations are carried out to (a) establish a histological diagnosis; (b) determine the histological boundaries of a lesion; and (c) establish whether the lesion comprises solid tumor tissue, isolated tumor cells within the parenchyma, or some other growth pattern.

Ultimate goals of MRI processing algorithms include accomplishing the preceding noninvasively. In this chapter, we cited most of the image-processing work related to this area and reviewed and illustrated the techniques with sound mathematical basis and highest potential for achieving these goals. We also showed an example in which biopsy samples were used to validate the image analysis results. Most of the techniques presented in this chapter are implemented in a user-friendly software package called EIGENTOOL, which runs on SUN workstations and is available to the researchers working in this field free of charge.

We presented a step-by-step methodology for the processing of brain tumor MRI studies. Recently, compound methods have been proposed for accomplishing some of these steps simultaneously. For example, it has been proposed to combine nonuniformity correction and image segmentation in a single iterative algorithm. Currently, these methods are much more computationally intense compared with the step-by-step procedures, and therefore their use is not clinically feasible.

Most of the literature on brain MRI processing and the examples presented here used gray level features for tissue segmentation and characterization. It is expected that future work will consider addition of other features (e.g., spatial connectivity, texture, and edge information) and methods (e.g., mathematical morphology and a priori knowledge) into the segmentation procedure. Segmentation results were presented as black-and-white cross-sectional pictures because of publication limitations. In practice, color-coded images and 3-D visualization are normally used to more efficiently present and use the segmentation results.

The methods presented in this chapter have generated promising results. However, future research work in both of the MRI acquisition and processing areas needs to be undertaken to generate faster, more accurate, and more reproducible segmentation and characterization of brain tumors. New MRI techniques such as magnetization transfer imaging, diffusion imaging, and perfusion imaging will generate additional information regarding anatomy and physiology of brain tumors useful for tissue segmentation and characterization. These images can be processed by the methods described in this chapter. However, because these new images may have different geometric distortion and resolution, using them along with standard spin-echo images requires specific preprocessing to adjust the resolution and correct their geometrical distortion. Magnetic resonance spectroscopy (MRS) and magnetic resonance spectroscopic imaging (MRSI) are also expected to play a significant role in MRI tissue characterization. Currently, the acquisition time and resolution of MRSI images are limiting factors for their use in clinical examinations. It is expected that by advancement of the MRI technology, these techniques will become clinically feasible in the future.

ACKNOWLEDGMENT

Development and evaluation of some of the techniques presented in this chapter have been supported in part by NIH under grants CA46124 and CA61263 and by

NSF under grant BES-9911084. Several of our colleagues at Henry Ford Hospital helped with the implementation and evaluation of the techniques. We would like to thank Donald Peck and Tom Mikkelsen for their assistance with testing and evaluation studies, as well as interpretation of the results. We also would like to thank Lucie Bower, Jalal Soltanianzadeh, and Tom Brusca for their help with programming and David Hearshen, Jeff Hasenau, Linda Emery, Tanya Murnock, Lisa Scapace, Holly Niggeman, and Tim Hickey for their help with data collection and analysis.

REFERENCES

1. PA Forsyth, PJ Kelly, TL Cascino, BW Scheithauer, EG Shaw, RP Dinapoli, EJ Atkinson. J Neurosurg 82(3):436–444, 1995.
2. PJ Kelly, C Daumas-Duport, DB Kispet, BA Kall, BW Scheithauer, JJ Illig. J Neurosurg 66(6):865–874, 1987.
3. PC Burger, P Kleihues. J Cancer 63(10):2014–2023, 1989.
4. PC Burger, BW Scheithauer, FS Vogel. Surgical Pathology of the Nervous System and Its Coverings. Churchill, Livingston, 1991.
5. H Soltanian-Zadeh, JP Windham, DJ Peck, AE Yagle. IEEE Trans Med Imag 11(3): 302–318, 1992.
6. JP Windham, MA Abd-Allah, DA Reimann, JW Froelich, AM Haggar. J Comput Assist Tomogr 12(1):1–9, 1988.
7. H Soltanian-Zadeh, JP Windham, JM Jenkins. IEEE Trans Med Imag 9(4):405–420, 1990.
8. DJ Peck, JP Windham, H Soltanian-Zadeh, JP Roebuck. Med Phys 19(3):599–605, 1992.
9. H Soltanian-Zadeh. Multi-dimensional signal processing of magnetic resonance scene sequences. PhD dissertation, University of Michigan, Ann Arbor, MI, 1992.
10. H Soltanian-Zadeh, JP Windham, AE Yagle. IEEE Trans Nuc Sci 40(4):1204–1212, 1993.
11. H Soltanian-Zadeh, JP Windham. J Magn Reson Med 31(4):465–466, 1994.
12. DJ Peck, JP Windham, L Emery, H Soltanian-Zadeh, DO Hearshen, T Mikkelsen. J Med Physics 23(12):2035–2042, 1996.
13. H Soltanian-Zadeh, JP Windham, DJ Peck. J IEEE Trans Med Imag 15(6):749–767, 1996.
14. MW Vannier, RL Butterfield, D Jordan, WA Murphy, RG Levitt, M Gado. J Radiology 154:221–224, 1985.
15. LP Clarke, RP Velthuizen, MA Camacho, JJ Heine, M Vaidyanathan, LO Hall, RW Thatcher, ML Silbiger. J Magn Reson Imag 13(3):343–368, 1995.
16. PA DeVijver, J Kittler, Pattern Recognition: A Statistical Approach. London: Prentice Hall International, 1982.
17. K Fukunaga. Introduction to Statistical Pattern Recognition. 2nd ed. San Diego: Academic Press, 1990.
18. G Biswas, AK Jain, RC Dubes. IEEE Trans PAMI 3(6):701–708, 1981.
19. K Fukunaga, WLG Koontz. IEEE Trans Comput 19:311–318, 1970.

20. H Soltanian-Zadeh, JP Windham. J Electronic Imag 1(2):171–182, 1992.
21. M Ozkan, BM Dawant. J IEEE Trans Med Imag 12:534–544, 1993.
22. LO Hall, AM Bensaid, LP Clarke, RP Velthuizen, MS Silbiger, JC Bezdek. IEEE Trans Neural Networks 3:672–682, 1992.
23. J Alirezaei, ME Jernigan, C Nihmias. Proc IEEE Conf Med Imag 1397–1401, 1995.
24. B Ashjaei, H Soltanian-Zadeh. A comparative study of neural network methodologies for segmentation of magnetic resonance images. Proceedings of the International Conference on Image Processing, Lausanne, Switzerland, 1996.
25. RL DeLaPlaz, PJ Chang, JV Dave. Approximate fuzzy C-means (AFCM) cluster analysis of medical magnetic resonance image (MRI) data. Proceedings of the IEEE International Conference on Systems, Man, and Cybernetics, 1987, 2:869–871.
26. RL DeLaPaz, EH Herskovits, V Di Gesu, WA Hanson, R Bernstein. J SPIE 1259:176–181, 1990.
27. A Simmons, SR Arridge, GJ Barker, AJ Cluckie, PS Tofts. J Magn Reson Imag 12:1191–1204, 1994.
28. MC Clark, LO Hall, DB Goldgof, LP Clarke, RP Velthuizen, MS Silbiger. J IEEE Eng Med Biol November/December: 730–742, 1994.
29. ME Brandt, TP Bohan, LA Kramer, JM Fletcher. J Comput Med Imag Graphics 18:25–34, 1994.
30. RP Velthuizen, LP Clarke, S Phuphanich, LO Hall, AM Bensaid, JA Arrington, HM Greenberg, ML Silbiger. J MRI 5:594–605, 1995.
31. WE Phillips, RP Velthuizen, S Phuphanich, LO Hall, LP Clarke, ML Silbiger. J Magn Reson Imag 13:277–290, 1995.
32. M Vaidyanathan, LP Clark, RP Velthuizen, S Phuphanich, AM Bensaid, LO Hall, JC Bezdek, H Greenberg, A Trotti, M Silbiger. J Magn Reson Imag 13:719–728, 1995.
33. B Ashjaei, H Soltanian-Zadeh. Adaptive clustering techniques for segmentation of magnetic resonance images. Proceedings of the ISRF-IEE International Conference on Intelligent and Cognitive Systems, Neural Networks Symposium, Tehran, Iran, 1996.
34. H Soltanian-Zadeh, JP Windham, L Robbins. Semi-supervised segmentation of MRI stroke studies. Proceedings of SPIE Medical Imaging 1997: Image Processing Conference, Newport Beach, CA, 1997.
35. WK Pratt. Digital Image Processing. New York: John Wiley & Sons, Inc., 1978.
36. KR Castleman. Digital Image Processing. Englewood Cliff, NJ: Prentice-Hall, Inc., 1979.
37. RC Gonzalez, P Wintz. Digital Image Processing. 2nd ed. Reading, MA: Addison-Wesley Publishing Company, Inc., 1987.
38. AK Jain. Fundamentals of Digital Image Processing. Englewood Cliffs, NJ: Prentice Hall, 1989.
39. JR Mitchell, SJ Karlik, DH Lee, A Fenster. J Magn Reson Imag 4(No 2):197–208, 1994.
40. PH Higer, B Gernot. Tissue Characterization in MR Imaging: Clinical and Technical Approaches. New York: Springer-Verlag, 1990.
41. M Just, M Thelen. J Radiology 169:779–785, 1988.
42. HK Brown, TR Hazelton, JV Fiorica, AK Parsons, LP Clarke, ML Silbiger. J Magn Reson Imaging 10(No 1):143–145, 1992.

43. HK Brown, TR Hazelton, ML Silbiger. Am J Anat 192(No 1):23–24, 1991.
44. H Grahn, NM Szeverenyi, MW Roggenbuck, F Delaglio, P Geladi. J Chemometrics Intell Lab Syst 5:311–22, 1989.
45. JP Windham, H Soltanian-Zadeh, DJ Peck. Tissue characterization by a vector subspace method. Presented at the 33rd Annual Meeting of the American Association of Physicists in Medicine (AAPM), San Francisco, CA, July 1991. Abstract Published in Med Phys 18(3):619, 1991.
46. JN Lee, SJ Riederer. J Magn Reson Med 5:13–22, 1987.
47. U Schmiedl, DA Ortendahl, AS Mark, I Berry, L Kaufman. J Magn Reson Med 4:471–486, 1987.
48. JR MacFall, SJ Riederer, HZ Wang. J Med Phys 13(3):285–292, 1986.
49. ER McVeigh, MJ Bronskill, RM Henkelman. J Magn Reson Med 6:314–333, 1988.
50. RO Duda, PE Hart. Pattern Classification and Scene Analysis. New York: John Wiley & Sons, 1973, pp 114–121.
51. GTY Chen, CA Pelizzari. J Comput Med Imag Graph 13(3):235–240, 1989.
52. MV Herk, HM Kooy. J Med Phys 21(7):1163–1178, 1994.
53. J Mangin, V Frouin, I Bloch, B Bendriem, J. Lopez-Krahe. Cereb Blood Flow Metab 14:749–762, 1994.
54. PA Van den Elsen, JB Antoine Maintz, ED Pol, MA Viergever. IEEE Trans Med Imag 14(2):384–396, 1995.
55. BA Ardekani, M Braun, BF Hutton, I Kanno, H Iida. J Comput Assist Tomogr 19(4):615–623, 1995.
56. AP Zijdenbos, BM Dawant, RA Margolin. J Comput Med Imag Graph 18(1):11–23, 1994.
57. A Chakraborty, LH Staib, JS Duncan. IEEE Trans Med Imag 15(6):859–870, 1996.
58. C Davatzikos, RN Bryan. IEEE Trans Med Imag 15(6):785–795, 1996.
59. Y Ge, JM Fitzpatrick, BM Dawant, J Bao, RM Kessler, RA Margolin. IEEE Trans Med Imag 15(4):418–428, 1996.
60. S Sandor, R Leahy. IEEE Trans Med Img 16(1):41–54, 1997.
61. G Henrich, N Mai, H Backmund. J Comput Assist Tomogr 3(3):379–384, 1979.
62. H Soltanian-Zadeh, JP Windham. Med Physics 24(12):1844–1853, 1997.
63. A Simmons, PS Tofts, GJ Barker, DAG Wicks, SA Arridge. Considerations for RF nonuniformity correction of spin echo images at 1.5 T, SMRM'92, Book of Abstracts, 4240.
64. A Simmons, PS Tofts, GJ Barker, SA Arridge. Improvement to dual echo clustering of neuroanatomy in MRI, SMRM'92, Book of Abstracts, 4202.
65. BR Condon, J Patterson, D Wyper, A Jenkins, DM Hadley. BJR 60(709):83–87, 1987.
66. DAG Wicks, GJ Barker, PS Tofts. Magn Reson Imag 11(2):183–196, 1993.
67. WM Wells, III, WEL Grimson, R Kikinis, FA Jolesz. IEEE Trans Med Img 15(4):429–442, 1996.
68. R Guillemaud, M Brady. IEEE Trans Med Img 16(3):238–251, 1997.
69. KO Lim, A Pfefferbaum. J Comput Assist Tomogr 13(4):588–593, 1989.
70. BM Dawant, AP Zijdenbos, RA Margolin. IEEE Trans Med Imag 12(4):770–781, 1993.
71. PA Narayana, A Borthakur. Magn Reson Med 33:396–400, 1995.
72. SK Lee, MW Vannier. Magn Reson Med 36:275–286, 1996.

73. CR Meyer, PH Bland, J Pipe. Retrospective correction of MRI amplitude inhomogeneities. N Ayache, ed. Proceedings of CVRMed'96, Berlin, Germany: Springer-Verlag, 1995, pp 513–522.
74. L Nocera, JC Gee. Robust partial volume tissue classification of cerebral MRI scans. Proceedings of SPIE Medical Imaging 1997: Image Processing Conference 3034, part one, pp 312–322, 1997.
75. H Soltanian-Zadeh, JP Windham, AE Yagle. Trans Imag Proc 14(2):147–161, 1995.
76. SM Kay. Modern Spectral Estimation Theory and Application, Englewood Clifs, NJ: 1988.
77. JL Devore. Probability and Statistics for Engineering and Science, Monterrey Books/Cole Publishing Co., 1987.
78. H Stark, JW Woods. Probability, Random Processes, and Estimation Theory for Engineers, Englewood Cliffs, NJ: Prentice-Hall Inc., 1986.
79. HL Van Trees. Detection, Estimation, and Modulation Theory. New York: John Wiley & Sons, Inc., 1968.
80. DG Brown, JN Lee, RA Blinder, HZ Wang, SJ Riederer, LW Nolte. Magn Reson Med 14(1):79–96, 1990.
81. JB de Castro, TA Tasciyan, JN Lee, F Farzaneh, SJ Riederer, RJ Herfkens. J Comput Assist Tomogr 12(2):355–362, 1988.
82. RB Buxton, F Greensite. Mag Res Med 18(1):102–115, 1991.
83. SL Meyer. Data Analysis for Scientists and Engineers. New York: John Wiley & Sons Inc., 1975, pp 39–48.
84. JL Jaech. Statistical Analysis of Measurement Error. New York: John Wiley & Sons Inc., 1985.
85. HC Andrews, CL Patterson. Singular Value Decomposition and Digital Image Processing, IEEE Trans. ASSP. ASSP-24:26–53, 1976.
86. TS Huang, PM Narenda. Image restoration by singular value decomposition. Appl Optics 14:2213–2216, 1975.
87. BR Hunt, O Kubler. Karhunen-Loeve Multispectral Image Restoration-Part I: Theory. IEEE Trans. ASSP. ASSP-32:592–599, 1984.
88. N Ahmed, KR Rao. Orthogonal Transforms for Digital Image Processing. New York: Spring-Verlag Inc., 1975, pp 189–224.
89. JT Tou, Gonzalez. Pattern Recognition Principles. 2nd ed. Reading, MA: Addison-Wesley Publishing Company Inc., 1977.
90. SA Zoharian, AJ Jarghaghi. Minimum mean-square error transformation of categorical data to target positions. IEEE Trans Signal Proc 40(1):13–23, 1992.
91. DG Luenberger. Optimization by Vector Space Methods, New York: John Wiley & Sons Inc., 1969.
92. S Wilks. Mathematical Statistics. New York: New York, John Wiley & Sons, 1962, pp 577–578.
93. JK Gohagan, EL Spitznagel. Multispectral analysis of MR images of the breast. Radiology 163(3):703–707, 1987.
94. HA Koenig, R Bachus, ER Reinhardt. Pattern Recognition for Tissue Characterization in Magnetic Resonance Imaging. Health Care Instrumentation (Siemens Med. Div., Erlangen, Frg.) 1(6):184–187, 1986.

95. JP Windham, AM Haggar, DO Hearshen, JR Roebuck, DA Reimann. Soc Mag Res Imag Book of Abstracts 2:1081, 1988.
96. DJ Peck, JP Windham, LL Emery, LM Scarpace, T Mikkelsen. Directed surgical biopsy using the eigenimage filter. Presented at the 5th Annual Meeting of the International Society for Magnetic Resonance in Medicine (ISMRM), Vancouver, BC, Canada, 1997.
97. Hamid Soltanian-Zadeh, Donald J Peck, Joe P Windham, Tom Mikkelsen. Brain Tumor Segmentation and Characterization by Pattern Analysis of Multispectral NMR Images. NMR in Biomedicine: Themed Issue Pattern Recognition Analysis of MR Data, 11(4/5):201–208, 1998.
98. GH Ball, DJ Hall. Behav Sci 12:153–155, 1967.
99. H Soltanian-Zadeh, JP Windham. Optimal feature space for MRI. Proceedings of the 1995 IEEE Medical Imaging Conference, San Francisco, CA, Oct. 1995.

13
Brain Tumor Imaging: Fusion of Scintigraphy with Magnetic Resonance and Computed Tomography

Richard J. T. Gorniak, Elissa L. Kramer, and Marilyn E. Noz
New York University School of Medicine, New York, New York

I. INTRODUCTION

Patients with intracranial diseases frequently undergo multiple imaging studies during the course of their evaluation and treatment. Although these studies individually can provide important information, combining studies acquired using two different modalities into one integrated image set may enhance the clinician's understanding of a patient's disease. Because each modality has characteristic imaging capabilities, fusion of complementary images from different modalities can result in a synergistic image that shows the correspondence of features depicted by each imaging method. This can be seen in the registration of ^{201}Tl single photon positron emission tomography (SPECT) and magnetic resonance (MR) images of the brain. Many functional modalities produce images showing radiopharmaceutical distribution, which demonstrate functional parameters of tissues but poorly display anatomy. On the other hand, conventional MR or computed tomography (CT) images demonstrate structural details well but offer little information about the physiology of these structures. By registering functional with structural images, the anatomical context of functional findings is enhanced. For example, areas of high-grade astrocytoma seen on ^{201}Tl SPECT could be localized to a specific position within a complex lesion depicted on a MR image. This could be useful in assisting in both diagnosis and neurosurgical or radiotherapy planning.

Several registration techniques have been developed to fuse images of the brain. In fact, image fusion has been studied more in the brain than any other body area. Fusion techniques attempt to find a mathematical transform that can be applied to an image, so that any point in the transform of that image corresponds exactly to the analogous point in another image. For brain images a three-dimensional (3D) rigid body transformation usually is used as the basis of the registration process. This transformation allows for linear movement along and rotation around each axis in three dimensions, resulting in six registration variables. Although this is an affine transformation that preserves the original relationships of all the structures involved, others may or may not allow scale. Nonrigid transformations, such as polynomial warping transformations, have more degrees of freedom allowing for scaling and shear. Although nonrigid transformations can be used more broadly than rigid transformations, the added computational complexity generally is not necessary for applications limited to the brain. For a good review of fusion techniques in the brain, see Van den Elsen et al. (1) and Maintz (2).

The use of a rigid body transformation assumes the pixel size is known in each image set, there is no uncorrected spatial distortion of the image sets, and the structures in the brain have not changed position relative to each other between image acquisitions. These assumptions are met in most brain images. Without a scaling parameter in the registration transform, accurate pixel sizes must be known for each image set. This information is usually determined during image acquisition. Spatial distortion, as might be seen in MR images, can be compensated for with postprocessing (3) or controlled with proper shimming. Although the position of structures in the brain may vary to a small degree with the pulsations of blood flow, short-term changes are not usually significant, unlike the chest or abdomen, where structures frequently move significantly in short periods of time.

II. TECHNICAL CONSIDERATIONS

Registration methods that calculate the six rigid body parameters by comparing structures in both images must consider a number of factors. Initially, structures to be used as the registration landmarks, such as the scalp or brain, must be identified in both image sets. Identifying these structures usually involves marking or segmenting structures manually or with an automated method. Then, based on the identified structures, an algorithm determines the six registration parameters that best fuse the landmark structures.

The determination of the six variables of the rigid body transformation is the key task of any rigid-body registration algorithm. The methods used can be classified into general categories such as (a) methods that take a global approach to the data set using surface-based techniques such as least squares search, principal axis, and moment-matching techniques; (b) methods that take a structural-based approach by defining objects within the image sets; and (c) methods that take a procedural approach. Any one of these methods may or may not introduce information into the study, such as external markers, that was not there intrinsically.

Surface-based methods have been used widely in the registration of CT, MR, positron emission tomography (PET), and SPECT images (4,5). Initially, surfaces visible in both image sets are extracted. The surfaces used depend on which two modalities are to be registered, because different structures are common to different combinations of images. For example, the brain surface is used in ^{99m}Tc fluorodeoxyglucose ^{18}PET or technetium ^{99m}Tc hexamethyl-polypropylene-oxime (HMPAO) SPECT/MR registration, whereas the scalp surface is used in ^{201}Tl SPECT/MR registration. These surfaces can be defined through semiautomated algorithms or manual outlining.

The sum of squares algorithm calculates the registration parameters from the extracted surfaces, using a search technique to minimize mismatch between the extracted surfaces (i.e., the sum of the squares of distances from points on surface A to the nearest points on surface B) (6). According to Pelizzari, this process is analogous to fitting a hat to a head. A major problem with this approach is that a large number of points (approximately 1,000–10,000) must be identified on the surface of each object to be matched. In addition, convergence of the search technique can be a problem if the relative difference in surface angulation is very large (20 degrees or more). Although registration parameter selection is automated, it is often necessary for a user to steer the process to obtain a sufficiently good match with reasonable convergence speed.

The eigenvalue decomposition approach to surface identification for registration finds the principal axes of the image. These represent orthogonal axes, about which the moments of inertia are at a minimum, and depend only on surface shape. Surface-matching techniques include the eigenvalue decomposition of scatter matrices (second-order moments) applied to the threshold version of the original images or to the surface data (7). Here again, a large number of points identifying the surfaces must be found (8,9). Another approach (10) uses single-value decomposition techniques to determine the eigenvalues.

Moment-matching techniques applied to surface matching use centroids and principal axes (11). The major problem with this technique is that the object (such as the brain) needs to be completely scanned for the registration accuracy to be acceptable. A more comprehensive discussion of principal axis and moment matching techniques contrasted with each other and with the sum of squares search technique has been reported by Rusinek and colleagues (12).

Algorithms that base registration on structures include a 2D global tracking algorithm based on Fourier phase correlation methods (13), cross-correlation using Fourier invariance properties, and logarithmic transforms to decouple the variables (14). Warping algorithms involving both internal and external landmarks have been used extensively in our laboratory for fusion in many parts of the body, including the brain (15).

Another approach is based on the pixel values of similar tissues in two studies being related to each other. The method used by Woods et al. (16,17), as modified for cross-modality registration, has been used with MR and ^{18}FDG or $H_2{}^{15}O$ PET registration. Once nonbrain structures are removed, the MR images are partitioned on the basis of pixel value into 256 regions. Ideally, areas with similar pixel values represent similar types of tissue. In PET, these areas of similar tissue ideally have similar PET pixel values. The algorithm seeks to maximize the uniformity of PET pixel values in each MR partition. Uniformity is defined by the weighted average of the standard deviation of the PET pixel values contained in the partitions defined on MR images. Once the MR images are edited so that only the brain remains, no user interaction is required. A different approach based on pixel values is to use the "mutual information" contained in the two images (18,19). Again, image preprocessing is necessary.

Yet other means take a procedural approach that requires the use of external devices, such as a stereotactic frame fixed to the head, at the time of image acquisition. This frame enforces reproducibility of positioning at the time of the acquisitions and thus permits the maintenance of geometric consistency between either intermodality or intramodality scans. Also, the stereotactic frame offers unambiguous, easy-to-discern landmarks. This allows for simple, fast, mostly automated registration with the accuracy needed for neurosurgical planning (20). Other methods that use external devices include a holder specifically molded to the patient's head (21,22) or a noncustom headholder (23,24). The headholder used by the PET group at the Karolinska Institute in Stockholm (21) provides, in the experimental setting, reproducible head localization to within 1 mm in all three planes between PET scans and CT scans. Clinically, however, serial PET scan may show significant mismatch (25) with this method. These problems also have been encountered by other researchers using this approach (24). Although necessary for certain applications, external markers have several disadvantages. The markers must be placed in the same position before every study, which can be difficult if the scans are done days or weeks apart or at different institutions. Also, application of invasive markers, such as a frame screwed to the skull, takes time, hospital resources, and personnel and is uncomfortable for the patient. A comprehensive discussion of the use of markers of different varieties has been published (1).

Use of an anatomical atlas is another example of a procedural approach to image registration. To date, atlases have only been constructed for the brain (23,26–31), although several full-body atlases are either currently being constructed or are planned (32). An anatomical atlas may be transformed to fit images obtained in any particular patient. Both an elastic transformation (29–31) and a warping algorithm (27) have been applied to this task. These methods require that corresponding curved surfaces be stretched or shrunk to effect the best fit possible. This requires the identification of exact edges. Because this is more easily accomplished with CT or MR, the atlas image is transformed to the structural patient image. This is then correlated with the functional image. The difficulty of edge detection has been a major challenge in the use of atlases for image registration. In an effort to overcome the problem of edge detection in using an atlas, one group has defined an atlas of regions of interest (ROI's) drawn at specific levels in the brain over specific structures (26). This atlas was developed from MR scans of normal subjects. The atlas regions of interest are reshaped to fit the patient's anatomy as defined by a structural study (e.g., MR scan). The method reported also incorporates a "Z"-shaped tube inserted into a headholder as a fiducial marker. Patient scans are aligned using the fiducial marker that is affixed to the headholder and then the ROIs are overlaid.

Although these methods have been reported to work well with many imaging modalities, many depend on the accurate selection of landmarks, which may not be possible on all images sets. Interactive methods overcome this by giving control of the registration process to an expert who directly manipulates the registration parameters based on a display of the image sets. Although interactive visual methods are broadly applicable, they depend on the skill of the user and the limitations of the original images (33). One study showed that translational misregistration of less than 2 to 3 mm and rotational misregistrations of less than 2 to 4 degrees were not visually detectable by an expert in ^{18}FDG-PET/MR registrations (34).

Interactive methods of registration combine the interpretive power of a human user with a computer based image manipulation and display program. With the interactive method currently used in our laboratory (35), scaled 2D and/or 3D images from both image sets are displayed simultaneously with contours from one image superimposed on the other. The user then visually assesses mismatches in analogous structures apparent in both images and, by adjusting the translation and/or rotation of one image set, attempts to correctly match them. The 2D and 3D images are redisplayed, interactively showing the adjustments of translation and rotation. The user then reassesses mismatch and continues to refine the registration parameters. This process is repeated until the user is visually satisfied that the best set of translation and rotation parameters have been selected.

With any method, understanding the accuracy of registration is vital to interpreting the registered image set. Ideally, registration would result in an exact mapping of the findings of one image set into the same anatomical location in the other. This perfect registration may not be achievable, even if the assumptions mentioned earlier for rigid body transformations are true. Error may be introduced in some methods during selection of the registration landmarks in each image set.

This is especially relevant with functional images, because the borders of structures can be less distinct in functional images, which can lead to inaccurate localization of the landmarks.

It is difficult to compare accuracy of the many registration methods because of the different combinations of image modalities used and the different methods used to measure accuracy. Registration based on external markers is considered the most accurate. For SPECT/MR, Erickson (36) reports an error of 3 mm using fiduciary markers and a brain phantom. In one study, we reported the accuracy of a variety of registration methods applied to the same CT/MR and PET/MR image sets (37). The image sets are acquired with a stereotactic frame in place. These images are registered based on the frame, resulting in the "gold standard" registration. The frame is edited from these images, and then the images are registered with a variety of retrospective techniques. We found the median error for PET/MR registration to be similar for all the techniques used (2–4.9 mm). Using similar methods to calculate accuracy, we calculated the median error for our interactive method applied to ^{201}Tl SPECT/MR registration to be 5.8 mm (38). Generally, registration accuracy is on the order of the voxel size of lowest resolution scan.

Registration error varies not only from patient to patient but also from pixel to pixel in the same set of images. Although translational error is constant from pixel to pixel, the component of error caused by error in the selection of rotation parameters varies with distance from the center of rotation. So areas distant from the center of rotation will have a greater error component caused by rotational misregistrations (see Fig. 1). A derivation of an equation that illustrates this spatial variation in error can be found in Appendix A of West et al. (37).

III. OUR METHOD

The registration method used in our laboratory (39) (validated in Ref. 38) for the 3D registration of data sets is implemented with the IBM Visualization Data Explorer (DX) software suite, which provides an object-oriented, graphical programming interface. The DX data model is discipline-independent (i.e., it can be used for any visualization application including medicine), self-describing, and supports regular and irregular grids with node and connection-dependent data. DX uses a data-flow driven client-server execution model, and runs on UNIX workstations from most leading manufacturers. Window content, layout, and access were structured for convenient use and ease of learning. Each image is fully annotated with variable names, display parameters, patient name, and scan date, which are automatically extracted from the image header.

For digital fusion and manipulation of 3D tomographic data, slices from each image modality must be transferred to a single computer system and con-

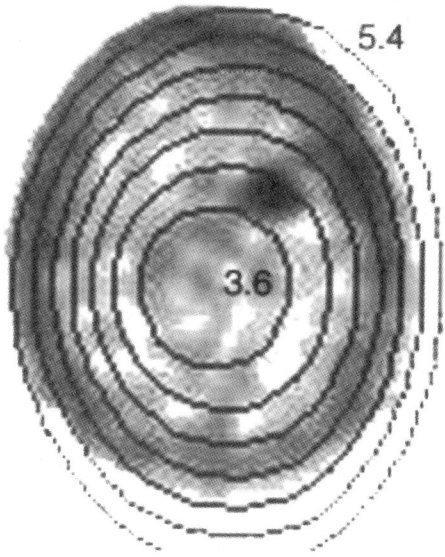

Fig. 1 ^{201}Tl SPECT axial image with contours showing the spatial variability of registration error. Error was determined by comparing registrations with and without a stereotactic frame. First, the "true" registration was determined by registering a SPECT image set with a MR image set using a stereotactic frame. The frame was edited from the images, then the images were registered three times by an expert user without the frame. The average absolute distances of the three registrations from the "true" registration were calculated at 800 points in the brain volume. Note that the error increases with distance from the axis of rotation (center of the innermost contour). Each contour represents a 0.3-mm increase in error.

verted to a common format. The transfer may be accomplished by any standard method. Interformat (40), a commercially available image conversion program, is used to do the conversion to the DX specific format "on the fly," or the images can be converted to an intermediate format, such as qsh (41), which is the standard AAPM format, subsequently known as the Interfile format (42). Because DX is flexible in allowing the user to write compiled program modules or scripts, qsh-formatted images are easily interpreted by DX using a simple AWK script or DX program module.

The features extracted from the 3D data sets are boundaries/surfaces of organs, tumors, bones, or high-radiation emission regions. These surfaces are key items used in registering radionuclidic functional images to structural images and are the anatomical references used in the interpretation of fused data. Two options are available for feature extraction, the isosurface option, and the multiscan composition option. The multiscan composition option for viewing different MR scanning sequences simultaneously is based on selecting regions with statistically similar values from each sequence. The pulse sequences used include T1-weighted, which shows increased signal from fat, protein-rich fluid, or subacute hemorrhage, T2-weighted, which shows increased signal in areas with high water content such as edema, infarction, inflammation, or tumor, and proton density (PD). Even though T1-weighted scans provide basic structural information, T1-weighted scans combined with T2-weighted and PD scans provide a clearer delineation of disease and surrounding tissue. In most cases, brain MR scans require an axial correction of data values to compensate for the magnetic field inhomogeneity, which can cause similar tissues to have different pixel values depending on their axial location.

The first step in the extraction of significant features using the multiscan composition option is to select a set of points in the ROI; points may be in more than one image, T1, T2, or PD. On the basis of these points, an average and sample covariance matrix are computed. Then at each point in the 3D data space, the Mahalanobis distance of the corresponding (T1, T2, PD) value is generated. (Mahalanobis distance is based on the sample mean and covariance. It is the euclidean distance from the mean with the inverse of the covariance matrix used as the metric.) A surface is then formed based on this distance. Note that points are not classified as lesion, CSF, etc. This method defines a surface about statistically similar tissues as defined by the user's selection based on T1, T2, and PD images.

To confirm that each of the point groups are coherent and disjointed, a 3D cluster plot can also be formed with ellipsoids surrounding the clusters, which correspond to the thresholds used for each surface. An advantage of this approach is that it compensates for anteroposterior intensity gradients. This is particularly valuable for large structures like the skin surface. Points can be selected around the head, and the Mahalanobis ellipsoid will be elongated radially from the origin of the T1-weighted, T2-weighted, and PD space.

Using the isosurface option, surfaces consisting of one specified pixel value can display the 3D distribution of emission activity in SPECT scans. For example, regions of abnormal activity can be displayed as an opaque 3D isosurface, and areas of normal scalp activity can be displayed as a transparent surface. The surfaces are extracted by selecting visually appropriate pixel levels. This simple method is also able to extract the scalp surface from the MR data. Contours can be displayed on opaque and/or transparent isosurfaces to improve shape perception and estimate the size of various regions.

Using the isosurface option or the multiscan composition option, surfaces can be formed corresponding to scalp surface, lateral ventricles, tumor, etc. In some cases extraneous surface segments are formed as a result of data artifacts or "poor" segmentation. The 3D image can be edited to keep only relevant surface segments (see Fig. 2).

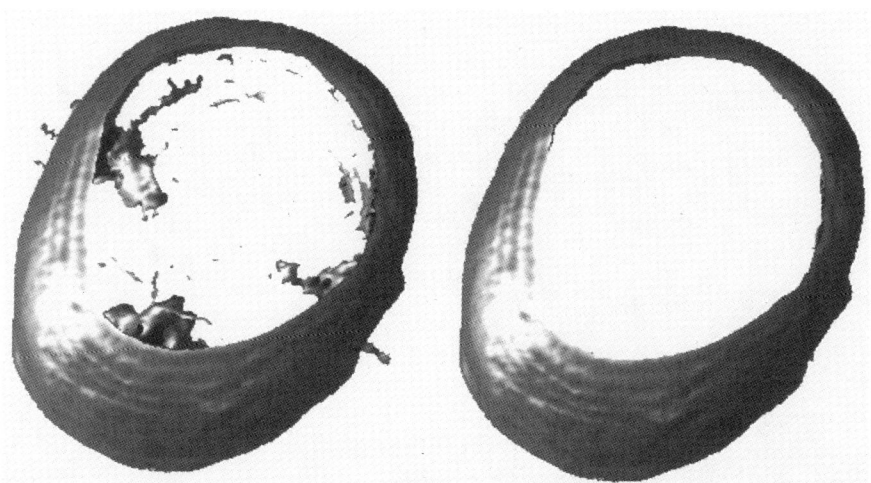

Fig. 2 (Left) Pixel value 70 isosurfaces extracted from a MR data set showing the scalp and nonscalp surfaces. (Right) Same pixel value 70 isosurface, but with the surfaces not continuous with the scalp removed.

Registration of the data sets is required before fusion and analysis can be performed. The coordinates of the functional data are translated and rotated relative to the structural coordinate system, so that a given 3D coordinate refers to the same anatomical location in both data sets. Two approaches are available for registration: direct 3D registration and iterative 2D/3D registration.

The direct 3D approach is based on aligning extracted structural and functional surfaces of the same anatomical region. For example, the structural and functional data of a patient can be registered based on aligning scalp surfaces. This approach relies on the ability to extract an appropriate surface from the functional data and can produce a repeatable registration. Fig. 3 illustrates a satisfactory fusion using a stereotactic frame. In our experience with SPECT images at NYU (43), direct 3D registration is consistently possible only when external fiducial markers are available on both image sets. In cases in which satisfactory surfaces cannot be obtained, an alternate approach is used based on 2D, as well as 3D, images.

In the iterative 2D/3D registration, 3D surfaces of the scalp are used for initial parameter selection. By use of the scalp surfaces as a guide, registration parameters are selected to roughly match the two images. This is accomplished by interactively entering a registration parameter and then seeing the effect of the newly chosen parameter on the location of the SPECT scalp surface. By viewing

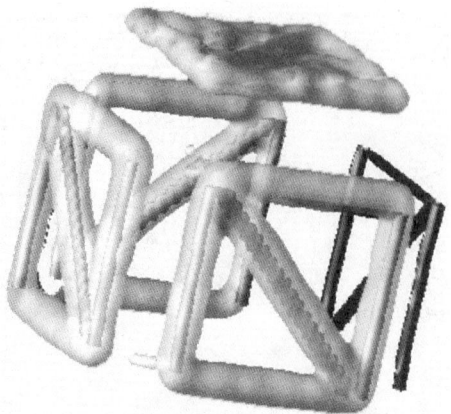

Fig. 3 An example of the direct 3D approach using a stereotactic frame as the basis of registration. The lateral and posterior portions of the frames are seen in both studies and are well registered. Black surface, stereotactic frame extracted from MR data. White surface, stereotactic frame extracted from SPECT data.

the surfaces from a variety of angles, the parameters that best match the entire surface are selected (Fig. 4).

Next, a coronal plane through the brain in both data sets is selected. This is displayed as a slice from each image set with isovalue contours from the SPECT slice superimposed over the MR slice. Axial and lateral translations and anteroposterior rotation of the 3D functional data set are then visually selected to align the scalp contours of the SPECT to scalp seen on MR. Then two axial images are formed, with the functional scan contours again placed over both images. It must be kept in mind that these data sets have already been preliminarily registered in the axial direction using 3D surfaces. The anteroposterior translation and axial rotation are now selected. Then a sagittal slice is used to select the lateral rotation. Once this estimate of the three translation and rotation parameters has been made, the 3D surfaces and 2D slices are used iteratively to fine tune the match. A second pass with the coronal, sagittal, and axial images is performed to make adjustments to the translations and rotations about all axes.

To confirm the registration, image pairs at other locations are compared using overlaid isocontours. The basic concept of the iterative 2D/3D approach is to adjust large registration disparities first, followed by smaller adjustments. This approach is well suited to SPECT/MR data, because even though the resolution of the SPECT data is low, the registration converges in one or two passes. Fig. 5

Fusion of Scintigraphy with MR and CT

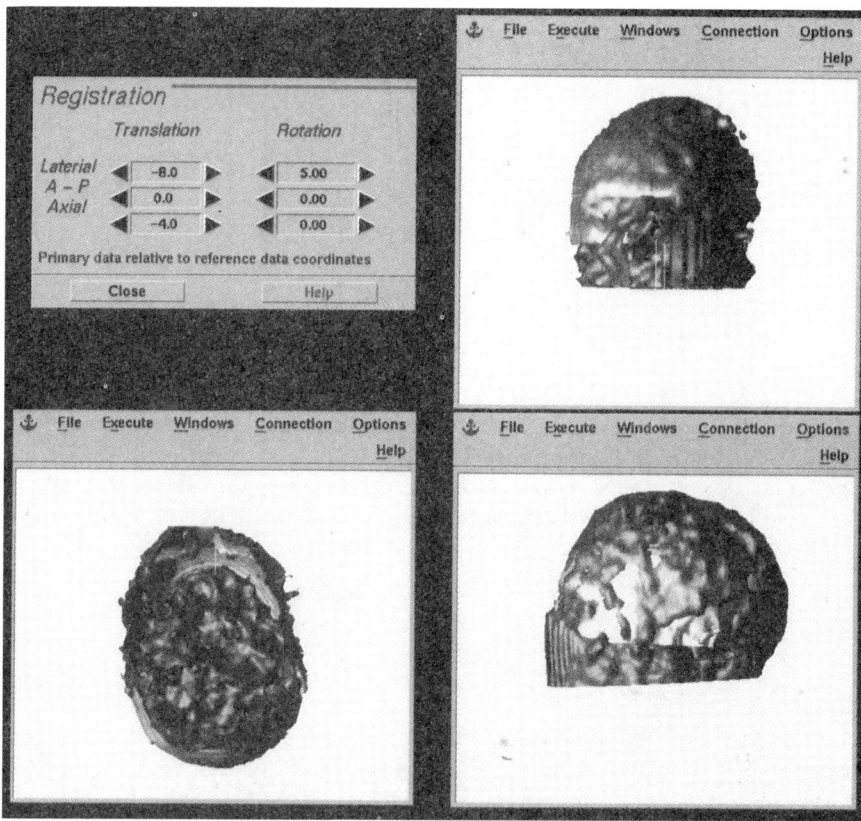

Fig. 4 The registration control panel used to input the registration parameters and three views of MR (gray) and SPECT (black) scalp surfaces after initial 3D registration.

shows various views from a completed registration using the iterative 2D/3D approach.

IV. CLINICAL APPLICATIONS

The use of registered image sets is clinically useful in assisting with diagnostic interpretation. Although visual comparison of separate images sets is adequate in many situations, registered images may provide further information in certain cases. Anatomical localization of functional findings may be difficult without reg-

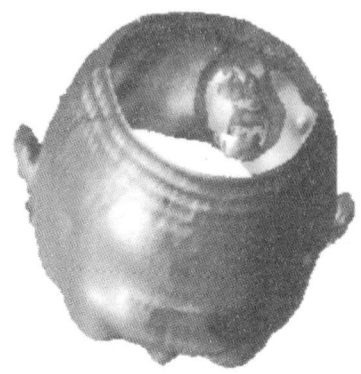

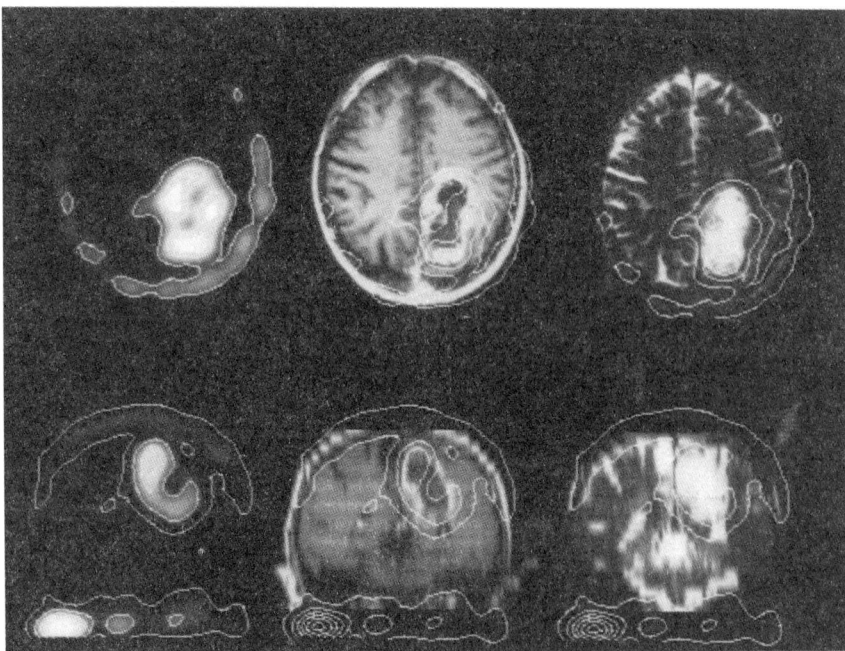

Fig. 5 (Top) Surfaces showing the spatial relationship of the tumor volume seen on MR and the volume of increased ^{201}Tl uptake. Gray surface, scalp surface extracted from MR data. White surface, tumor volume extracted from MR data. Black surface, volume of abnormal thallium uptake. (Middle) axial sections of ^{201}Tl SPECT, T1-weighted MR, and T2-weighted MR with isovalue contour (white) extracted from the SPECT data superimposed on the MR images, showing increased ^{201}Tl uptake around the lesion, but not at the center (bottom) coronal images.

Fusion of Scintigraphy with MR and CT

istration when the usual anatomy is distorted or displaced by disease or prior surgery. Registration may also assist in interpreting studies when the effects of partial voluming distort functional images. For example, tracer uptake may appear less evident in a small (less than twice the full width of half maximum) high-grade tumor or a tumor surrounded by necrotic areas. Registration also can be particularly useful in interpreting areas of increased uptake adjacent to locations normally showing some uptake, such as gray matter with ^{18}FDG PET or scalp with ^{201}Tl SPECT. Without precise placement in the anatomical context of a MR or CT image, such lesions could be overlooked as normal background uptake. One study of the clinical usefulness of registration showed that in 19 of 24 examinations, registration of MR and PET images was found to be important in distinguishing recurrent tumor from necrosis based on ^{18}FDG uptake (44). Registration was useful in all nine patients who had contrast-enhancing lesions close to the cerebral cortex. Interpretation of the PET scan was not assisted by registration in cases in which patients showed large diffuse regions of abnormal uptake or when the shape of the area of FDG uptake was obviously similar to the shape of the region with contrast enhancement. We have found a similar situation in ^{201}Tl SPECT performed in patients with primary brain tumors or central nervous system lymphoma. In these patients, lesions adjacent to the skull tend to merge with the normally intense scalp activity. An example of this is shown in Fig. 6. In this case, fusion helped demonstrate that activity resides within the lesion. By clarifying those functional scans that are sometimes difficult to interpret, registered im-

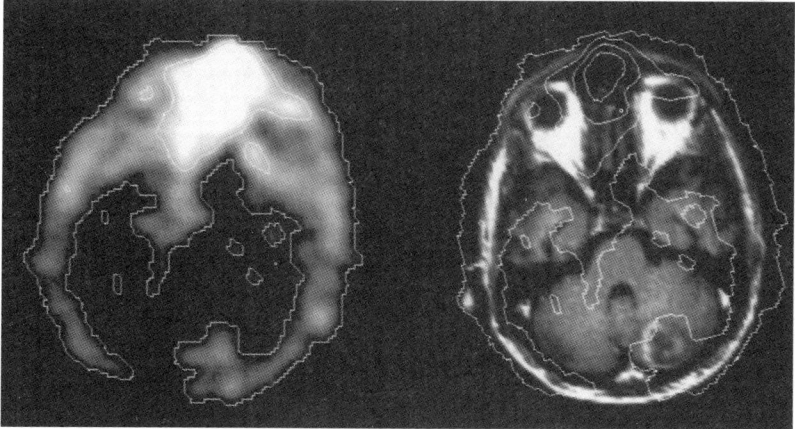

Fig. 6 The cerebellar lesion is clearly shown on the MR image (right). An area of uptake adjacent to the posterior scalp is seen on ^{201}Tl SPECT (left) but without registration the significance of this area would be uncertain. With the SPECT contour (white) superimposed on the MR image, it can be seen that the ^{201}Tl activity clearly corresponds to the ring-enhancing lesion.

ages may increase the sensitivity and specificity of functional studies. This is applicable particularly in the follow-up of cancer patients for recurrence or malignant transformation, in differentiating tumor recurrence from radiation necrosis in previously treated patients, or in differentiating lymphoma from opportunistic infections in immunosuppressed patients.

As well as assisting in the visual interpretation of images, registration enables more sophisticated methods of image analysis. Pixel-by-pixel calculations can be made involving both image sets. Parameters such as oxygen extraction rate can be calculated from registered PET scans showing oxygen metabolism and cerebral blood flow (45). Registered image sets have also been used to better define regions of interest used to calculate uptake indices in ^{201}Tl SPECT images (46).

In biopsy planning, registration enables targeting based on functional and anatomical characteristics. This has been shown to increase the yield of diagnostic biopsies (47,48). Because functional imaging, unlike MR or CT, can differentiate tumor from reactive gliosis or radiation necrosis (49), selecting areas of a lesion that show increased radionuclide uptake as biopsy sites increases the chance of sampling tumor. Fig. 7 shows an example in which biopsy planning may benefit from registration. By targeting the areas of ^{201}thallium uptake in the large lesion, the chance of sampling tumor might be increased.

In one study, 55 sites were targeted based on registered ^{18}FDG PET images and 35 were based on CT images alone. Of these biopsies, histological diagnoses were made on all 55 of the ^{18}FDG PET–targeted biopsies, whereas CT-based targets failed to yield a diagnosis (47,48). Not only is yield increased, but because functional imaging has been shown to differentiate between high- and low-grade astrocytoma (50,51), biopsies based on functional images may be more likely to

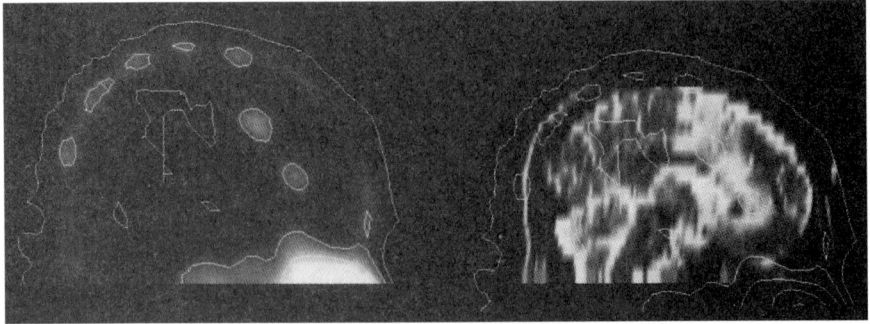

Fig. 7 (Left) a sagittal section of a ^{201}Tl SPECT scan showing two areas of increased uptake located anteriorly. (Right) a sagittal MR section reconstructed from axial images with a large T2 abnormality (white). The areas of increased thallium uptake (white contours) correspond to only a portion of the MR abnormality.

sample the highest grade portion of a tumor. This is critical for prognostic information and appropriate treatment planning.

Registration could also be useful in planning therapeutic interventions. The ability to localize highly malignant portions of a large mass seen on a MR image may enable a neurosurgeon to confidently remove less brain, reducing possible postsurgery neurological deficits (52,53). This may be especially useful in patients with prior radiation therapy, because radiation necrosis can be differentiated from tumor with PET or SPECT but not with MR. Alexander et al. (53) found registered ^{201}Tl SPECT/CT images useful in 37 reoperations after radiosurgery or brachytherapy. Another study showed the usefulness of registered ^{11}C-methionine PET/MR images (52) in tumor localization and H$_2$^{15}O-PET/MR registration to locate motor areas. With these images, the extent of tumor into the motor area could be detected. Of the 16 patients examined, 12 patients underwent radical resection, whereas 4 did not, because resection would have been impossible without functional deterioration. Although useful, there are limitations to this application. The limited resolution of functional images does not allow the detection of microtumor infiltration. Also, once the brain is manipulated during the operation, soft tissue relationships can be greatly altered, so the previously acquired images no longer represent the spatial relationship of structures in the brain of the patient during the operation.

Similarly, in radiation therapy planning it may be possible to deliver a high dose to tumor with increased activity as depicted on the functional image while sparing other areas. In a study of eight postresection patients with malignant gliomas, registered ^{18}FDG PET/functional MR cerebral blood volume/CT images were used to evaluate patients before, during, and after radiation therapy (54). In two patients, conventional radiation therapy planning was altered because of the added functional information. In one patient, a region with high functional activity was targeted for a higher than conventional dose boosted with proton beam therapy. In another patient, less radiation than usual was delivered to a hypometabolic area of brain and brain stem. Registration could be also useful in pretherapy SPECT or PET radioimmunoimaging, providing information about tumor localization of the therapeutic agent. Registration has also been used to calculate the absorbed dose of radioimmunotherapy. By superimposing PET images of iodine ^{124}I labeled 3F8 antibody with MR images, the patient-specific assessment of the target normal tissue absorbeddose ratio could be calculated for therapeutic administration of iodohippurate sodium ^{131}I or iodohippurate sodium ^{125}I labeled 3F8 (55). Such information could be useful in dosimetry and 3D treatment planning.

Clearly, very specific applications for image fusion of functional neuroimaging and brain MR or CT exist. Its transition to a routine clinical tool has been somewhat slowed by the difficulties in accomplishing the fusion in the clinic. These difficulties increasingly are being overcome on a more routine basis. Commercial file formats are becoming standardized, making the transfer of images across hardware and software platforms simpler. More powerful computer workstations that provide the computing power for manipulating large image files are more commonly available in the clinic. Not only is storage capacity increasing, but the time required for manipulating large data sets has decreased because of more efficient processors. The availability of network connectivity has made the actual access to and transfer of images a routine matter. All of this makes fusion a less time-intensive process that uses a smaller fraction of the available computing capacity. In addition, our comfort level with these registration processes has increased, and automation of these processes has become more prevalent, so that operator interaction with the images is reduced. Although in many situations registration is certainly a useful adjuvant for diagnosis and intervention planning, there are limitations to the routine clinical use of fusion techniques. Ensuring the accuracy of the registration in each patient is difficult. Without quality control, the use of registered images, especially in interventional planning, will remain experimental. Even with accurately registered images, the actual clinical meaning of registered scans has not been fully studied. Although it would seem that registration would increase the sensitivity and specificity of functional imaging studies, this has not been proven. Even with these limitations, clinicians are becoming convinced of the necessity for image fusion in the assessment and treatment of brain tumors. These algorithms have started to make their way into the everyday practice of neurooncology.

ACKNOWLEDGMENT

We thank Ed Farrell for his collaboration in the development of registration tools using the IBM Visualization Data Explorer (DX) software suite.

REFERENCES

1. PA Van den Elsen, EJD Pol, MA Viergever. Medical Image Matching—a Review with Classification. IEEE Eng Med Biol EMB 40:26–39, 1993.
2. JBA Maintz. Retrospective registration of tomographic brain images, Doctoral Thesis, University of Utrecht, The Netherlands, Helmholtz Institute, School for Autonomous Systems Research.
3. H Chang, JM Fitzpatrick. A technique for accurate magnetic resonance imaging in the presence of field inhomogeneities. IEEE Trans Med Imag 11:319–329, 1992.
4. TG Turkington, RJ Jaszczak, KL Greer, RE Coleman, CA Pelizzari. Correlation of SPECT images of a three-dimensional brain phantom using a surface fitting technique. IEEE Trans Nucl Sci 39(5):1460–1463, 1992.

5. BL Holman, RE Zimmerman, KA Johnson, PA Carvalho, RB Schwartz, JS Loeffler, E Alexander, CA Pelizarri, GTY Chen. Computer-assisted superposition of magnetic resonance and high-resolution technetium-99m-HMPAO and thallium-201 SPECT images of the brain. J Nucl Med 32(8):1478–1484, 1991.
6. CA Pelizarri, GTY Chen, DR Spelbring, RR Weichselbaum, CT Chen, Accurate three-dimensional registration of CT, PET and/or MR images of the brain. J Comput Assist Tomogr 13:20–26, 1989.
7. TL Faber, EM Stokely. Orientation of 3-D structures in medical images. Trans Pattern Anal Machine Intell PAMI-10:626–633, 1988.
8. M Mosfeghi, H Rusinek. Three-dimensional registration of multimodality medical images using the principal axes technique. Philips J Res 47(2):81–97, 1992.
9. KD Toennies, JK Udupa, GT Herman, IL Wornom III, SR Buchman. Registration of 3D objects and surfaces. IEEE Comput Graph Appl 10(3):52–62, 1990.
10. CR Meyer, GS Leichtman, JA Burnberg, RL Wahl, RL Quint. Simultaneous usage of homologous points, lines and planes for optimal, 3D, linear registration of multimodality imaging data. IEEE Trans Med Imag 14:1–11, 1995.
11. A Gamboa-Aldeco, LL Fellingham, GTY Chen. Correlation of 3D surfaces from multiple modalities in medical imaging. Proc SPIE, 626:467–473, 1986.
12. H Rusinek, W-H Tsui, AV Levy, ME Noz, MJ DeLeon. Principal axes and surface fitting methods for three-dimensional image registration. J Nucl Med 34(11):2019–2024, 1993.
13. E DeCastro, C Morandi. Registration of translated and rotated images using finite Fourier transformation. IEEE Trans Pattern Anal Machine Intell, PAMI-9:700–703, 1987.
14. A Apicella, JS Kippenhan, JH Nagel. Fast multimodality image matching. Medical Imaging III: Image Processing 1092:252–263, 1989.
15. GQ Maguire Jr, ME Noz, H Rusinek, J Jaeger, EL Kramer, JJ Sanger, G Smith. Graphics applied to image registration. IEEE Comput Graph Appl 11:20–29, 1991.
16. RP Woods, SR Cherry, JC Mazziotta. Rapid automated algorithm for aligning and reslicing PET images. J Comput Assist Tomogr 16(4):620–33, 1992.
17. RP Woods, JC Mazziotta, SR Cherry. MRI-PET registration with automated algorithm. J Comput Assist Tomogr 17:536–546, 1993.
18. C Studholme, DL Hill, DJ Hawkes. Automated three-dimensional registration of magnetic resonance and positron emission tomography brain images by multiresolution optimization of voxel similarity measures. Med Physics 24(1):25–35, 1997.
19. F Maes, A Collignon, D Vandermeulen, G Marchal, P Suetens. Multimodality image registration by maximization of mutual information. IEEE Trans Med Imag 18(2):187–197, 1997.
20. CR Mauer, JM Fitzpatrick, MY Wang, RL Galloway, RJ Maciunas, GS Allen. Registration of head volume images using implantable fiducial markers. IEEE Trans Med Image 16(4):447–461, 1997.
21. M Bergstrom, BJ Boethius, L Eriksson, T Greitz, T Ribbe, L Widen. Head fixation device for reproducible position alignment in transmission CT and positron emission tomography. J Comput Assist Tomogr 5(1):136–141, 1981.
22. PT Fox, JS Perlmutter, ME Raichle. A stereotactic method of anatomical localization for positron emission tomography. J Comput Assist Tomogr 9(2):141–153, 1985.

23. AC Evans, C Beil, S Marrett, CJ Thompson, A Hakim, Anatomical-functional correlation using an adjustable MRI-based region of interest atlas with positron emission tomography. J Cereb Blood Flow Metab 8:513–530, 1988.
24. PG Spetsieris, V Dhawan, S Takikawa, D Margoulef, D Eidelberg. Imaging cerebral function. IEEE Comput Graph Appl 13(1):15–26, 1993.
25. GQ Maguire Jr, ME Noz, EM Lee, JH Schimpf. Correlation methods for tomographic images using two and three dimensional techniques. In: SL Bacharach, ed. Information Processing in Medical Imaging. Dordrecht, The Netherlands: Martinus Nijhoff Publishers, 1986, pp 266–279.
26. C Bohm, T Greitz, D Kingsley, BM Berggren, L Olsson. Adjustable computerized stereotaxic brain atlas for transmission and emission tomography. Am J Neuroradiol 4(3):731–733, 1983.
27. T Greitz, C Bohm, S Holte, L Eriksson. A computerized brain atlas: Construction, anatomical content and some applications. J Comput Assist Tomogr 15(1):26–38, 1991.
28. S Marrett, AC Evans, L Collins, TM Peters. A volume of interest (VOI) atlas for the analysis of neurophysical image data. Proc SPIE, 1092:467–477, 1989.
29. R Bajcsy, R Lieberson, M Reivich. A computerized system for the elastic matching of deformed radiographic images to idealized atlas images. J Comput Assist Tomogr 7:618–625, 1983.
30. R Dann, J Hoford, S Kovacic, M Reivich, R Bajcsy. Evaluation of elastic matching system for anatomic (CT, MR) and functional (PET) cerebral images. J Comput Assist Tomogr 13:603–611, 1989.
31. R Bajcsy, C Broit. Matching of deformed images. IEEE Proc Sixth International Conference on Pattern Recognition. October, 1982, pp 351–353.
32. DR Masys. Visible human project. National Library of Medicine.
33. U Pietrzyk, K Herholz, WD Heiss. Three-dimensional alignment of functional and morphological tomograms. J Comput Assist Tomogr 14(1):51–59, 1990.
34. JCH Wong, C Studholme, DJ Hawkes, MN Maisey. Evaluation of the limits of visual detection of image misregistration in a brain fluorine-18 fluorodeoxyglucose PET-MRI study. Eur J Nucl Med 24:642–650, 1997.
35. EJ Farrell, RJT Gorniak, EL Kramer, ME Noz, GQ Maguire Jr, DP Reddy. Graphical fusion of multiple 3D image sets in radiology. J Med Syst 21(3):155–172, 1997.
36. BJ Erickson, CR Jack. Correlation of single photon emission CT with MR image data using fiduciary markers. Am J Neuroradiol 14:713–720, 1993.
37. J West, JM Fitzpatrick, MY Wang, BM Dawant, CR Maurer Jr, RM Kessler, RJ Maciumas, C Barillot, D Lemoine, A Collignon, F Maes, P Suetens, D Vandermeulen, PA van den Elsen, S Napel, TS Sumanaweera, B Harkness, PF Hemler, DLG Hill, DJ Hawkes, C Studholme, JBA Maintz, MA Viergever, G Malandain, X Pennac, ME Noz, GQ Maguire Jr, M Pollack, CA Pelizzari, RA Robb, D Hanson, RP Woods. Comparison and evaluation of retrospective intermodality brain image registration techniques. J Comput Assist Tomogr 21(4):554–566, 1997.
38. RJT Gorniak, EJ Farrell, EL Kramer, GQ Maguire Jr, ME Noz, DP Reddy. Accuracy of an interactive registration technique applied to thallium-201 SPECT and MR brain images. Med Physics 24(8):1354, 1997.

39. R Gorniak, EL Kramer, ME Noz, EJ Farrell, A Litt, M Gruber. Interactive 3-dimensional registration of MR and 201 thallium SPECT brain images. In RL Arenson, RM Friedenberg, eds. SCAR 96, Computer Applications to Assist Radiology. Symposium Foundation, Carlsbad, CA. Denver, Colorado, June 6–8 1996, pp 422–429.
40. DP Reddy, GQ Maguire Jr, ME Noz, R Kenny. Automating image format conversion—twelve years and twenty-five formats later. In: HU Lemke, K Inamura, CC Jaffee, R Felix, eds, Computer Assisted Radiology—CAR'93. Berlin, West Germany: Springer-Verlag, 1993, pp 253–258.
41. ME Noz, GQ Maguire Jr. QSH: A minimal but highly portable image display and handling toolkit. Comput Meth Prog Biomed 27(11):229–240, 1988.
42. GQ Maguire Jr, ME Noz. Image formats: Five years after the AAPM standard format for digital image interchange. Med Physics 16(5):818–823, 1989.
43. LG Brown, GQ Maguire, ME Noz. Landmark-based 3D fusion of SPECT and CT images. Proceedings of the SPIE Sensor Fusion VI Conference. SPIE—The International Society for Optical Engineering, Boston, 2059:166–174, September 1993.
44. SJ Nelson, MR Day, PJ Buffone, L Wald, et al. Alignment of volume MR images and high resolution [^{18}F] fluorodeoxyglucose PET images for the evaluation of patients with brain tumors. J Comput Assist Tomogr 21(2):183–191, 1997.
45. U Pietrzyk, K Herholz, A Schuster, HM Stockhausen, H Lucht, WD Heiss. Clinical applications of registration and fusion of multimodality brain images from PET, SPECT, CT, and MR. Eur J Radiol 21:174–182, 1996.
46. R Rubinstein, H Karger, U Pietrzyk, T Siegal, JM Gomori, R Chisin. Use of ^{201}thallium brain SPECT, image registration, and semi-quantitative analysis in the follow-up of brain tumors. Eur J Radiol 21:188–195, 1996.
47. B Pirotte, S Goldan, LM Bidaut, A Luxen, et al. Use of positron emission tomography (PET) in stereotactic conditions for brain biopsy. Acta Neurochir 134:79–82, 1995.
48. M Levivier, S Goldman, B Pirotte, JM Brucher, et al. Diagnostic yield of stereotactic brain biopsy guided by positron emission tomography with [^{18}F]fluorodeoxyglucose. J Neurosurg 82:445–452, 1995.
49. Schwartz RB, Carvalho PA, Alexander E III, et al. Radiation necrosis vs high-grade recurrent glioma: differentiation by using dual-isotope SPECT with 201Tl and 99mTc-HMPAO. Am J Neuroradiol 12(6):1187–1192, 1991.
50. Black KL, Hawkins RA, Kim KT, et al. Thallium-201 (SPECT): a quantitative technique to distinguish low grade from malignant brain tumors. J Neurosurg 71:342–346, 1989.
51. N Oriuchi, M Tamura, T Shibazaki, C Ohye, et al. Clinical evaluation of thallium-201 SPECT in supratentorial gliomas: relationship to histologic grade, prognosis and proliferative activities. J Nucl Med 34:2085–2089, 1993.
52. T Nariai, M Senda, K Ishii, T Maehara, et al. Three-dimensional imaging of cortical structure, function and glioma for tumor resection. J Nucl Med 38:1563–1568, 1997.
53. E Alexander, JS Loeffler, RB Schwartz, et al. Thallium-201 technetium-99m HM-PAO single-photon computed tomography (SPECT) imaging for guiding stereotactic craniotomies in heavily irradiated malignant glioma patients. Acta Neurochir 122:215–217, 1993.

54. FS Pardo, HJ Aronen, D Kennedy, G Moulton, et al. Functional cerebral imaging in the evaluation and radiotherapeutic treatment planning of patients with malignant glioma. Int J Radiat Oncol Biol Phys 30:663–669, 1994.
55. G Sgouros, S Chiu, KS Pentlow, LJ Brewster, et al. Three-dimensional dosimeyrt for radioimmunotherapy treatment planning. J Nucl Med 34:1595–1601, 1993.

14
Image Registration in the Thorax, Abdomen, and Pelvis

Candice L. Aitken
Harvard Medical School, Boston, Massachusetts

Marilyn E. Noz and Elissa L. Kramer
New York University School of Medicine, New York, New York

I. INTRODUCTION

With advances in nuclear medicine, imaging techniques using radiolabeled substances, such as single photon emission computed tomography (SPECT) and position emission tomography (PET), have added significantly to the diagnosis and evaluation of tumors. In particular, the use of radiolabeled antitumor antibodies or tumor receptor ligands to detect abnormal concentrations of tumor-associated antigens or receptors in tumors and metastases has increased. Imaging modalities that give structural details, such as computed tomography (CT) or magnetic resonance imaging (MRI), do not provide the functional or tissue-specific information provided by SPECT or PET scans. For the most part, CT and MRI will show only deformation or displacement of normal structures or space-occupying lesions within normal structures, albeit with extraordinary detail.

PET relies on radioisotopes like fluorine Fluorine-18, Nitrogen-13, and Oxygen-15, that are incorporated readily into metabolic substrates like fluorodeoxyglucose (FDG) and naturally occurring molecules like water or amino acids. It provides tomographic images of the distribution of these molecules as they are incorporated into metabolic processes. PET tumor imaging is based on alterations in metabolism in the pathological states being studied. SPECT uses more conventionally available radioisotopes, like I-123 and I-131 or radiometals like technetium Tc-99m sulfur colloid and In-111 attached to pharmaceuticals, peptides, or proteins to identify unusual tissue characteristics. Both modalities can provide data in a tomographic format through any plane depending on the angle of reconstruction. This tomographic presentation of emission data provides enhanced contrast and improved localization. Tomographic emission images are more easily compared with other transectional data like CT or MRI. With radiolabeled antibodies for radioimmunodetection, as with most tumor-seeking radiopharmaceuticals, the use of SPECT has increased the sensitivity for the detection of abnormal concentrations of tumor-associated episopes or receptors both in the abdomen and chest (1–5). When combined with structural imaging, radiolabeled tracer images can delineate the nature of a residual mass in a treated patient by identifying tissue characteristics associated with pathology (e.g., tumor). They can also identify abnormal tissue within structures that shows no evidence of enlargement, destruction, or deformation on CT or MRI.

The problems associated with SPECT images are severalfold. SPECT images provide very little anatomical detail; determining the transaxial level of a particular SPECT slice is often difficult. Similarly, the normal landmarks needed in evaluating SPECT images may not be easily identifiable. It may be difficult to identify the anatomical structure in which there is an abnormal localization of radiotracer, especially if that structure is enlarged or of abnormal configuration. This makes the use of PET and SPECT for the staging of tumors and surgical planning more difficult. The persistence of blood pool activity can obscure a finding. In areas with high blood pool activity, areas of abnormality may be masked by the persistence of blood pool activity. There may also be nonspecific localization of the radiopharmaceutical in normal tissue that cannot be differentiated from or might mask specific tumor uptake. Organs normally involved in the excretion or clearance of a radiopharmaceutical (i.e., liver, kidney or bowel) may accumulate radioactivity. Nonspecific liver uptake may then obscure intrahepatic tumor activity; similarly, nonspecific bowel uptake that is focal may be difficult to differentiate from specific tumor uptake. Without anatomical landmarks, it may be difficult to know whether uptake is specific or nonspecific (6).

CT and MRI, on the other hand, provide exquisite anatomical detail. Abnormal structures (e.g., masses) can be located relative to anatomical landmarks. The determination of transaxial level is facilitated by the richness of detail. Both abnormal masses and enlarged lymph nodes can be identified. In some cases, millimeter sized masses or abnormalities are detectable.

The difficulties presented with CT are in characterizing the abnormality. Abnormal masses cannot be characterized precisely in terms of cause; in a treated patient they can represent recurrence or fibrosis at the site of a previously known tumor or abscess (6,7). Alteration or distortion of normal anatomy by surgery or prior disease can make the identification of an abnormality precarious. Certain structures are variable in their appearance or positioning (8). For instance, loops of small bowel may be confused with soft tissue masses even when oral contrast is used. Lymph nodes cannot be considered abnormal until they measure more than 1 cm. This may lead to a false-negative diagnosis on CT. False-positive results occur when a hyperplastic lymph node is present. The CT cannot differentiate between an inflamed or hyperplastic lymph node and metastatic disease. In the mediastinal staging of lung cancer, this can be a common problem.

The structural detail provided by CT, when combined with the functional information provided by SPECT or PET, can be complementary (1,3,5,9–11). Image registration or fusion can add spatial accuracy to the combination of structural and functional imaging (6,12). The fusion of functional information with structural images can help identify the location of a focus of uptake. This may help distinguish normal from abnormal biodistribution of radiopharmaceuticals. Similarly, it may help to identify a structure as either a normal variant, scar, or residual disease. These fused images can help precisely identify structures that contain increased uptake of the radiopharmaceutical and help identify the metabolically active portion of a structure. They also localize otherwise occult sites of disease. The precise margins on CT or MRI may be used to identify boundaries for measurements of activity on PET and SPECT (i.e., for generating regions of interest for further analysis). Image registration has applications in cancer diagnosis and staging, surgical planning, and radiation treatment planning.

II. TECHNICAL CONSIDERATIONS

Image fusion in the trunk presents technical difficulties not encountered in registration of images of the head or brain (7,13). The size of organs can change (e.g., bowel can distend and deflate) or be constantly in motion (e.g., respiratory motion). Also, organs can change in position relative to each other simply because of the degrees of freedom of motion possible in the trunk. Pelvic rotation is the most extreme example of this, but changes in curvature of the spine that occur with differences in positioning may be equally problematic. When images for fusion are acquired prospectively, differences in positioning may be reduced. Because of the malleability of the trunk, the ability to stretch, warp, or deform images is critical to fusion of body images.

A. General Considerations in Image Registration

Almost all fusion algorithms require the identification of corresponding points or surfaces in the two image sets to be fused. When both images display a normal structure, corresponding identifiable points or surfaces on this entity may be identified. Otherwise, external fiducial systems may be used. However, the decision to use fiducials must be made before acquiring the study. Fiducial markers both increase the number of landmarks identified and are more easily identified. Although we prefer to use fiducial markers, many methods of registration are successful using internal landmarks alone.

Once the images are acquired, some attention needs to be paid to file formats. Hardware and software must be capable of displaying the file formats involved. For digital fusion and manipulation of three-dimensional (3D) tomographic data, slices from each different image modality must be transferred to a single computer system and converted to a common format. The transfer may be accomplished by any standard method such as file transfer protocol (FTP) over a network or by reading magnetic tapes, floppy disks, etc. Interformat (14), a commercially available image conversion program may be used to convert a specific input file format into any number of specific output formats. For the algorithm used in this laboratory, the images are converted into *qsh* (15), which is the standard AAPM format, subsequently known as the Interfile format (16). The image file format associated with *qsh* provides two files: a header file as text in the form of sets of standard key-value pairs comprising the nonpixel data and a second separate file composed of the N-dimensional array of numeric values (image data) that comprise the actual pixel values. The header information (the key-value pairs) is stored as ASCII character strings. Thus, the header files can be easily interpreted by any software package using a simple script, such as one written in AWK or PERL. These header files can be used as a database to store a history of the image processing or by other processes to read values from the header file, answer requests for values, add new key-value pairs, and update image header files. This provides facilities similar to environment variables with the added capability of updating these values and sharing them between separate processes.

To date, several algorithms have been used to fuse SPECT or PET with CT or MRI. In general, these algorithms may be categorized as "two-dimensional (2D)" or "three-dimensional." A 2D algorithm generally deals with two dimensions or one image slice at a time. The operator must identify the correct slice pair from each image set and then perform in-plane matching. In contrast, with 3D images, volume images are created from each image set and these volumes are registered. In middle ground the operator has the ability to reslice 3D data sets to permit matching of the slice level and angles of reconstruction and then perform in-plane alignment.

There is vast literature describing attempts to perform image registration, both automatically and semiautomatically, for the head. Several good review articles (17–19), give insight into the problems and to many proposed solutions. Common to most attempts at image registration are the difficulties encountered in attempting image registration in areas of the body other than the head (e.g., the po-

Registration in the Thorax, Abdomen, and Pelvis

tential for changes in organ shape and movement of one structure relative to another) (7,13). There is a great deal of emphasis on submillimeter accuracy that might be necessary for neurosurgery but is not always necessary for cancer diagnosis and treatment. This level of accuracy is not attainable with functional images that have a pixel size great than 1 mm. Most registration methods and algorithms that claim to be fully automatic actually incorporate a mechanism for user interaction (20) or require preprocessing (21). An algorithm used for image fusion should be applicable anywhere in the body, not need fiducial markers, and be applicable retrospectively.

The objective of this section is to present an overview of the methods used fusing SPECT and/or PET with CT and/or MRI scans, particularly as they apply to the thorax, abdomen, and pelvis. The methods used in our laboratory will then be described.

1. Technical Approaches to Image Registration

Two major approaches to image transformation are commonly used. The first is affine transformation involving the operations of translation, rotation, and scale, which preserves the original relationship of all the structures involved. The second uses warping, which performs the preceding three operations, as well as skew.

Approaches to determining transformation coefficients fall into three major categories: (a) analytical with respect to structure; (b) analytical with respect to surfaces; and (c) procedural. Two other approaches, although analytical in nature, introduce data external to the studies. One of these is the use of an anatomical atlas and the other is the use of external markers. It should be noted that these approaches are not mutually exclusive and may be used in conjunction with each other.

a. Fourier Analysis Methods

One of the solutions for the problem of structure identification is to determine translation, rotation, and scaling transformations using Fourier analysis methods. One group has approached the problem by using a 2D global tracking algorithm based on phase correlation Fourier methods (22). Another solution uses a cross-correlation that uses Fourier invariance properties and logarithmic transforms to decouple the variables. Although this eliminates the iterative nature of the algorithm and reduces the computational expense, as with the first method, the images must be preprocessed (23,24).

b. Polynomial-based Warping

Identification (of structure) that involves translation, rotation, scaling, and skew can be implemented with a polynomial-based warping algorithm. These techniques have been applied to correlate serial thallium heart scans (25) and have been used extensively in our laboratory (6,12,26,27). A linear and nonlinear polynomial warp using interactively specified 3D landmarks was proposed for correlating CT, MRI, and PET (28). Promising results were obtained with rigid objects (an artificial fixed geometry scene and a cadaver), but when nonlinear distortion is present, problems with oscillation occur unless enough landmarks are specified in a well-distributed manner over the entire 3D surface.

c. Surface Identification

Surface identification is another method that has been used to register images. There are three major approaches to surface identification: the least squares search technique, eigenvalue decomposition, and moment matching techniques. The first approach (20,29–35) uses a search technique to minimize "mismatch" between the surfaces (i.e., the sum of squares of distances from points on surface A to nearest points on surface B). The second approach finds the principal axes, because these depend only on the shape and represent orthogonal axes about which the moments of inertia are minimum. Implementation of this technique involves the eigenvalue decomposition of scatter matrices (second-order moments) applied to the threshold version of the original images (36) or to the surface data (37,38). In the third approach, surface fitting is accomplished by moment-matching techniques (39). All of the preceding approaches to surface matching work well on structures with bony outlines such as the head but are less successful with structures composed of soft tissues such as in the abdomen. Their application to parts of the body other than the head is limited, because the presence of well-defined contours is necessary. Scott et al. and Kolbert et al. (34,35) have used the approach of outlining particular organs, such as the liver, on all the slices (drawing contours or regions of interest) and then applying the least squares search method.

d. Procedural Approach

The procedural approach to image registration is based on accurate and reproducible positioning of the body part at the time of the study acquisitions. Erdi et al. (40) have used a body cast to immobilize the body and help ensure accurate repositioning. Two different ways of accomplishing this, currently available only in the head, are to use a stereotactic frame and to use an anatomic atlas, (Chapter 13).

e. Landmark Identification

Methods of registration involving landmark selection do not require rigid structures and, therefore, are applicable in all parts of the body. Landmarks are homologous points that appear on both image sets to be registered or fused. The relative position between the landmarks in one image and those corresponding in the second image can be used in the registration algorithm. Landmarks can be defined geometrically to locate corresponding points in the two different objects (i.e., using the relations between lines, planes, and angles) or topologically (i.e., using only the connections between objects to identify them) (13,41). Ideally, one would like to determine the landmarks automatically, but it is typical to identify them manually or to use a combination of these methods in which an operator, after examining the automatically chosen landmarks, is able to adjust them.

Choosing landmarks to match two images has distinct advantages over edge or surface definition. Primarily, fewer points need to be designated. Theoretically, in a plane, only three landmark point pairs need be identified. In practice, eight to twelve point pairs should be chosen. (Fig. 1.) By applying linear regression techniques to the complete set of landmark pairs, the errors inherent in each individual landmark pair are minimized in a least squares sense by averaging over the whole set of landmarks (26). This number of landmark points is still considerably less than the number of points needed for surface-fitting algorithms. This approach permits

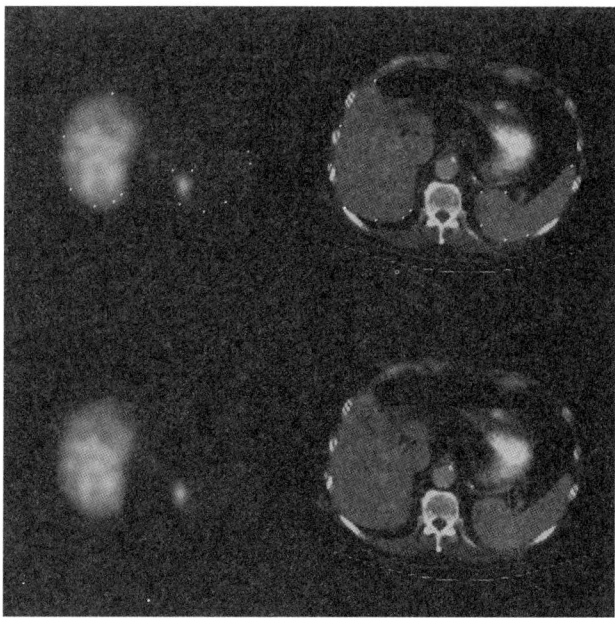

Fig. 1 After matching the transaxial level, corresponding landmarks have been identified by the user using the configuration of the border of the liver and spleen. Eleven pairs of landmarks were identified. It is important to identify these point pairs in as widely displaced a distribution as possible.

local registration and global registration. This means that whole image slices can be matched or objects within the image slice can be matched separately. Landmarks may be selected before or after image acquisition and in all parts of the body so that the method may be applied retrospectively.

Landmarks may relate to intrinsic anatomy depicted in the image but may also be identified with an anatomical atlas or external physical devices. Often a combination of techniques are used (42).

f. Internal Landmarks

The identification of internal landmarks requires the identification of anatomical sites within an image. This is rarely a problem on structural studies. More often, the anatomy depicted on functional images is less complete and will depend on the biodistribution and metabolism of the radiopharmaceutical administered. For instance, in studies using In-111 chelate–conjugated tumor-specific antibodies, blood pool activity, and localization of released In-111 in bone marrow provides anatomical information from skeletal structures and great vessels (6). Body edges often can be identified on SPECT scans from scatter; this has been applied in technetium Tc-99 sulfur colloid–labeled antibody fragment SPECT studies of the thorax in patients with lung cancer (12,43). Edges and contours of normal organs can be used when these organs accumulate the radiopharmaceutical as the liver does in blood pool SPECT studies for liver hemangiomas (27).

A more novel approach to anatomical landmark matching has been reported by Liehn et al. and Perault et al. (44,45), who have injected technetium Tc-99m diphosphonate and simultaneously imaged the In-111–labeled antibody and the bone scanning agent using multiple energy windows. The simultaneous acquisitions provide two image sets, a technetium Tc-99m diphosphonate image set and an In-111 labeled antibody image set, which have the same size and orientation. The bone scan image offers improved definition of skeletal anatomy on SPECT scan for matching with the CT.

External Landmarks. External markers using point (46) or line sources (12,26), sometimes in a "N" configuration (also referred to as "Z" configuration) (40,47–48), have been used to provide additional points for referencing between two image sets. For a discussion of different markers systems see Van den Elsen et al. (18). For SPECT we have used point source markers containing a radionuclide with an emission of lower energy than the radiopharmaceutical being used. For instance, in In-111–labeled antibody imaging, Co-57 sources are imaged in a separate 5% window centered at 122 keV avoiding overlap with a 15% to 20% window centered on the 173 and 247 keV photopeaks of In-111. This provides two separate but completely matched image sets that may be viewed separately or together as one image. These point sources are placed at key and reproducibly identifiable anatomical landmarks to define external landmarks (e.g., the umbilicus for the abdomen and in the thorax at the sternal notch, coracoid processes, and xyphoid process) (12). For MRI, vitamin E capsules or an air-filled tube are commonly used (18,26). For CT, the small metal markers used for radiation treatment planning or an iodinated contrast filled tube may be used. Because selected sites are often readily identifiable on CT or MRI, it is not always necessary to use markers on the CT or MRI. To ensure reproducibility between studies, the point of placement may be marked with ink or dye on the patient.

Strings or belts of skin markers provide an alternative to individual points. Each marker string would consist of alternating sets of markers appropriate to the modalities being used (e.g., for PET, Gallium-68; for SPECT, Co-57; for CT, metallic "BBs"; and for MRI, vitamin E capsules). Optimally, patients would undergo the different imaging studies without removing and replacing the marker belts. This method of external markers has been successfully used for external narrow-beam radiotherapy planning in primary brain tumors (49). It is the method preferred by our group (6,12) and several groups active in the field of image registration or fusion (47,50,51). The use of external markers is flexible and adaptable to all body locations; however, in parts of the body other than the head, where skin may be relatively slack, marker location may not be reproducible in relation to internal anatomy. One approach to overcoming this difficulty has been to use immobilization devices to better approximate patient position from one study to another. Aquaplast, plaster, or alpha cradle immobilization, common techniques used in radiation oncology, could be used. The external markers are then placed on the immobilization device. This has all the inherent weaknesses of procedural approaches to registration caused by difficulty in repositioning the trunk. Another method that uses external landmarks has been to use a 3D space digitizer system. This may be used to acquire data about the patient's outer skin surface and its relation to the scanner. Markers on the patient's surface can be included easily as part of this data set. A number of different devices are available that use magnetic, optical, and ultrasonic methods for acquisition of this 3D information. Each system reacts differently to operation near large metallic objects such as gamma cameras and CT scanners or in the presence of large magnetic fields. The spatial resolution of these systems is constantly improving as new developments improve the technology.

2. Display Requirements

When images that are obtained at different times or from contrasting modalities, such as PET and CT, are to be viewed side by side, it is useful to have the ability to give each image its own background and saturation values, as well as color scale. This is important for comparative studies to allow optimal interpretation of images and identification of features within the image. Frame buffers based on the

X11 windowing system and/or the Motif graphical user interface provide this facility.

3. Matching Geometry

Once the images are available, the differences in the geometry of the two images must be accounted for. The differences in the center-to-center interslice distance of the two different image sets must be considered. One approach has been to try during acquisition or reconstruction to match slice thickness of the various image sets as closely as possible. We have taken two simple approaches to this problem. The first is to tailor the CT or MRI slice acquisition so that the thickness matches the SPECT slice thickness or a multiple thereof. The other is to choose two slices that represent the same distance from a fiduciary marker or anatomical landmark. Slices must also be matched for size within the plane of reconstruction. The dimensions of the pixel matrices of the two images must be the same. Typically SPECT images are acquired in a 64×64 or 128×128 matrix, and CT and MRI images are acquired generally in a 256×256 or 512×512 matrix. In practice, we have interpolated all our images to a matrix size of 128×128 for subsequent matching. The difference in the size represented by a pixel in one image compared with the other is compensated for through the "warping" algorithm (described later), which allows translation, rotation, scale, and skew. Once the matrix dimensions match and the transaxial level corresponds, corresponding landmarks must be identified on each image. This can be done using several different methods.

B. Examples of Methods

Three broad categories of image registration approaches are: 2D combined with 3D, rigid body 3D, and 3D with warping. In the first approach, only two dimensions (i.e., one plane) are manipulated at one time. The entire volume of the acquisition is available for manipulation, and any plane may be adjusted. In the second approach, rigid body 3D, a three-step procedure involving feature extraction, registration, and fusion with quantification is performed to graphically fuse SPECT with CT or MRI scans. The third approach is an attempt to combine the landmark/warping method used in the 2D/3D combined method with 3D display.

1. Combined 2D–3D Method

To render the images coplanar, an oblique reconstruction (52) or tilt algorithm is used to obtain an oblique slice from the CT and/or MRI image set that most closely aligns with the PET or SPECT image (53). (Fig. 2) A transaxial slice is displayed, and the levels for sagittal and coronal reconstruction, which form the (x,y) coordinate of the pivot point, are chosen on this slice. The sagittal and coronal

Registration in the Thorax, Abdomen, and Pelvis

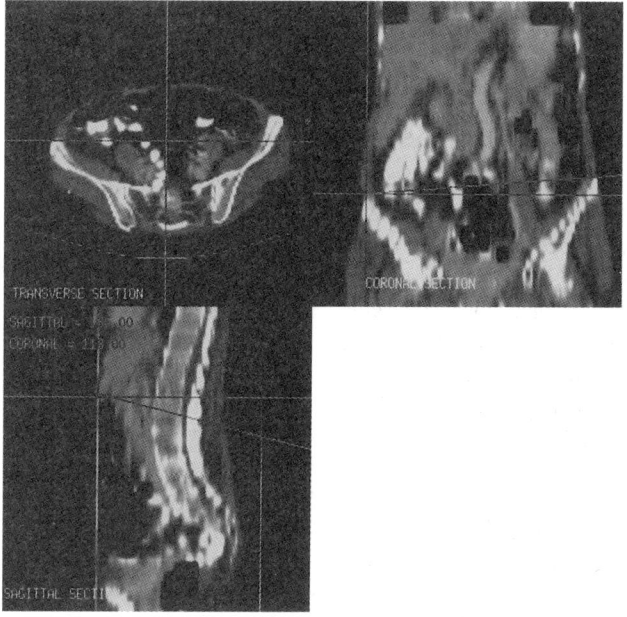

Fig. 2 Particularly when the area of interest is in the pelvis or lower abdomen, differences in the angle of the plane of reconstruction between the CT and SPECT scan may occur. This demonstrates a display for reorienting the plane of reconstruction of the CT scan. On the transaxial view (top, left), a sagittal and coronal plane are chosen using line cursors. The chosen coronal section is displayed (top, right), and the correct angle for the transaxial plane of reconstruction is chosen. Usually the angle that is perpendicular to the patient's vertical midline axis is chosen. Similarly, the sagittal plane is displayed and a plane of reconstruction that mimics the SPECT is chosen. The entire volume of data is then reoriented along these new planes.

views are then reconstructed and displayed. A cursor on the coronal view (along with its coordinates) is displayed and moved through the coronal view for the purpose of obtaining the z coordinate of the pivot point. A line on the coronal view at this z level is rotated until the desired tilt is obtained in the x-z plane. Then a line on the sagittal view at the correct z height is rotated until the tilt in the y-z plane is selected. The values of the pivot point and angles are stored in the image header file. The oblique reconstruction is then performed. Most commercial SPECT processing software packages provide some oblique angle reconstruction capabilities, but only a few provide the ability to tilt in all three planes. Most do not permit reorientation within the coronal plane, so it is important to provide this capability within the fusion software. It may be preferable to perform this oblique angle reconstruction while displaying both image sets.

Landmarks are chosen on the reference image and on the image to be registered. Each landmark from the reference image is cross-correlated with the corresponding landmark from the other image. A frame buffer used as a raster display is used for viewing images simultaneously, thus aiding the comparison of the relative positions of features on each image and the measurement of their respective coordinates. Usually between 10 and 20 pairs of landmarks are chosen (54). These point pairs (or landmarks) may correspond to external markers placed on identifiable and reproducible external anatomical landmarks. Depending on the distribution of radiopharmaceutical, other anatomical landmarks depicted in both images may be used to match corresponding points. For instance, in the In-111–labeled monoclonal antibody studies where some activity accumulated in the skeleton, we found that we could use skeletal landmarks such as the sacral promontory or the posterior aspect of the sacroiliac joint on both the SPECT image and on the CT of the pelvis. Yet another type of landmark that we have found useful is edge or surface matching. Very often on the SPECT study, either the scatter will help depict the body edge or one can use the edge of the functioning organ as the functional image landmark. In matching SPECT of the thorax after administration of Tc-99m–labeled antibody, the edge of the scatter on the image which corresponds to body surface is matched with the body surface on CT. Similarly, the configuration (edge) of the liver on the SPECT study of an In-111–labeled antibody scan could be matched with the liver edge on the CT scan. The shape of the respective edges provides landmarks that can be matched. At the end of this procedure, sets of coordinate pairs (x,y; u,v) that relate the respective locations of the anatomical landmarks in the two images are produced, (Fig. 3A, B).

Once corresponding points, edges, or surfaces are identified, an algorithm is applied that describes the relationship between the corresponding sites. Our approach to this has been to use a polynomial warping algorithm (55). A linear regression analysis is performed on the landmarks, followed by a Gauss Jordan

Fig. 3 A CT scan (A, top right) in this man with a history of colon cancer and an elevated serum carcinoembryonic antigen (CEA) level. He underwent a SPECT study 72 hours after infusion of 5 mCi In-111–labeled CEA-specific monoclonal antibody (ZCE025, Hybritech, Inc., San Diego, CA). The CT scan showed a solitary abnormality in the spleen, which is marked here with the region of interest. This region of interest was warped from its original size and location onto the SPECT (A, top left) using the image registration parameters generated from the algorithm. The warped region of interest is seen to overlay the "hot spot" on the SPECT (A, bottom left). This SPECT study showed a second focus of uptake in the left upper quadrant of the abdomen. After warping, a region of interest generated over the second focus (B, left) showed that this unexpected focus of uptake overlaid an unremarkable area in the spleen on CT (B, right). Some months later, a follow-up CT showed a splenic lesion in that location. A region of interest generated over the liver on the CT is warped and overlaid on the SPECT as a quality control.

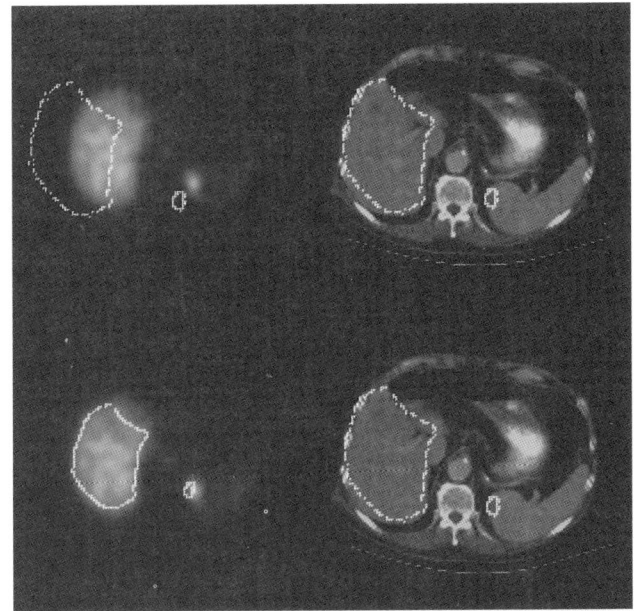

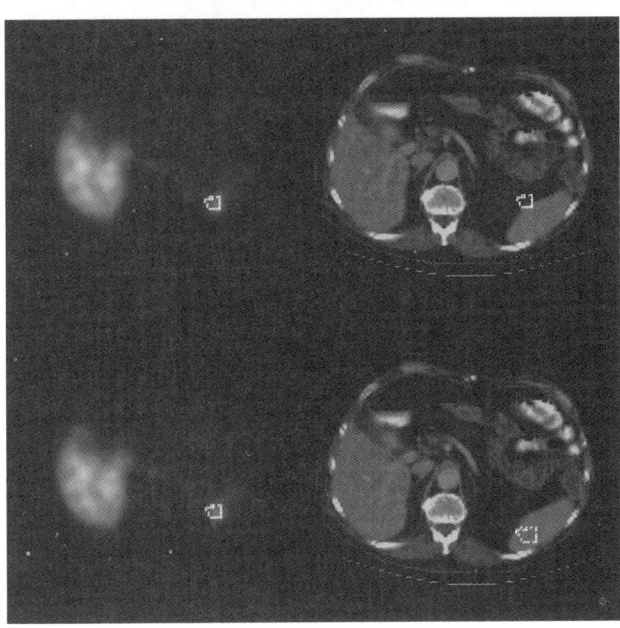

matrix inversion to find the eigenvalues of the matrix that form the transformation coefficients (56). Either first- or second-order polynomials are used, depending on the severity of the transformation. These eigenvalues are then used together with a resampling technique to determine the new coordinates for each pixel in the image to be moved. The alteration achieved by the application of the algorithm may be performed on either the images themselves or on a region of interest (ROI) that describes an outline of a structure on the CT or MRI or on a concentration of radioactivity on the SPECT.

a. Validation Studies

To determine the relative accuracy of our registration methods, studies have been performed using a Jaszczak phantom filled with 925 MBq (25 mCi) of Tc-99m pertechnetate with a ring of 5.55 kBq (150 µCi) I-123 pills fixed to the phantom at the level of the spheres in the phantom. A dual-energy window acquisition was used with one energy window centered about the 159 keV peak of I-123 and the other centered about the 140 keV peak of technetium Tc 99m. Two projection data sets were generated, one that demonstrates the activity in the markers (I-123) and one that demonstrates the activity in the phantom (Tc-99m). A CT scan of the phantom filled with iodinated radiographic contrast and an MRI scan with the phantom filled with water and with a ring of vitamin E capsules fixed to the phantom in place of the I-123 capsules were also acquired. Registration of the SPECT with the CT, as checked by placing a cursor on the corresponding pixels, was achieved within one SPECT pixel, or ±3.2 mm. The five width or half maximum (FWHM) of the SPECT scanner used was 1.2 cm in all three planes (26). This may limit the accuracy of the match compared with what could be achieved in registering CT with MRI.

In a project to assess the sensitivity, specificity, and accuracy of Tc-99m–labeled red blood cell SPECT imaging versus MRI in the diagnosis of hepatic cavernous hemangiomas, functional information as seen by SPECT was correlated with anatomical information derived from MRI or CT (27). Thirty lesions were fused using SPECT-MRI and 20 using SPECT-CT. To assess the accuracy of the fusions, two statistical models were developed. One examined the center-to-center match of two ROI over each of the registered images. The other examined the percent overlap between the ROI. Fusing was accurate within an average of 1.5 ± 0.8 (SD) pixels. The technique enabled diagnostic confirmation of hemangiomas as small as 1 cm in diameter (Fig. 4). These clinical results are consistent with the phantom data. They also are comparable to the results others have obtained in the abdomen (13).

Qualitatively, registration of SPECT from radiolabeled tumor-specific antibody studies with CT has been performed both in the abdomen and chest (6,12). Unexpected foci of activity on the antibody SPECT have been identified anatom-

Registration in the Thorax, Abdomen, and Pelvis

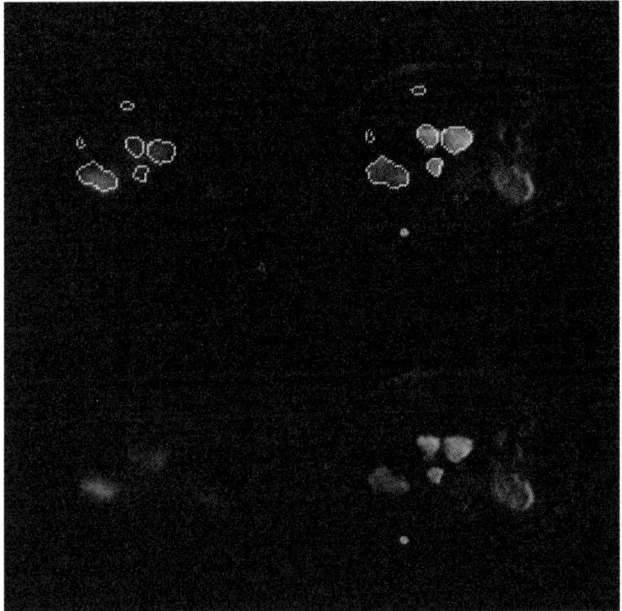

Fig. 4 This patient had multiple abnormalities on CT in the liver. An MRI was performed. This image from a T1 sequence shows multiple high-density lesions throughout the liver. A SPECT study performed in this patient $1\frac{1}{2}$ hours after intravenous administration of 30 mCi of technetium Tc 99–labeled red blood cells demonstrates increased blood pool accumulation in several sites. Regions of interest were generated on the MRI slice and warped onto the SPECT, showing correspondence between the high-intensity foci in MRI and the high-uptake foci on SPECT.

ically by fusion with CT and confirmed at surgery. It is anticipated that this technique may be applied systematically to analyze CT, MRI, and SPECT in tumor staging and identification.

Understanding the errors involved in misregistration is critical in quantitative analysis of functional images. To date, this has been studied in PET, where quantitative data are usually provided. As quantitative SPECT becomes more common, understanding the kinds of errors and their magnitude will be increasingly important. We have looked at the effect of remaining differences in tilt between two image sets after oblique reconstruction. The oblique projection algorithm already described was used to tip the structural image set (in this case, the CT of the brain) from three different very well-matched normal study pairs. Three different angulations, ±4 degrees, ±8 degrees, and ±12 degrees, out of the sagittal plane (an angular difference of 15 degrees or greater would be noticeable on the CT scout film) were used. Regions of interest were drawn on the resulting slices on the left and right caudate and putamen. These ROIs were then overlaid on the corresponding fused PET slices. The nCi/cm3 were calculated for each ROI derived from the untilted slice (zero degrees) and for each of the six angular displacements. The differences in nCi/cm3 between the tilted and the untilted slices ranged from +4% to −16%, suggesting that small mismatches in tilt in the sagittal plane would not invalidate measures of asymmetry (57). As an extra check on the accuracy of our anatomist, we presented her with each of the untilted slices and with the ±12-degrees tilts. The slices were presented in a random order, and each slice was presented more than once. She then outlined the right and left caudate and putamen on each slice. An analysis of variance test was performed on the measurements taken at these three angles. In no case was a statistically significant difference in means found. We can conclude that the ROI outlines drawn at the three different angles are statistically comparable and, therefore, that the results of our original study are not due to the anatomist. The phantom study previously discussed validates the transformation methods.

2. 3D Rigid Body Method (58,59)

The objective of this work is to use a three-step procedure for graphically fusing SPECT with CT and/or MRI scans. The steps are feature extraction, registration, and fusion with quantification. The resulting fused 3D images provide additional insight into the nature and extent of disease and its relation to normal adjacent structures. The tools developed to accomplish our goal have proven to be useful in clinical situations. At each step in the procedure, there are options appropriate for the organ, scan mode, and pathology.

Feature extraction yields 3D boundaries/surfaces of organs, bone, and high/low radioactive emission regions that are then used to register the radionuclide data to structural scans. The registration is accomplished with routine diagnostic scans without reliance on a head frame or fiducial markers and is based on visualizing 3D shapes and 2D images. With registered data sets, 2D and 3D images from SPECT and CT/MRI can be displayed in the same image (i.e., fused). Interactive graphical methods can then be used to measure (a) the relative position, size, and shape of regions of interest and (b) the magnitude and distribution of radioactivity. Quantitative geometric and radioactive emission information are of particular interest.

Although scans using tumor-avid pharmaceuticals are obtained for the purpose of identifying sites of active tumor, information such as tumor size and even exact anatomical tumor location is difficult to obtain from the functional study alone. The visualization tools that we used focus on geometric measurements by allowing anatomical information derived from the structural (CT/MRI) data to be registered with the functional SPECT data. Of particular interest is the ability to integrate into one image information from different MRI sequences, T1-weighted (T1,

Registration in the Thorax, Abdomen, and Pelvis

a scanning sequence that has short time of signal repetition and thus emphasizes certain particular tissue characteristics), T2-weighted (T2, a scanning sequence that has a long echo time and thus emphasizes certain particular tissue characteristics that are different from those emphasized in T1-weighted images), and proton density (PD, a scanning sequence that produces an image in which the brightest signal reflects the highest density of protons). In characterizing tumors, particularly brain tumors, each MRI imaging sequence contributes different information.

For this purpose we have used the IBM Visualization Data Explorer (DX) (IBM Visualization Data Explorer, International Business Machines Corporation, Yorktown Heights, NY) software suite, which provides an object-oriented, graphical programming interface (Figs. 5A, B). The DX data model is discipline-independent (i.e., it can be used for any visualization application including

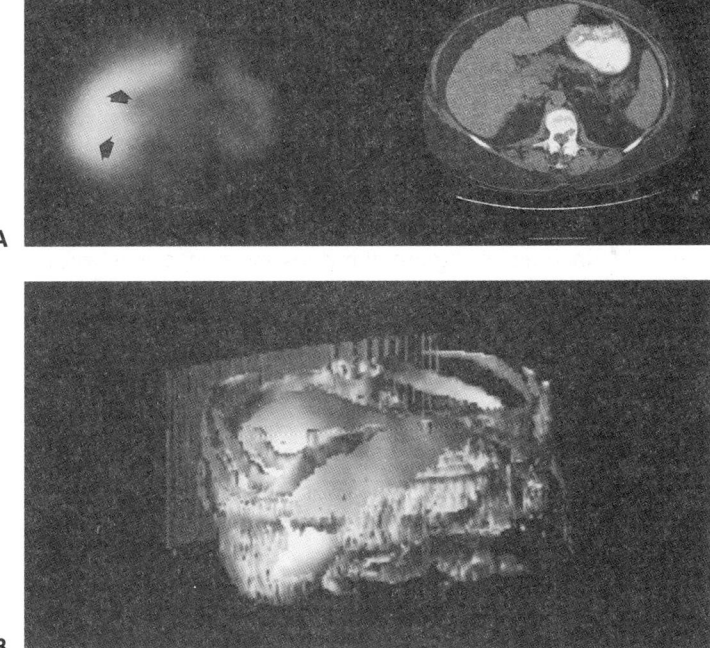

Fig. 5 In this patient with a history of breast carcinoma, a SPECT scan using Indium-111 BrE-3 antibody, specific for a tumor-associated epitope of breast epithelial mucin, shows areas of increased activity in the liver that (A, left, arrows) corresponded to apparently normal areas in the liver on the CT scan (A, right). However, follow-up CT some months later demonstrated metastatic lesions at these sites. The lower image (B) demonstrates the use of DX, a 3D registration program to align the CT with a radiolabeled antibody SPECT study in all directions. For analysis of the abnormalities on the SPECT and CT, 2D displays are used.

medicine), self-describing, and supports regular and irregular grids with node and connection-dependent data. DX uses a data-flow–driven client-server execution model and runs on UNIX workstations from most leading manufacturers. Window content, layout, and access were structured for convenient use and ease of learning. Each image is fully annotated with variable names, display parameters, patient name, and scan date. The latter data are automatically extracted from the image header.

The visualization programs are structured to minimize execution time. Data volume is a key factor. In some cases, images can be interpolated to reduce size without loss of relevant data for quick visualization and determination of parameters. Where appropriate, data can be rescaled to 1 byte to reduce memory requirements. Caching and paging behavior are also important design considerations. DX provides the option to cache results at each process step. When a display parameter is changed, only those steps affected by the change are recomputed, with minimal computation and rapid response. However, excessive caching may result in paging, thus reducing response time. The selection of which nodes are cached and paging behavior was included in the overall program design analysis.

a. Feature Extraction

The features extracted from the 3D data sets are boundaries or surfaces of organs, bone, and high-radiation emission regions. These surfaces are key items used in registering radionuclide functional to structural images and are the anatomical references used in the interpretation of fused data. We have found isosurface rendering to be more useful than volume rendering for feature extraction. For the isosurface rendering, the image consists of solid pixels, all of which have a specified pixel value and transparent pixels having a different specified pixel value.

A surface consisting of only one specified pixel value, an isosurface, can display the 3D distribution of emission activity in SPECT scans by displaying regions of abnormally high or low activity as an opaque 3D isosurface and of normal activity as a transparent surface. For tumor-avid SPECT images, the transparent surface often corresponds to the surface of the involved organ. The opaque surface corresponds to the localized abnormal accumulation of radioactivity within the organ. Contours can be displayed on the opaque and/or transparent isosurfaces to improve shape perception and estimate the size of various regions.

On the basis of MRI, CT, and SPECT 3D data sets, isosurfaces are formed corresponding to skin surface, brain lateral ventricles, tumor, lung surfaces, bone, etc. In some cases extraneous isosurface segments are formed as a result of data artifacts or poor segmentation. The 3D image can be edited to keep only relevant surface segments.

The first step in the extraction of significant features is to select a set of points in the ROI; points may be in more than one image set. Points are selected first in one or two image sets. Based on these points, an average and sample covariance matrices are computed. Then at each point in the 3D data space, scan region, the Mahalanobis distance of the corresponding value is generated. The Mahalanobis distance is based on the sample mean and covariance. It is the euclidean distance from the mean with the inverse of the covariance matrix used as the metric. An isosurface is then formed based on this distance. Note that points are not classified as lesion, cerebrospinal fluid, etc. This method defines an isosurface about statistically similar tissues as defined by the user.

After selecting several key regions of anatomical interest, contours are displayed in 2D image sets. To confirm that each of the point groups is coherent and disjoint, a 3D cluster plot can also be formed with ellipsoids surrounding the clusters that correspond to the thresholds used for each surface. An advantage of this approach is that it compensates for anteroposterior intensity gradients. This is particularly valuable for large structures like the skin surface. Points can be selected around the head, and the Mahalanobis ellipsoid will be elongated radially from the origin of the T1-weighted, T2-weighted, and PD space.

b. Registration

Registration of the data sets is required before fusion and analysis can be performed. The coordinates of the functional data are translated and rotated relative to the structural coordinate frame to ensure that a given 3D coordinate refers to the same anatomical location in both data sets. Two approaches are available for registration: direct 3D registration and iterative 2D/3D registration. The direct 3D approach is based on aligning structural and functional surfaces of the same anatomical region. For example, the structural and functional data of a patient can be registered based on aligning skin surfaces, one opaque and one transparent. It is possible to visualize the 3D surfaces from several viewpoints. This approach relies on the ability to extract an appropriate surface from the functional data and can produce a repeatable registration even with very ill-defined surfaces. In our experience with SPECT images at New York University, however, direct 3D registration is always possible only when external fiducial markers are available on the functional images (41). In cases in which satisfactory surfaces cannot be obtained, an alternate approach is used based on 2D and 3D images.

In the iterative 2D/3D registration, 3D surfaces are used for the initial parameter selection. Most frequently, the coronal views are used to define the anterior, middle, and posterior extent of a significant organ or tissue. During the registration process, the 3D surfaces are continuously updated, thus giving a visual display of the results of each operation of rotation and translation.

The first step is to select a data plane through the 3D SPECT data set based on identifiable features. Interactive 3D rotation is key to positioning this plane. Next, a comparable plane is selected for the structural, in this case CT, data.

Because these images have clear structures, a 3D liver surface is not needed to select the coronal plane. Axial and lateral translations of the 3D functional data set, and the anteroposterior rotation, are then visually selected to align the contours to anatomical features in the structural image. The two axial slices at the same axial location are formed, with the functional scan contours again placed over both images. It must be kept in mind that these data sets have already been preliminarily registered in the axial direction using 3D surfaces. The anteroposterior translation and axial rotation are now selected. Then a sagittal slice is used to select the lateral rotation. Once this rough estimate of the three translation and rotation parameters has been made, the 3D surfaces and 2D slices are used iteratively to fine tune the match. A second pass with the coronal, sagittal, and axial images is performed to make adjustments to the translation values and rotations about all axes.

To confirm the registration, image pairs are compared using overlaid isocontours (2D) of isosurfaces (3D) for different plane locations and directions. The basic concept of the iterative 2D/3D approach is to adjust large registration disparities first, followed by smaller adjustments. This approach is well suited to SPECT/CT data, because even though resolution of the SPECT data is low, the registration converges in one or two passes.

c. Fusion with Quantification

With registered data sets, 3D surfaces from functional data can be fused with surfaces from the structural data sets. Also planes of functional and structural images can be displayed with the 3D isosurfaces. The 2D slice images provide detailed information in a plane, whereas the 3D isosurfaces present the global relationships.

The width, height, and depth of 3D regions can be obtained using the surface contours, along with a clear interpretation of shape. After registration, these surfaces are merged with CT structures. The CT structures often used include the spine, ribs, and descending aorta. Because the CT, which is a routine clinical scan, has slice thickness of 15 mm in the axial direction, the bone surfaces have a very irregular shape. An original CT slice is included in the presentation. In addition to the three standard directions, the user can pick any three surface points to define a plane and display a 2D slice from either data set. This allows the user to obtain detailed spatial information about objects of special interest that may not be aligned along conventional planes.

In DX, an interactive "Pick" module is used to extract pixel values (representing relative radioactivity accumulation) at selected points, to measure distances between points, or to view an emission profile plot along a selected line segment. Also, the volume enclosed by a surface is evaluated with a "Measure" module. This can be the entire isosurface or just a segment like a hot spot near the spine. The ability to calculate volume is particularly important when using a radiolabeled tumor-avid agent to identify a tumor. This volume calculation for a tumor enables one to follow the tumor over the course of therapy for response and is useful for radiation dose calculations in radioimmunotherapy.

d. Validation

This method has been validated both by comparing the results obtained with known results previously obtained and by clinical follow-up on particular patients. We have also studied a group of 33 brain tumor images, nine of which had stereotactic frames, and we compared the results obtained including and not including the frame. The average 3D difference between the standard registration and registration without a stereotactic frame was 5.8 ± 2.9 mm. The average 3D difference was determined by applying the two sets of registration parameters to an 800-pixel sample of each patient's brain volume, then calculating the average distance between the corresponding pixels of each trial (60). This validation has not yet been performed for the body.

3. 3D Warping Method

We are currently collaborating with the Radiation Physics Institute of the Karolinska Institute in Stockholm, Sweden, to produce a registration system that combines our landmark/warping approach with the 3D visualization techniques previously described. We are developing visualization programs in which landmarks will be chosen on one or more axial slices while the 3D image and the sagittal and coronal slices will be displayed for reference. These 3D landmarks will then be used directly in the polynomial warping algorithm described earlier. Essentially, this will eliminate the oblique slice projection and will allow the user to page back and forth through the entire image set.

III. CLINICAL APPLICATIONS OF IMAGE REGISTRATION

A. Applications in the Thorax

The application of image registration or fusion to the chest presents less difficulty than the abdomen, because there are fewer degrees of motion possible. Respiratory motion may introduce discrepancies, because CT is obtained with breath holding at deep inspiration and SPECT with quiet respiration. The position of the arms will also have an influence on the relative expansion of the chest. Nonetheless, differences in rotation can usually be accounted for either by careful positioning or by rotation of images after the acquisition. As in other parts of the body, image fusion in patients with suspected tumors has been used to give anatomical meaning to SPECT or PET images, especially in the mediastinum. When there is other underlying disease and the relative expansion or collapse of a particular part of the lung may distort the usual anatomy, fusion will help in surgical planning.

Image fusion has also been invaluable in differentiating tumor from other disease in the lung.

Image registration has been used in lung perfusion studies to accurately determine the location of perfusion abnormalities. A composite image is formed by the superimposition of the Tc-99m macroaggregated albumin SPECT and chest CT images (61). The precise localization of lung segments allowed by image registration helps to quantify perfusion abnormalities and changes. Perfusion lung images have long been used in conjunction with pulmonary function testing (FEV_1) to predict regional pulmonary function after lobectomy or pneumonectomy. The actual borders of lung segments or lobes seen on the CT may be superimposed on the SPECT depiction of the distribution of pulmonary perfusion. This will provide a better understanding of the clinical impact of resecting a lobe or wedge of lung on pulmonary function.

Image registration of radiolabeled antibody studies with chest CT in lung carcinoma may be used for the staging of non-small cell lung carcinoma (NSCLC) as an integral part of determining the approach to treatment. Thoracic CT scans were registered with Tc-99m–labeled IMMU-4 anti-carcinoembryonic antigen Fab' antibody fragment SPECT scans in 14 patients with NSCLC (43). All of the patients had biopsy proven NSCLC, stages IIb–IV. A landmark-based algorithm was used to fuse the two modalities. External fiducials (Co-57) were placed on prominent superficial anatomical landmarks: the coracoid process, the sternal notch, and the xiphoid process. Accuracy of registration was based on two measurements: center-to-center distance and the overlap of ROIs. The accuracy of the registration was determined to be within 1.3 ± 0.8 pixels. Although the SPECT alone provided information about abnormal accumulation of tumor antigens, registration of the images allowed differentiation of abnormal uptake caused by tumor in the mediastinum from normal blood pool activity in the great vessels and thus added specificity (Fig. 6).

In this series, 40 pairs of structural-functional images were registered. The registered images differentiated areas of tumor and mediastinal lymphadenopathy from blood pool in 7 of 14 patients. Fusion of Tc-99m IMMU-4 SPECT with CT helped distinguish necrotic tumor from viable tumor in three treated patients. In two of three patients who had undergone a prior surgical resection, image fusion of the radiolabeled antibody SPECT with the CT demonstrated that the postoperative changes on the CT at the surgical site represented recurrence. In a third of those three patients, fusion of the two image types confirmed the presence of scar. This illustrates that image registration is especially useful in differentiating recurrence from fibrosis at the postsurgical site. Eight of the 14 patients showed mediastinal or hilar lymphadenopathy on CT. In seven of these eight patients, fusion of the radiolabeled antibody SPECT with CT localized increased activity to the enlarged lymph nodes. In six of these seven positive fusion cases, tumor was confirmed. In the eighth patient, where fusion showed ab-

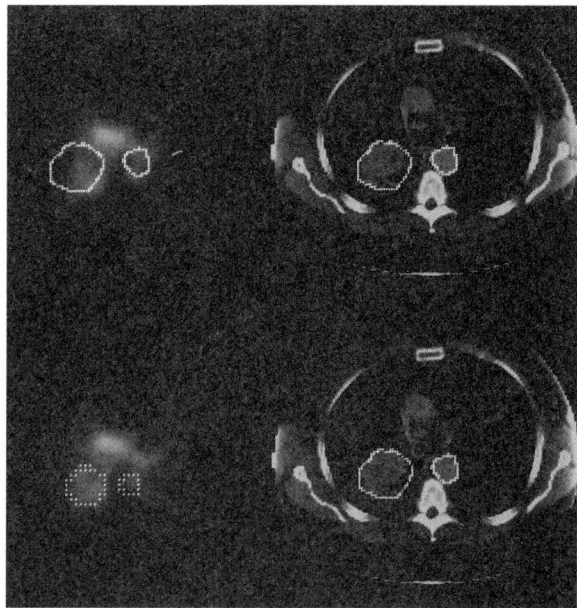

Fig. 6 This patient with an abnormal chest x-ray was believed to have primary lung carcinoma. A chest CT performed as part of his staging workup showed a large irregular mass in the right posterior medial lung field. A technetium T 99m IMMU-4 Fab' CEA-specific monoclonal antibody study (CEAscan, Immunomedics, Morris Plains, NJ) was performed including SPECT of the chest. This showed increased uptake in the right lung but also in the mediastinum. A region of interest drawn over the right lung mass on the CT warps onto the increased uptake on the SPECT study. Similarly, a region of interest generated over the descending aorta warps onto a SPECT focus of uptake corresponding to blood pool, not lymph nodes.

sence of antibody accumulation in the enlarged lymph nodes, a biopsy revealed benign sinus histiocytosis. Therefore, image registration allowed differentiation of lymph nodes enlarged because of metastasis or another process, in this case, benign sinus histiocytosis. This demonstrates that image registration can be useful in the staging of NSCLC.

In another similar study (12) using fusion of technetium Tc 99m NR-LU-10 Fab antibody SPECT with chest CT, characterization of nodules was enhanced, (Fig. 7A, 7B). NR-LU-10 Fab antibody is specific for an adenocarcinoma-associated glycoprotein. As in the previously described study, fusion of these two types of studies was helpful in identifying the viable portion of lung tumors (e.g., within postobstructive pneumonias). It was also helpful in establishing the true negative

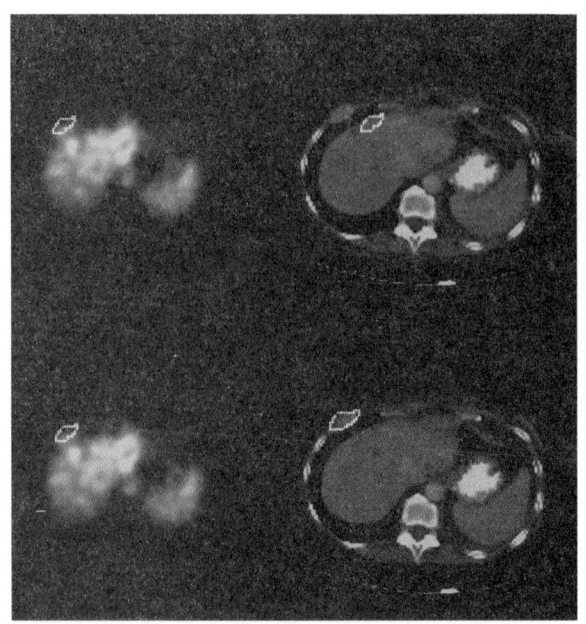
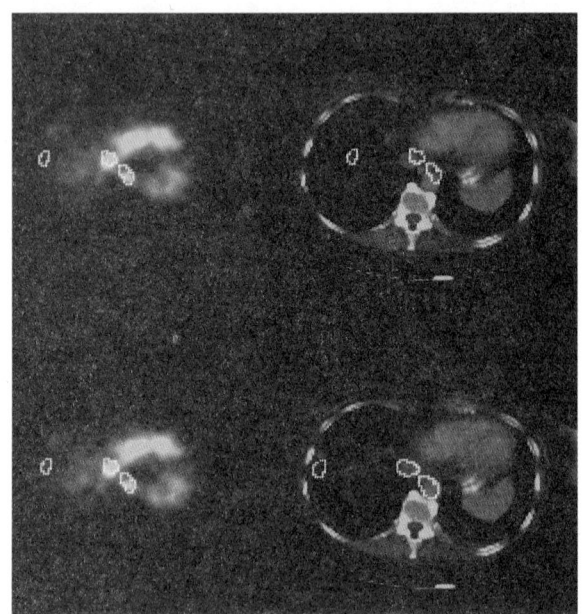

nature of a nodule. Often the background "noise" associated with a SPECT reconstruction of the lungs makes the interpretation of radiolabeled antibody concentration difficult, especially if target/background ratios are low. Although that was not a problem in this series of patients, it has been a problem more often with pulmonary metastases. Also, in small tumors partial volume effects may decrease the tumor to background ratios and make interpretation of SPECT images difficult. Fusion helped confirm that the absence of uptake at the site of a lesion on the CT represented an inflammatory process. In addition, image registration helped localize mediastinal lymphadenopathy to specific sets of lymph nodes.

Recently, Fluorine-18 FDG PET for the evaluation of lung cancer has been officially approved for clinical use. As with monoclonal antibody SPECT, clinical usefulness in the chest may be enhanced by registration with CT. Applying Pelizzari's surface-fitting algorithm to pleural surfaces, Yu et al. (62) have used image registration of CT and PET to evaluate the extent of disease and mediastinal invasion. By use of this technique, the authors found easier characterization of lung lesions as pneumonia, consolidation, or scar vs. tumor. This method used an automated segmentation method based on thresholding of both the CT and PET at 50% of the soft tissue value. The accuracy based on phantom data was within 2 to 3 mm in this study, although some axial displacement between the CT and PET was identified.

A method of image registration using dual isotope SPECT and CT scans has been applied to thyroid and carcinoid tumors involving the thorax by Perault et al. (45). In this retrospective study, 13 patients underwent SPECT scans with Tc-99m hydroxymethylene diphosphonate (bone SPECT scans) and either In-111 pentetreotide, Iodene-131, or I-131 metaiodobenzylguanidine (antibody SPECT scans). The bone scan was registered to the CT using internal landmarks, (e.g., the spine, sternum, xiphoid process) and a Sun-4 computer. The transformations used to align the bone scan SPECT with the CT were then applied to the antibody SPECT image, so that it could be superimposed onto the CT scan once corresponding slices were determined. The algorithm used to register the images was a spatially varying geometric transformation. An operator

---

Fig. 7 (A) This woman with metastatic nonsmall cell lung carcinoma underwent a Tc-99m IMMU-4 Fab' CEA-specific monoclonal antibody study. This SPECT scan showed both liver metastases and a slightly less intense and exophytic focus just at the "anterior surface of the liver." Fusion with CT showed that the region of interest generated over this superficial uptake actually corresponded to an expansile bony metastasis in the rib. (B) In this same patient, a region of interest generated over a small focus above the liver on the SPECT projected over a metastatic lung nodule on CT. Regions of interest over central blood pool–containing structures (inferior vena cava and aorta) warp onto these same structures on the CT. These provide a "check" on the accuracy of the match.

had to choose slices from the antibody SPECT scans that corresponded to slices from the CT. These decisions were based partly on the sternum-to-spine distance and the width of the thoracic cage. In eight of these patients, at 10 sites, abnormal uptake was anatomically localized and histologically confirmed through follow-up. The root mean square (RMS) error between homologous points was used to gauge the accuracy of the registration process. The average error was 7.0 ± 1.6 mm.

Scott et al. (63) have also fused images in patients with metastatic thyroid cancer. They have reported one patient with a hepatic metastasis of a thyroid carcinoma in which image registration provided confirmation. Fusion in this case showed I-131 activity at the site of the lesion in the liver on CT confirming that this represented a functioning thyroid metastasis rather than another malignancy or benign lesion. As with other fusion studies performed by their group, an external fiducial band was fitted around the upper abdomen, surfaces were outlined manually, and Pelizzari's algorithm applied for registration.

B. Applications in the Abdomen and Pelvis

Registration of images in the abdomen has been limited thus far because of the more fluid anatomy and the potential for changes in the configuration of normal anatomical structures. This problem has been overcome in part by the use of several approaches: intrinsic landmarks, (e.g., blood pool in the aorta), surface anatomy of the liver, and external fiducials (e.g., Co-57 markers placed on easily identifiable surface anatomy, such as the xiphoid process, and anterior superior iliac spines). Fusion is helpful in differentiating nonspecific from specific uptake on SPECT or PET in the abdomen. Also, unfilled loops of small bowel may mask subtle pathological anatomical findings on the CT scans. Fusion may reveal abnormal tumor among these small bowel loops.

Registration of SPECT and CT scans or MR images in the abdomen has been used by Birnbaum et al. (27) to confirm the diagnosis of hepatic hemangiomas in 20 patients with 35 known hepatic hemangiomas. This study was designed to test the registration software on a patient population with intrahepatic lesions and assess its accuracy. Hepatic hemangiomas were studied because they represent well-defined regions on SPECT scans. Tc-99m–labeled red blood cells were used for the SPECT scans and iodinated intravenous contrast for the CT scans. Registration was performed off-line using a Sun 3/180 workstation. Intrinsic anatomical structures were used to register the images, which included the splenic tip, liver edge, inferior vena cava, and aorta. Regions of interest were then drawn around normal anatomical structures, such as the liver, spleen, or aorta, to test the accuracy of the landmarks and the registration. The accuracy of registration with this technique was determined to be ±1.3 pixels using a phantom study. Regions of interest were then drawn around the hepatic hemangiomas on the CT scan or the MR image. These ROIs were then "warped" and projected onto the registered SPECT image. The ROI from the SPECT was then analyzed for blood pool activity (see Fig. 4). This procedure also worked in reverse: a ROI could be drawn on an area of the SPECT that represented a high concentration of labeled red blood cells. Quantitative measures were designed to measure the accuracy of image registration: ROI center-to-center distance and ROI overlap. The accuracy of these registrations was 1.5 ± 0.8 pixels.

Thirty-four of 35 suspected hemangiomas were confirmed with image registration. The smallest hemangioma detected was 1 cm, with a range of sizes from 1 cm to 11 cm. Image registration was valuable in differentiating between a hemangioma and a branching blood vessel. The advantages of this method include the side-by-side display of the different modalities and the use of intrinsic anatomical markers for the registration algorithm. A disadvantage is that accuracy depends on accurate landmark identification and placement. There were 50 registered pairs, 20 CT-SPECT and 20 MR-SPECT in 12 patients with 20 hemangiomas and 10 MR-SPECT in 8 patients with 15 hemangiomas. Thirty-four of 35 hemangiomas correlated with hot spots on axial SPECT images. Hemangioma blood pool activity existed in 48 of 50 registered pairs.

In another study of eight subjects with suspected or known colorectal adenocarcinoma, SPECT scans were registered with CT scans of the abdomen (6). SPECT scans were completed using In-111–labeled anti-carcinoembryonic antigen (anti-CEA) monoclonal antibodies. External fiducials were placed for the SPECT scans at the sternal notch, xiphoid process, umbilicus, or the anterior superior iliac spines. Oral contrast was administered before the CT scans. The images were transferred off-line to a Sun 3/180 workstation. External fiducials and internal landmarks (liver, aorta, sacrum, femoral vessels) were used to correlate slices from the CT with slices from the SPECT. The SPECT was translated and rotated using linear regression.

The SPECT scans identified known tumor sites in seven patients with known tumors. Seven additional sites were identified as a result of image registration. One subject had no known tumor but underwent testing because of an elevated CEA level. The image registration showed a single focus that later was identified histologically as adenocarcinoma. CT alone identified six known abdominal tumors and also identified hilar and parenchymal lung disease in the seventh patient. In one patient, CT missed a synchronous neoplasm in the cecum (Fig. 8). However, the CT identified lymphadenopathy in one patient that was not identified on the SPECT. Six areas of increased uptake on the SPECT could not be anatomically localized using side-by-side correlation of the two modalities. With image registration, four of the six were identified as tumors. Fusion helped identify two SPECT foci as false positives; registration of the images identified the uptake as inferior vena cava blood pool activity and irregular liver uptake, respectively. In one patient without known disease, an area of increased uptake

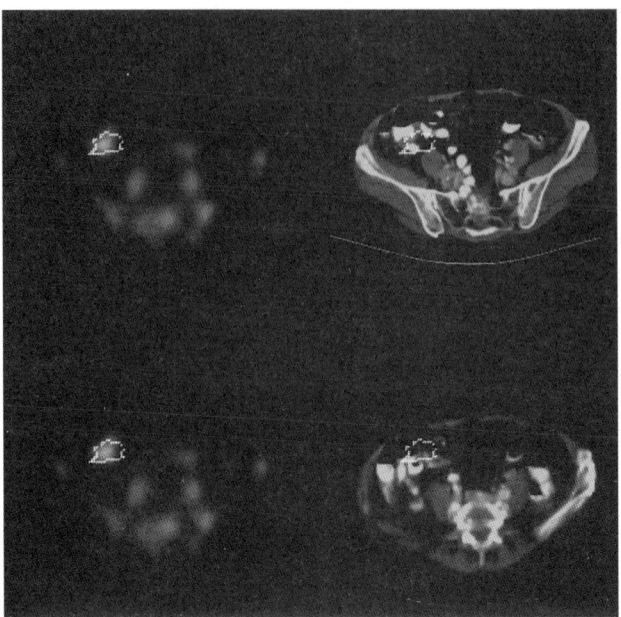

Fig. 8 This woman was seen with complaints of blood-streaked stools. A sigmoidoscopy showed a sigmoid colon lesion (not shown). Radiolabeled CEA-specific antibody studies (ZCE025, Hybritech, Inc., San Diego, CA) demonstrated a second focus of uptake in the right lower quadrant of the abdomen in addition to uptake in the sigmoid lesion. Although the CT was initially interpreted as negative in the right lower quadrant, a region of interest generated over the right lower quadrant "hot spot" and warped onto the CT overlaid an area of thickening of the wall of the cecum. At laparotomy for resection of the sigmoid lesion, a second synchronous primary tumor was discovered in the cecum at this site.

demonstrated tumor that was localized subsequently using the CT. This CT was initially read a negative. In one patient fusion added no additional information.

SPECT and CT images were registered from eight patients with known or suspected colorectal carcinoma (12). The SPECT images were obtained 3 or 4 days after the infusion of In-111-ZCE025, a CEA-specific monoclonal antibody. External Co-57 markers were placed at the umbilicus, the anterior superior iliac spines, and 3 cm inferior to the umbilicus. In the postsurgical patient, definitive determination of whether a mass represents scarring or fibrosis or tumor recurrence may be difficult using the CT alone. In this study, the fusion of the images helped to detect a recurrence at the site of a previous surgery; an abnormal area of increased uptake corresponded exactly to this site. The variable position of the loops of small bowel complicates the interpretation of small soft tissue density structures on CT alone. These loops of bowel may obscure small masses or may be wrongly identified as a mass. In one case, the registration of SPECT and CT images helped to determine that several small metastases were localized in and around the small bowel. A third patient demonstrated increased activity that localized to the liver. In this patient, the CT alone was difficult to read because of previous wedge biopsies and distortion of the normal liver shape (Fig. 9). These hot spots were later confirmed as liver metastasis at biopsy. In another patient, the fusion of the CT with the SPECT helped determine that the increased uptake represented normal blood pool activity in the inferior vena cava rather than a lymph

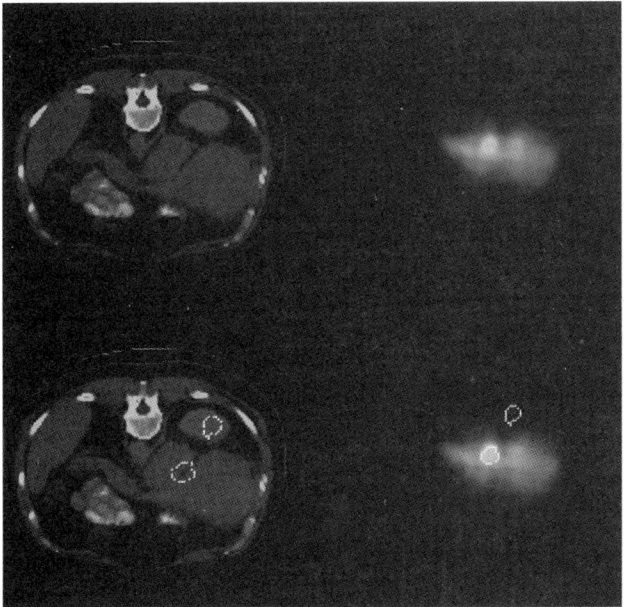

Fig. 9 This patient had undergone multiple hepatic wedge resections for colon carcinoma metastases. Follow-up with both MRI (not shown) and CT (right) showed a markedly distorted liver configuration. On this particular slice, a soft tissue density projected out from the surface of the liver posteriorly (posterior region of interest). Although his serum CEA level was rising, the appearance of the liver had been interpreted as hepatic regeneration. The patient underwent In-111 CEA-specific antibody imaging (ZCE025, Hybritech, Inc., San Diego, CA). The SPECT study (right) showed a focus of increased uptake within the liver. The region of interest generated over this "hot spot" (top left) warped onto an unremarkable area in the liver on the CT. This was confirmed as a metastasis. In contrast, a region of interest placed within the more posterior soft tissue density on CT was warped onto an area without increased activity on the SPECT. This soft tissue density represented an irregular area of regenerating normal liver.

node or the right adrenal gland. In another patient, a second unsuspected focus of uptake could be clearly localized as abnormal (see Fig. 3A, B).

Superimposition of CT or MR scans with F-18 FDG-PET scans have been used to help differentiate pancreatic cancer from mass-forming pancreatitis (MFP) by Kato et al. (64). These two clinical situations can be difficult to differentiate, because they share some gross pathological features, including cyst formation, pancreatic enlargement, ductal dilation, and ascites. This study of 24 patients registered the scans from different modalities in most of the cases by drawing the levels of the CT or MR slices on the patient's abdomen. These lines were used as a guide for the planes of the PET scans. Regions of interest were drawn on the superimposed images along isocontours at 70% to 80% of the peak count of PET. Differential absorption ratios (DAR = tissue tracer concentration/injected dose/body weight) over these ROIs were calculated 50 minutes after infusion. There was a slightly different range of values that helped differentiate between pancreatic carcinoma (mean, 4.64 ± 1.94) and MFP (mean, 2.84 ± 2.22). In the study there were two false positives (tubular adenocarcinoma) and one false negative (mucinous adenocarcinoma).

Image registration involving two subsets of patients receiving I-131 CC49 was completed by Scott et al. (65) for radioimmunotherapy and radioimmunodiagnosis. In the first set, there were 10 patients undergoing radioimmunodiagnosis for suspected recurrence of their colorectal cancer. The second group of 14 patients were involved in a phase I radioimmunotherapy study of I-131 CC49. Registration of I-131 CC49 SPECT with either CT or MR increased the accuracy of the localization of abnormal accumulation of the radiopharmaceutical and improved the staging of the cancer. CT and MR images were first digitized. No external markers were used for the SPECT. Surface contours were drawn around the liver on SPECT slices. The registration algorithm used was the surface-fitting algorithm developed by Pelizzari. With this method, surface-fitting mean accuracy was determined in a phantom study to be 3.6 mm for the liver and 1.8 mm for intrahepatic tumors. In the I-131 CC49 studies, the mean accuracy was 0.92 cm and 0.79 cm for metastatic lesions in the radioimmunotherapy and radioimmunodiagnosis trials, respectively.

Image registration was found to be especially useful in distinguishing normal blood pool activity from nearby sites (e.g., paraaortic lymph nodes, omentum, and bone metastasis). In three of the patients in the phase I trial, the SPECT scans were negative, probably because of an inadequate dose of antibody. Overall, in 11 of 24 cases, the registered images helped localize abnormal accumulations of the radiopharmaceutical. In these cases, the SPECT alone was insufficient to accurately determine the location of the abnormal uptake. In the patients undergoing radioimmunodiagnosis, registration helped localize areas of abnormal uptake on the SPECT. Metastatic disease was found at surgery in six of nine patients that had foci of increased uptake in the liver and two patients with extrahepatic disease. Although all of the lesions greater than 1 cm were detected on the CT scan (13), the registration helped localize smaller lesions that appeared on the SPECT alone. In one patient, image registration localized one lesion to the adrenal gland and a second to the liver. In this patient, the CT scan was negative in the liver until 7 months later, when a lesion on the CT localized to the same location in the liver that was shown in the registered SPECT. In the radioimmunotherapy trial, registered images identified all liver masses >1.5 cm on the CT or MR scan. In this study, the image registration helped differentiate disease near blood pool activity from actual blood pool activity. In 8 of 14 patients, registration helped localize metastatic disease. These cases included patients with numerous liver metastasis, tumor necrosis, and paraaortic or omental disease. One patient had an enlargement of the left adrenal gland that did not correspond to an area of increased uptake on the SPECT. This lesion was later determined to be benign.

In a study of three patients with colorectal cancer, Erdi et al. (40) performed image registration of CT or MR with SPECT scans. The SPECT studies used either Tc-99m–labeled 88BV59 IgG (two patients) or I-131–labeled 16.88 IgM (one patient). This study used a customized body cast to match slice positions of the different image types. This body cast had a "N"- or "Z"-shaped rubber tube attached to it that was filled with Tc-99m pertechnetate for the SPECT scan, contrast dye for the CT scan, and manganese for the MR scans. This cast also served to immobilize the patients. This is a unique approach to image fusion in the body. The images were fused using a new computer graphics program that aligned the external fiducials. Accuracy was assessed by calculating the center-to-center distance between markers on the registered scans; accuracy was 3 to 4 mm and 6 to 8 mm for axial and sagittal registrations, respectively. In the first patient, uptake in the SPECT correlated to the pancreas on CT, which was later discovered to be metastatic disease of the biliary tree. This method eliminates much of the movement that can occur because of the nonrigid anatomy of the abdomen.

Seventeen patients with colorectal carcinoma were evaluated by Welt et al. (66) using CT/SPECT registration in a phase I study of I-131–labeled monoclonal antibody F19, an antibody that binds fibroblast activation protein. Surfaces were drawn on the CT and SPECT images and registered using Pelizzari's algorithm on a DEC Micro VAXII computer. Image registration helped anatomically localize areas of increased uptake on the SPECT. There was one patient in whom this technique was especially useful. This patient had had previous surgery for colorectal cancer and rising serum CEA levels. SPECT showed increased uptake at the site of the previous surgery, whereas the CT scan was difficult to interpret. In addition, the SPECT showed metastasis to both lobes of the liver; the mass in the right lobe was visible on CT, whereas the left lobe of the liver appeared normal on the CT. Both of the liver masses and the mass at the site of previous surgery were later shown to be tumor. Image registration was also useful in determining disease in extrahepatic portal lymph nodes.

Liehn et al. (44) have taking an interesting approach, registering CT with SPECT using the internal anatomy provided by the bony pelvis. Ten patients with suspected cancer recurrence underwent both antibody SPECT scans, using in In-111 antibody and bone scan SPECT using Tc-99m HMDP. Five patients with recurrent ovarian carcinoma underwent antibody SPECT with in In-111–labeled OC125 antigen, whereas the five patients with recurrent colorectal carcinoma were given In-111–labeled monoclonal antibodies to CEA. In-111 antibody SPECT and Tc-99m HMDP bone scan SPECT studies were acquired simultaneously. All of the patients had abnormal CT scans that were interpreted as recurrence, scar fibrosis, or equivocal; however, after the registration, all cases were discovered to be recurrence as confirmed either by surgery, biopsy, or the rapid increase in size of an abnormal mass on CT. The purpose of the bone SPECT was to help in the alignment of the antibody SPECT with the CT. The pelvic bones identified on bone scan served as internal landmarks; they were used to register the bone SPECT with the CT. The same transformation was then used to align the antibody SPECT with the CT scan. The mean accuracy of the registration was determined to be less than 1 cm based on the bone scan SPECT/CT fused images.

"Anatometabolic fusion," registration of F-18 FDG-PET with CT or MRI has been performed by Wahl et al. (67) in 10 patients with visceral carcinomas. These images were digitally fused on a Sun-4 workstation with MIT X-windows using a rigid rotate translate scale. Both external fiducials, containing fluorine F 18 FDG, and internal anatomy, such as the carina and the lung apices, were used in the fusion. The mean error magnitude of fusion was 5.0 ± 0.8 mm across fiducial markers. Nine of 10 patients were successfully registered. In the tenth patient, respiratory motion affected the quality of the PET scan.

Registration of the PET with the MRI demonstrated that the increased uptake corresponded to a focal tumor in a rib rather than a lymph node, as originally suspected. In one patient, an abnormal mass on the MRI corresponded to a cold spot on the PET scan. Months later, the mass was unchanged and was determined to represent scarring caused by aggressive chemotherapy. In another patient, an area of increased activity on the PET scan corresponded to a collapsed central portion of the right lower lobe of the lung. In another case, the hot spots on the PET scan corresponded to normal-sized lymph nodes; months later, these nodes were found to be positive for cancer. Problems encountered in this method include changes in position between imaging studies caused by different patient position or range of respiratory motion, and the fullness of distensible organs such as the bowel or bladder.

C. Applications in Dosimetry

At Memorial Sloan-Kettering Cancer Center, a method of registration of PET or SPECT images with CT/MRI was developed for radioimmunotherapy treatment planning. In one report (68) they describe its application to two patients, one of which had a retroperitoneal tumor mass. The PET images used i I-124–labeled 3F8 antibodies. PET contours of areas of activity were superimposed without interpolation on a CT or MR slice. The CT or MR slice was chosen based on its axial value. The contour from the PET scan was then manually interpolated to fit the area on the CT or MRI slice. This transformation was then performed on the rest of the PET slices. This new area was used to calculate the appropriate dose. This method uses patient-specific anatomy provided by CT to calculate absorbed dose rate or total dose to a defined target region.

The registration of MR images with SPECT images also has applications in dosimetry. It has been used by Pohjonen et al. (69) at Helsinki University Central Hospital to improve the determination of liver and spleen volume and activity in radioimmunotherapy dosimetry. The researchers found that no previously tested SPECT segmentation method provided the accuracy that they needed. This study both tested the registration system on volunteers and evaluated the transfer of outlines drawn on the borders of the spleen and liver from the MR to the SPECT in a radiolabeled platelet study. SPECT images of three male volunteers were obtained at two separate sessions: for the first set of images indium In-111–labeled platelets were used, and 2 days later, the second was acquired after injection of Tc-99m–labeled colloids. External markers consisted of tubes filled with coconut butter for MRI and either In-111 or Tc-99m for SPECT. They were placed on the sacrum, thoracic spine, umbilicus, xiphoid process, and the lateral margin of the twelfth rib. The registration was performed with a Sun-5 workstation and noniterative least squares algorithm. The accuracy of the registration was determined by the RMS error. In the two patients whose MR was a fast scan, the average RMS error was 11 mm and 14 mm for single and dual detector gamma cameras, respectively. The third patient had a slower MRI sequence than the other two patients; his residual error values were 18 mm and 15 mm, for the two cameras. In dosimetry, great accuracy in volume and activity determination is necessary. The authors found that activity measures improved with the registration of the MR with the SPECT image. This provides a prototype for future radioimmunotherapy work.

In a subsequent study, Kolbert et al. (35) describe further implementation of the method described by Sgouros et al. (68). The SPECT/PET images and the CT/MR images are registered by use of the method developed by Pelizzari and Chen and then transferred to a 3D internal dosimetry program (3D-ID) to define ROIs on the fused image. The software uses Interactive Data Language (IDL) and

C and is platform independent. This kind of integration of image fusion for region of interest analysis with dosimetry calculation represents the logical next step in the use of image registration for treatment planning.

In a study by Parsai et al. (70), registration of SPECT and CT scans has been used to provide an anatomical context for the uptake of P-32 colloids in infusional brachytherapy for the treatment of neoplasms. P-32 colloids are directly injected into the tumor using P-32 Bremsstrahlung SPECT and CT guidance. Registration of the CT with a SPECT backscatter image, obtained using external Tc-99m sources, allows the visualization of the anatomical areas in which the P-32 accumulates. The Tc-99m backscatter SPECT is used to obtain the body contour, whereas the P-32 SPECT determines the localization of the colloid. Image registration was performed using a 3D software program (MCO, from the Medical College of Ohio) that aids in the planning of radiation therapy on a DEC Alpha AXP UNIX workstation. A surface-fitting algorithm developed at MCO was used to map the surface contour of the SPECT onto the CT. Once the Tc-99m backscatter SPECT was mapped onto the CT, the same transformation was applied to the Bremsstrahlung SPECT to register it with the CT. The AVS (Advanced Visual System) software was used to determine the accuracy of the registered images. The registration accuracy was determined to be 3 to 4 mm. The patients in this study had pancreatic cancer (one patient), liver metastasis (two patients), and lung cancer (one patient).

Koral et al. (71) propose a method using fusion of CT and SPECT images in dosimetry of lymphoma patients with monoclonal antibody therapy. I-131 SPECT was performed in six patients: three had MB1 monoclonal antibody and three had anti-B1 antibody therapy. External markers composed of glass–fiber paper soaked with I-131 were placed at the intersections of lines drawn on the abdomen and were used for the SPECT, whereas lead markers were used for the CT. These lines represented the slices for the CT scans and the location of the tumor. Superimposition of the markers using a computer program designed to minimize the RMS distance between corresponding markers was achieved. Superimposition of CT on SPECT allows for patient-specific attenuation correction, making SPECT quantitative as well as qualitative. Attenuation coefficient maps were derived by a three-range energy extrapolation based on a two-range technique developed by Nickoloff. In addition, calculation of the mean absorbed dose based on time-activity curves of daily SPECT scans and tumor volume from CT is possible. This method improves the accuracy of dosimetry. In this study of four tumors in three patients with non-Hodgkins lymphoma, the mean absorbed dose correlated well with the prognosis. The tumor-specific absorbed dose with anti B-1 therapy was 1.4 to 1.7 mGy/MBq. This method uses the same pixels for the activity and volume measurement. The mean dose for the entire tumor or organ is determined, and there is less bias toward high-uptake tumors. It is thought that this method should provide a correct estimate of the actual uptake of the radiolabeled antibody.

Problems associated with this method include the fact that the ink marks used in the placement of markers disappear. In addition, nonrigid movements of body are not accommodated in this algorithm.

IV. CONCLUSION

There have been various approaches that have been successful in fusing the functional information provided by SPECT or PET with the rich anatomical details of CT or MRI. This fusion may be accomplished despite the freedom of motion possible in the chest, abdomen, and pelvis and the changeability of the organs within. Liehn et al. (44,45) have used bone scan SPECT to register antibody-SPECT with CT. Erdi et al. (40) have developed a device that helps to restrict patient movement in their registration of SPECT with CT or MRI. Kolbert et al. (35) have made advances in radioimmunotherapy using registration. At New York University, we use a combination of internal landmarks and external fiducials to perform registration. Surface-fitting algorithms, especially when warping is possible, show particular promise.

Image registration enhances diagnosis, confirmation, follow-up, and treatment planning of cancer patients. The functional information provided by SPECT or PET is put into an anatomical context provided by CT or MRI. In addition, image registration helps distinguish between specific (i.e., tumor) and nonspecific (i.e., blood pool) activity in the SPECT or PET. Image registration allows for characterization of soft tissue masses on CT scans and allows recurrent tumor to be differentiated from a surgical scar.

For image registration to be truly useful in a clinical setting, we need to concentrate on data compatability issues, for example, ensuring that registration is possible even if images are acquired at different centers and on different types of machines. The registration methods should be performed without too much advanced preparation, so that images can be fused even if the need for fusion was not recognized before the images were acquired. The image registration should be easy to perform in a clinical setting. It should not be a complicated process that takes hours to complete and is reserved for a select few. The display of the images should be optimized to provide the maximum information. Registration should not obscure detail or information from either data set.

Much progress has been made in manipulating data from multiple modalities and sources. More powerful computing tools enable the processing of even larger data sets. Time requirements are lessening. We look forward to increased automation and the inclusion of greater amounts of information, such as 3D displays and increased numbers of isosurfaces or volumes. Maturation of image fusion tools will most certainly enhance the clinical integration of both functional (SPECT/PET) and structural (CT/MRI) imaging.

REFERENCES

1. EL Kramer, JJ Sanger, C Walsh, H Kanamuller, MW Unger, C Halverson. Contribution of SPECT to imaging of gastrointestinal adenocarcinoma with 111In-labeled anti-CEA monoclonal antibody. Am J Roentgenol 151:697–703, 1988.
2. C Berche, JP Mach, JD Lumbroso, C Langlais, F Aubry, F Buchegger, S Carrel, P Rougher, C Parmentier, M Tubiana. Tomoscintigraphy for detecting gastrointestinal and medullary thyroid cancers: first clinical results using radiolabelled monoclonal antibodies against carcinoembryonic antigen. BMJ 285:1447–1451, 1982.
3. A Bischof-Delaloye, B Delaloye, F Buchegger, W Gilgien, A Studer, S Curchod, JC Givel, F Mosimann, J Pettavel, JP Mach. Clinical value of immunoscintigraphy in colorectal carcinoma patients: a prospective study. J Nucl Med 30:1646–1656, 1989.
4. P Peltier, JP Dutin, JF Chatal, P Fumoleau, P Bourguet, JC Liehn, JP Vuillez, JY Herry, A Loboguerrero. Usefulness of imaging ovarian cancer recurrence with In-111-labeled monoclonal antibody (OC 125) specific for CA 125 antigen. The INSERM Research Network (Nantes, Rennes, Reims, Vuillejuif, Saclay.) Ann Oncol 4:307–11, 1993.
5. AC Perkins, MC Powell, ML Wastie, IV Scott, A Hitchcock, BS Worthington, EM Symonds. A prospective evaluation of OC125 and magnetic resonance imaging in patients with ovarian carcinoma. J Nucl Med 16:311–316, 1990.
6. EL Kramer, ME Noz, JJ Sanger, AJ Megibow, GQ Maguire. CT-SPECT fusion to correlate radiolabeled monoclonal antibody uptake with abdominal CT findings. Radiology 172: 861–865, 1989.
7. RL Kaplan, LC Swayne. Composite SPECT-CT images: technique and potential applications in chest and abdominal imaging. Am J Roentgenol 152:865–866, 1989.
8. LG Strauss. Fluorine-18 deoxyglucose anf flase-positive results: a major problem in the diagnostic of oncological patients. Eur J Nucl Med 23:1409–1415, 1996.
9. JF Chatal, P Fumoleau, JC Saccavini, P Thedrez, C Curtet, A Bianco-Arco, A Chetanneau, P Peltier, M Kremer, Y Guillard. Immunoscintigraphy of recurrences of gynecologic carcinomas. J Nucl Med 28:1807–1819, 1987.
10. EL Kramer, ME Noz, L Liebes, S Murthy, S Tiu, DM Goldenberg. Radioimmunodetection of non-small cell lung cancer using technetium-99m-anticarcinoembryonic antigen IMMU-4 Fab' fragment. Preliminary results. Cancer 73: 890–895, 1994.
11. EM Pitcher, PH Stevens, ER Davies, PR Goddard, PC Jackson. Transfer and combination of digital image data. Br J Radiology 58:701–703, 1985.
12. EL Kramer, ME Noz. CT/SPECT Fusion for Analysis of Radiolabeled Antibodies: Applications in Gastrointestinal and Lung Carcinoma. Int J Radiat Appl Instrum Part B 18:27–42, 1991.
13. CR Meyer, GS Leichtman, JA Burnberg, RL Wahl, RL Quint. Simultaneous Usage of Homologous Points, Lines and Planes for Optimal, 3D, Linear Registration of Multimodality Imaging Data. IEEE Trans Med Imaging 14:1–11, 1995.
14. DP Reddy, ME Noz, GQ Maguire Jr, JJ Sanger, D Garza, S Horiwitz, S. In: HU Lemke, K Inamura, CC Jaffee, MW Vannier, eds. Computer Assisted Radiology—CAR'95. On-demand Conversion of Proprietary Image Formats to DICOM 3.0. Berlin: Springer-Verlag, 1995, pp 1339–1345.

15. ME Noz, GQ Maguire Jr. QSH: A Minimal but Highly Portable Image Display and Handling Toolkit. Computer Methods Programs Biomed 27:229–240, 1988.
16. GQ Maguire Jr, ME Noz, Image Formats: Five Years after the AAPM Standard Format for Digital Image Interchange. Med Phys 16:818–823, 1989.
17. LG Brown. A Survey of Image Registration Techniques. ACM Computing Surveys 24:325–376, 1992.
18. PA Van den Elsen, EJD Pol, MA Viergever, Medical Image Matching—a Review with Classification. IEEE Eng Med Biol 40:26–39, 1993.
19. JBA Maintz. Retrospective registration of tomographic brain images. Doctoral Thesis, University of Utrecht, Utrect, The Netherlands, 1996.
20. CA Pelizarri, GTY Chen, DR Spelbring, RR Weichselbaum, CT Chen. Accurate Three-dimensional Registration of CT, PET and/or MR Images of the Brain. J Comput Assist Tomogr 13:20–26, 1989.
21. RP Woods, JC Mazziotta, SR Cherry. MRI-PET Registration with Automated Algorithm. J Comput Assist Tomogr 17:536–546, 1993.
22. E DeCastro, C Morandi. Registration of Translated and Rotated Images Using Finite Fourier Transformation. IEEE Trans Pattern Anal Mach Intel 9:700–703, 1987.
23. A Apicella, J Nagel, R Duara. Fast Multimodality Image Matching. Phys Med Biol 33S1:391, 1988.
24. A Apicella, JS Kippenhan, JH Nagel. Fast Multimodality Image Matching, Medical Imaging III: Image Processing SPIE 1092:252–263, 1989.
25. M Singh, W Frei, T Shibita, GH Huth, NE Telfer. A Digital Technique for Accurate Change Detection in Nuclear Medicine Images-with Application to Myocardial Perfusion Studies Using Thallium 201. IEEE Trans Nucl Sci 26:565–575, 1979.
26. GQ Maguire Jr, ME Noz, H Rusinek, J Jaeger, EK Kramer, JJ Sanger, G Smith. Graphics Applied to Image Registration. IEEE Comput Graphics Appl 11:20–29, 1991.
27. BA Birnbaum, ME Noz, J Chapnick, JJ Sanger, AJ Megibow, GQ Maguire Jr., JC Weinreb EM Kaminer, EL Kramer. Hepatic Hemangiomas: Diagnosis with Fusion of MR, CT, and Tc-99m-labeled Red Blood Cell SPECT Images. Radiology 181: 469–474, 1991.
28. C Schiers, U Tiede, KH Hohne. In: HU Lemke, ML Rhodes, CC Jaffee, R Felix, eds. Computer Assisted Radiology CAR '89. Interactive 3D Registration of Image Volumes from Different Sources. Berlin: Springer-Verlag, 1989, pp 666–670.
29. RL Siddon. Prism Representation: a 3D Ray-tracing Algorithm for Radiotherapy Application. Phys Med Biol 30:817–824, 1985.
30. GTY Chen, M Kessler, S Pitluck. Structure transfer between sets of Three-Dimensional Medical Imaging Data. Proceedings of the National Computer Graphics Association, Dallas, TX, 171–177, 1985.
31. CA Pelizzari, GTY Chen. In: IAD Brunvis, et al., eds. The Use of Computers in Radiation Therapy. Registration of Multiple Diagnostic Imaging Using Surface Fitting. Amsterdam: Elsevier Science, 1987.
32. CT Chen, CA Pelizzari, GTY Chen, MD Cooper, D Levin. In: CN de Graaf, MA Viergever, eds. Information Processing in Medical Imaging. Image Analysis of PET data with the Aid of CT and MR Images. New York: Plenum Press, 1988, pp 601–611.

33. DN Levin, X Hu, KK Tan, S Galhotra, CA Pelizzari, GTY Chen, RN Beck, CT Chen, MD Cooper, JF Mullan, J Hekmatpanah, JP Spire. The Brain: Integrated Three-Dimensional Display of MR and PET Images. Radiology 172:783–789, 1989.
34. AM Scott, H Macapinlac, JJ Zhang, H Kalaigian, MC Graham, CR Divgi, G Sgouros, SJ Goldsmith, SM Larson. Clinical Applications of Fusion Imaging in Oncology. Int J Radiat Appl Instrum, Part B 21:775–784, 1994.
35. KS Kolbert, G Sgouros, AM Scott, JE Bronstein, RA Malane, J Zhang, H Kalaigian, S McNamara, L Schwartz, SM Larson. Implementation and evaluation of patient-specific three-dimensional internal dosimetry. J Nucl Med 38:301–308, 1997.
36. TL Faber, EM Stokely. Orientation of 3-D structures in Medical Images. IEEE Trans Pattern Anal Mach Intel 10:626–633, 1988.
37. M Moshfeghi. Registration of 3D medical images from multiple modalities using landmarks or surfaces. Preprint. Registration of 3D Medical Images from Multiple Modalities Using Landmarks or Surfaces. Philips Laboratories, Briarcliff Manor, NY 1988.
38. KD Toennies, JK Udupa, GT Herman, IL Wornom III, SR Buchman. Registration of 3D Objects and Surfaces. IEEE Comput Graphics Appl 10:52–62, 1990.
39. A Gamboa-Aldeco, LL Fellingham and GTY Chen. Correlation of 3D Surfaces from Multiple Modalities in Medical Imaging. Proc SPIE, 626:467–473, 1986.
40. YE Erdi, BW Wessels, R DeJager, AK Erdi, L Der, Y Cheek, R Shiri, E Yorke, R Altemus, V Varma, LE Smith, MG Hanna Jr. A new fiducial alignment system to overlay abdominal computed tomography or magnetic resonance anatomical images with radiolabeled antibody single-photon emission computed tomographic scans. Cancer 73:923–931, 1994.
41. LG Brown, GQ Maguire Jr, ME Noz. Proceedings of the SPIE Sensor Fusion VI Conference. Landmark-Based 3D Fusion of SPECT and CT Images. SPIE—The International Society for Optical Engineering, Boston, 2059:166–174, 1993.
42. PG Spetsieris, V Dhawan, S Takikawa, D Margoulef, D Eidelberg. Imaging Cerebral Function. IEEE Comput Graphics Appl 13:15–26, 1993.
43. SS Katyal, EL Kramer, ME Noz, D McCauley, A Chachoua, A Steinfeld. Fusion of Immunoscintigraphy Single Photon Emission Computed Tomography (SPECT) with CT of the Chest in Patients with Non Small Cell lung Cancer. Cancer Res (Suppl) 55:5759s–5763s, December 1995.
44. JC Liehn, A Loboguerrero, C Perault, L Demange. Superimposition of Computed Tomography and Single Photon Emission Tomography Immunoscintigraphic Images in the Pelvis: Validation in Patients with Colorectal or Ovarian Carcinoma Recurrence. Eur J Nucl Med 19:186–194, 1992.
45. C Perault, C Schvartz, H Wampach, JC Liehn, MJ Delisle. Thoracic and abdominal SPECT-CT image fusion without external markers in endocrine carcinomas. The Group of Thyroid Tumoral Pathology of Champagne-Ardenne. J Nucl Med 38:1234–1242, 1997.
46. ME Noz, EL Kramer, GQ Maguire Jr, SA McGee, JJ Sanger. An Integrated Approach to Biodistribution Radiation Absorbed Dose Estimates Anatomical-Functional Correlation Using an Adjustable MRI-based. Eur J Nucl Med 20:165–169, 1993.
47. AC Evans, C Beil, S Marrett, CJ Thompson, A Hakim. Region of Interest Atlas with Positron Emission Tomography. J Cereb Blood Flow Metab 8:513–530, 1988.

48. K Sj(oe)green, M Ljungberg, K Erlandsson, L Floreby, SE Strand. In: JS Duncan, GR Gindi, eds. Information Processing in Medical Imaging. Registration of Abdominal CT and SPECT Images using Compton Scatter data. Berlin: Springer-Verlag, 1997, pp 232–244.
49. LR Schad, R Boesecke, W Schlegel, GH Hartmann, V Sturm, LG Strauss, WJ Loren. Three Dimensional image correlation of CT, MR, and PET studies in radiotherapy treatment planning of brain tumors. J Comput Assist Tomogr 11:948–954, 1987.
50. S Marrett, AC Evans, L Collins, TM Peters. A Volume of Interest (VOI) Atlas for the Analysis of Neurophysical Image Data. Proc SPIE 1092:467–477, 1989.
51. E Deisenhammer, K Hoell, C Luft, H Steinhaeusl, A Brugger. Analysis of Distribution of I-123 IMP and Tc-99m HMPAO with early and late SPECT in Cerebrovascular Disease. J Nucl Med 28:591, 1987.
52. JD Foley, A Van Dam, SK Feiner, JF Hughes. The Systems Programming Series: Fundamentals of Interactive Computer Graphics. 2nd ed. Reading, MA: Addison Wesley, 1990.
53. ML Rhodes, WV Glenn, YM Azzawi. Extracting oblique planes from serial CT sections. Extracting Oblique Planes from Serial CT Sections. J Comput Assist Tomogr 4:649–657, 1980.
54. EL Hall. Computer Image Processing and Recognition. New York: Academic Press, 1979, pp 186–189; 468–554.
55. GQ Maguire Jr, ME Noz, EM Lee, JH Schimpf. In: SL Bacharach, ed. Correlation Methods for Tomographic Images Using Two and Three Dimensional Techniques Information Processing in Medical Imaging. Dordrecht, The Netherlands: Martinus Nijhoff Publishers, 1986, pp 266–279.
56. SH Pizer, VL Wallace. To Compute Numerically. Boston: Little, Brown & Company, 1983, pp 182–204.
57. GQ Maguire Jr, J Jaeger, L Farde, ME Noz. Use of Graphical Techniques for Error Evaluation. J Med Sys 11:277–286, 1987.
58. EJ Farrell, EL Kramer, GQ Maguire Jr, ME Noz. Proceedings of the SPIE Medical Imaging 1995. Quantitative 3D Visualization in Nuclear Medicine. SPIE—The International Society for Optical Engineering 2431:54–64, 1995.
59. EJ Farrell, RJT Gorniak, EL Kramer, ME Noz, GQ Maguire Jr, DP Reddy. Graphical Fusion of Multiple 3D image Sets in Radiology. J Med Syst 21:155–172, 1997.
60. RJT Gorniak, EJ Farrell, EL Kramer, GQ Maguire Jr, ME Noz, DP Reddy. Accuracy of an Interactive Registration Technique Applied to Thallium-201 SPECT and MR Brain Images. Med Phys 24:1354, 1997.
61. GW Moskowitz, JC Vaugeois, RG Schiff, LM Levy. Improvement of SPECT lung perfusion physiology with CT high resolution structural anatomy. J Nucl Med 27:1038, 1986.
62. JN Yu, FH Fahey, HD Gage, CG Eades, BA Harkness, CA Pelizzari, JW Keyes Jr. Intermodality, retrospective image registration in the thorax. J Nucl Med 36:2333–2338, 1995.
63. AM Scott, H Macapinlac, J Zhang, F Daghighian, N Montemayor, H Kalaigian, G Sgouros, MC Graham, K Kolbert, SDJ Yeh, E Lai, SJ Goldsmith, SM Larson. Image Registration od SPECT and CT Images Using an External Fiduciary Band and Three-Dimensional Surface Fitting in Metastatic Thyroid Cancer. J Nucl Med 36:100–103, 1995.

64. T Kato, H Fukatsu, K Ito, M Tadokoro, T Ota, T Isomura, S Ito, M Nishino, T Ishigaki. Fluorodeoxyglucose postiron emission tomography in pancreatic cancer: an unsolved problem. Eur J Nucl Med 22:32–39, 1995.
65. AM Scott, HA Macapinlac, CR Divgi, JJ Zhang, H Kalaigian, K Pentlow, S Hilton, MC Graham, G Sgouros, C Pelizzari, G Chen, J Schlom, SJ Goldsmith, SM Larson. Clinical Validation of SPECT and CT/MRI image registration in radiolabeled monoclonal antibody studies of colorectal carcinoma. J Nucl Med 35:1976–1984, 1994.
66. S Welt, CR Divgi, AM Scott, P Garin-Chesa, RD Finn, M Graham, EA Carswell, A Cohen, SM Larson, LJ Old, WJ Rettig. Antibody targeting in metastatic colon cancer: a phase I study of monoclonal antibody F19 against a cell-surface protein of reactive tumor stromal fibroblasts. J Clin Oncol 12:1193–1203, 1994.
67. RL Wahl, LE Quint, RD Cieslak, AM Aisen, RA Koeppe, CR Meyer. "Anatometabolic" tumor imaging: Fusion of FDG PET with CT or MRI to localize foci of increased activity. J Nucl Med 34:1190–1197, 1993.
68. G Sgouros, S Chiu, KS Pentlow, LJ Brewster, H Kalaigian, B Baldwin, F Daghighian, MC Graham, SM Larson, R Mohan. Three-dimensional dosimetry for radioimmunotherapy treatment planning. J Nucl Med 34:1595–1601, 1993.
69. HK Pohjonen, SE Savolainen, PH Nikkinen, VO Poutanen, ET Korppi-Tommola, BK Liewendahl. Abdominal SPECT/MRI fusion applied to the study of splenic and hepatic uptake of radiolabeled thrombocytes and colloids. Ann Nucl Med 10: 409–417, 1996.
70. EI Parsai, KM Ayyangar, RR Dobelbower, JA Siegel. Clinical fusion of three-dimensional images using Bremsstrahlung SPECT and CT. J Nucl Med 38:319–324, 1997.
71. KF Koral, KR Zasadny, ML Kessler, JQ Luo, SF Buchbinder, MS Kaminski, I Francis, RL Wahl. CT-SPECT fusion plus conjugate views for determining dosimetry in iodine-131-monoclonal antibody therapy of lymphoma patients. J Nucl Med 35: 1714–1720, 1994.

Index

Abdomen, 392
Adaptive histogram equalization (AHE), 121
   contrast-limited, 122
   interpolative, 122
Adaptive neighborhood contrast enhancement (ANCE), 222
   case study, 224
Additive tolerance region growing, 216–219
Affine transformation, 371
Anatomical
   atlas, 350
   model, 283
Angle image, 319
Area test, 175

Background
   structure, 195
   suppression, 256
Band-pass filtering, 196

Bayesian risk, 74–76
Bi-lateral
   asymmetry, 205
   subtraction, 204, 207
BI-RAD
   scale, 170
   standard, 22
Bivariate test, 175
Bonferroni correction, 228
Brain
   MRI, 295–297, 353
      feature extraction, 316
      preprocessing, 302–313
      registration, 348, 352
   tumor, 359–362
      segmentation, 323
Breast
   boundary detection, 191–192
   cancers
      masses, 187–189
   correspondence, 204

[Breast]
   mass
      detection (examples), 206–208
      features, 196–202
      peripheral enhancement, 193–194
      thickness (correction for), 193–194, 206
      thresholding for segmentation, 191
      tissue segmentation, 191–192

CAD (*see* Computer Aided Detection/Diagnosis)
Calcification,
   (*also see* Microcalcification)
   appearance, 12
   defined, 8–9
Calibration, 194
Cancer(s)
   breast, 132, 187
   colon, 393
   colorectal, 397
   interval, 224–225, 235
   lung, 2, 388
   ovarian, 398
   pancreatic, 396
Chest
   radiography, 244
   x-rays (contrast enhancement), 246
Classification 40
   defined, 3
   region, 203
Classifiers, 144–145, 324
   supervised, 326
   unsupervised, 334
Clinical implementation
   abdomen/pelvis, 392–398
   chest radiography, 64
   dosimetry, 399
   image display, 57–58
   mammography, 63
   prompting, 56–57
   registered brain images, 357–362
   thorax, 387–392

Clinical testing, 33–34
Clustering (fuzzy), 282
CNR (contrast-to-noise ratio), 313
Colon cancer, 393
Color scale, 109
Colorectal cancer, 397
Computer-aided detection
   algorithms (mammography), 189–190
   breast tissue, 55
   case studies, 37–43
   challenges, 148
   chest radiography, 55
   clinical evaluation, 33–34
   computation time, 147
   diagnosis (CAD), 245
   evaluation, 19–42, 56
   in mammography, 132–135
   influence on image search, 59–62
   lung nodules, 255
   masses in mammograms, 188–189
   microcalifications, 132–135
   performance, 148
   prompting (cueing), 26, 48–54, 59
   ROC study, 174–181
   test data, 35–36, 38
   training and testing, 35, 38
Computed tomography (CT), 6, 367
   helical, 261
   spiral scan, 271, 274, 289
   thoracic, 261
Confidence
   level of, 173
   threshold, 173
Contextual region, 117–125
   edge-shadowing, 119–120, 124
Contrast
   object, 149
   radiographic, 149
   to noise ratio (CNR), 313

Index

Contrast enhancement, 103, 107, 111–128, 135–139
    adaptive, 117–124, 157, 214–215, 222–223
    of chest x-rays, 246
    global, 112–117
    histogram transformation, 112–117
    in MRI, 313
    incorporating object structure, 124–126
    intensity windowing, 112–117
    lung nodules, 246–255
    microcalcifications, 136, 216
    non-linear, 161–164
        function, 215
    peripheral (breast), 193–194
    pulmonary (nodule), 246–255
    quality of, 126–128
    ROC studies, 215–216
    unsharp masking, 120–121, 125
    x-ray, 246
Contrast-limited adaptive histogram equalization (CLAHE), 122, 124
Correlation
    cross, 349, 371
    filter, 198
Correspondence (breast), 204
Cross-correlation, 349, 371
Curvature
    tumor detection (use in), 286–287

Denoising, 163
DICOM GrayScale Standard Display Function, 107, 111
Difference of gaussians filter, 136, 196
Difference image, 251
Digital mammogram databases
    DDSM, 2, 155, 165
    MIAS, 25

Digital mammography, 147–148, 156, 194
Discriminant analysis, 322
Display
    color, 109
    digital, 110–111
    gray, 109
    hardware, 168
    intensity, 105
    perceived intensity, 105, 108
    pseudocolor, 109–110
    qualitative, 102–109
    scales, 101–111
    sensitivity, 106
Dosimetry, 399
Dual-Energy Imaging, 251–255

Edge
    detection, 202
    gradient orientation, 258
    shadowing effect, 119–120, 124
    tracking, 305
Eigen image filtering, 331–332
Exposure correction, 246
External markers, 375
Endobronchial lesions, 286
Enhancement (*see* contrast enhancement)

False negative fraction, 172–173
False positive fraction, 20, 105, 172–173
False positive rate, 145
Feature
    domain representation, 298
    extraction, 384
        brain (MRI), 316
    spaces, 298
Filter
    banks, 158
    correlation, 198
    cross correlation (normalized), 198

[Filter]
  Eigen imaging, 331–332
  gaussian, 136, 196
  matched, 198
  maximized minimum absolute
      CNR (MMAC), 313
  maximum CNR, 313
  prewhitened matched, 79
  statistical difference, 121
  steerable, 147
  Wiener, 309
Fourier (registration) methods, 371
Fractals, 139
Free response receiver-operator
    characteristic (FROC), 190,
    206–208
Fusion (of imaging modalities), 347
Fuzzy
  C-means, 335
  clustering, 282

Gaussian
  filters, 196
    difference of, 136, 196
  noise, 85, 94
Gram-Schmidt orthogonalization,
    323, 329
Graphical user interface (GUI),
    164–169
Gray level
  normalization, 194–195
  rebinning, 138
  thresholding, 141
Gray scale, 109
Ground truth (Gold standard), 21–25

Hepatic hemangiomas, 392
Histogram
  equalization, 115
    adaptive, 118, 121–124
    sharpened, 126
  transformation, 112–117

Hotelling
  observer, 73, 77–79
  trace, 79
Hough transform, 143, 199, 200

IBM Visualization Data Explorer,
    352, 383
Image(s)
  angle, 319
  discriminant analysis, 322
  fusion,
    brain, 347
    trunk, 367–370
  optimal transforms, 319
  registration
    brain, 348–352
    examples (SPECT, CT, MRI),
        376–387
    trunk, 369
Image enhancement, 135–139
  adaptive, 142–143, 214–215,
      222–223
  multiscale, 156
  non-linear, 161–164
  piecewise linear, 162
  region-based, 214–215
Image differencing (subtraction),
    204, 207, 251
Image interpretation, 14–15, 23
  BI-RADS standard, 22
Image intensity correction, 193
Imaging
  anatomical
    defined, 5–6
  dual-energy, 251–255
  functional
    defined, 5–6
  geometry, 6–7
  MRI, 4
  MRS, 4
  radionuclide, 4
  ultrasound, 4
  x-ray, 4

Index

Intensity windowing, 112–117
   mixture-modeling based, 114
Interactive (registration), 351
Interval Cancer, 224–225, 235
ISODATA algorithm, 335

Just noticeable difference
   defined, 105
   of CRTs, 106–107

Knowledge-based methods, 282–286

Landmarks, 372–375, 378
Laplace of gaussian filters, 196
Lesion(s)
   endobronchial, 286
   stellate (masses), 200–202
Level of confidence (LOC), 173
Look up table, 247
Lung(s)
   cancer, 388
      diagnosis, 243–244
      screening, 272
   nodules, 244
      enhancement, 246–255
   perfusion in lung (registration), 388
   segmented regions (photos), 256

Magnetic Resonance Imaging (MRI), 367
   brain, 295, 297, 353
      feature extraction, 316
   preprocessing, 302–313
Magnetic Resonance Spectroscopy (MRS), 341
Mahalanobis distance, 354
Mammogram(s)
   appearance, 204
   asymmetry, 204

[Mammogram(s)]
   databases, 155
   dense, 169
   digitization, 165, 168
   masses detection, 187–211
   microcalcification detection, 132–135
   of healthy tissue, 188–189
   preprocessing, 135–139, 191–195
   segmentation, 139–143
Mammographic screen-film systems
   characterization curve, 142
Mammographic screening, 165, 208, 224
Mammography
   algorithms (computer-aided detection), 189–190
   digital, 58
   digitized film, 133–135
   features, 10
   pixel size, 134
   resolution, 132
   screening, 208, 224
Markov random fields, 143
   model, 202
Mass(es)
   computer-aided detection in mammograms, 188–189, 206–208
   in breast, 187–189
      features, 196–202
   signs of malignancy, 188–189
   spiculated, 195
   stellate lesions, 200–202
Matched-filtering, 198
Maximized minimum absolute CNR (MMAC), 313
Maximum Likelihood Detector, 77
McNemar test of symmetry, 227, 230, 235
Median filters, 138
Metastases, 1

Microcalcifications, 55
　appearance, 140–141
　cause, 132
　cluster
　　defined, 131
　detection, 38–43, 132–135
　enhancement, 136, 216
　features used in detection,
　　143–144
　image properties, 164
Misrepresentation errors, 381
Moment-matching, 349
Morphological operators, 137
MRI, 367
　brain, 295, 297, 353
　　feature extraction, 316
　　preprocessing, 302–313
　imaging, 4
　signature vectors in, 301
MRS (Magnetic Resonance
　　Spectroscopy), 341
MUSICA™, 121, 215
Multiple views, 204–206, 207
Multiplicative tolerance region
　　growing, 219
Multiresolution
　pyramid, 305
　segmentation, 202
Multiscale
　analysis, 157, 198
　image contrast amplification
　　(MUSICA™), 121, 215
　reconstruction, 157
　representations, 157
Multiscale Image Contrast
　　Amplification (MUSICA™),
　　121, 215
Mutual information, 350

Neoplasm
　defined, 1–2
Neural networks, 145–147

Nipple location, 192
Nodules
　lung (enhancement), 246–255
　pulmonary, 244, 246–255
Noise, 96
　exponential, 86
　gaussian, 85, 94
　Laplacium, 90, 97
　Poisson, 88
　suppression, 309–313
Nonuniformity correction, 307
Normalized cross-correlation, 198

Observer
　examples, 85–98
　Hotelling, 73, 77–79, 95
　ideal, 73–77
　likelihood ratio, 73, 76
　linear, 77, 94–95
　mathematical, 73
　performance, 79–84
　test statistic, 73, 79
Optimal transforms, 319
Ovarian cancer, 398

Pancreatic cancer, 396
Partial volume estimation, 327
Pectoral muscle location, 192
Pelvis, 392
Perception
　and feedback, 51
　satisfaction of search, 62–63
　visual search, 62–62
Perceived dynamic range
　color scales, 109–110
　defined, 105
　of CRTs, 106–107
Peripheral enhancement (breast),
　　193–194
PET (positron emission
　　tomography), 349, 360, 367
Polynomial warping, 348, 371, 378

Index

Positron emission tomography (PET), 349, 360, 367
Preprocessing
 of mammograms, 191–195
 in brain (MRI), 302–313
Prewhitened matched filter, 79
Principal component analysis, 299, 318
Processing time, 167
Pulmonary nodule, 14, 244, 277
 enhancement, 246–255
 segmentation, 278–286

Radiologist
 diagnostic performance, 156
 dual-reading, 53
 eye position, 49–50, 61
 gaze duration, 49–50, 61
 impact of, 15, 48
 observer studies, 226
 performance, 48, 53, 59, 233
 variations in, 23, 34
Receiver operating characteristic (ROC), 80–81, 133, 171–174
 area under the curve (AUC), 27, 30–33, 80–81
 case study, 41
 free response receiver operating characteristic (ROC), 27
  case study, 39, 42
  defined, 27–28, 29
  mammographic case study, 155–157, 169–181
Recursive median filter, 136–137
Region segmentation, 202–203
 classification, 203
 growing, 202, 216–221
Registration, 204, 302
 2D-3D (combined), 376
 3D rigid body, 382
 brain, 348, 352
 image, 348–352

[Registration]
 direct 3D, 355
 Fourier (methods), 371
 image
  examples (SPECT, CT, MRI), 376–387
 in brain imaging, 357–362
 in lung perfusion, 388
 interactive, 351
 2D/3D, 355
 thorax, 387–392
 trunk (image), 369–387
Rockit software, 175

Screening, 15–16, 23, 33
 computation time, 147
 lung cancer, 272
 mammography, 131, 182, 187–189, 208, 224
Segmentation
 brain tumors, 323
 breast tissue, 191–192
 intracranial, 307, 309
 knowledge/rule-based, 282–286
 lung (thresholding), 281
 multiresolution, 202
 pulmonary nodules, 278–286
 region, 202–203
 vasculature, 276–278
Sensitivity, 20, 172, 188
Sigmoidal function, 158, 162–163, 182
Signal-to-noise ratio (SNR), 328
 defined, 73, 78, 79
 related to AUC, 83–84
Signature vectors (in MRI), 301
Single photon positron emission tomography (SPECT), 347, 360, 367
Single view, 195–203
Skeletonization
 of vascular tree, 278

Software
  Rockit, 175
Specificity, 20, 145, 172
SPECT (Single photon positron emission tomography), 347, 360, 367
Spiculated mass(es), 195
  wavelet expansion of, 161
Spiculation measures, 203
Spicule detection, 200–202
Staging, 3
Statistical decision theory, 71–72
  examples
    BKE, 95–98
    NKE, 98
    SKE, 93–98
    SKE/BKG, 85–93
Statistical difference filter, 121
Steerable filter, 147
Stellate
  lesions (masses), 200–202
  speculated, 12
Stereotactic frame, 350, 355
Subband reconstruction, 167
Subtraction
  bilateral, 204, 207
  image differencing, 204, 207, 251
Supervised classifiers, 326
Suppression
  background, 256
  noise, 309–313
Surface-matching, 349, 372
Symmetry, McNemar's test of, 227, 230, 235

Template matching, 196–198
Texture features, 200
Threshold
  confidence, 173
    level of (LOC), 173

Thresholding, 162, 202
  segmentation
    for breast, 191
    for lung, 281
Thorax
  clinical implementation, 387–392
  registration, 387–392
Tissue
  inhomogeneities, 308
  parameter-weighted images, 318
Tolerance region growing
  additive, 216–219
  multiplicative, 219
Tomography
  computed (CT), 367
    helical, 261
    positron emission (PET), 349, 360, 367
    single photon positron emission (SPECT), 347, 360, 367
    thoracic, 261
TPF test, 176
Tracking (edge), 305
Transformation
  affine, 371
  histogram (contrast enhancement), 112–117
  optimal, 325
True negative fraction, 172–173
True positive fraction, 20, 105, 172–173
Tumor(s)
  appearance, 3–11
  brain, 359–362
    segmentation, 323
  breast cancer, 11–13
  defined, 1–2
  detection (curvature), 286–287
  features, 11–14
  growth factors, 8
  imaging
    reasons for, 2–3

[Tumor(s)]
   isointense, 3–4
   lung cancer, 14–15
   matrix, 3
   model, 71
   stellate (speculated), 12
   visualization, 10, 15
Two-alternative forced-choice (2AFC) experiment, 81

Unsharp masking, 120–121, 125, 136, 214, 249
Unsupervised classifiers, 334

Variable conductance diffusion (VCD), 125–126
Vasculature (segmentation), 276–278
Visualization Data Explorer (IBM), 352, 383

Wavelets, 137–138, 156, 198
   expansion of spiculated masses, 161
   quadratic spline, 160
   thresholding, 163–164
   transform, 158